AF615351

Springer Series in Pharmacologic Science

Ronald J. Tallarida, *Editor*

Ronald J. Tallarida
Robert B. Raffa
Paul McGonigle

Principles in General Pharmacology

With 88 Illustrations

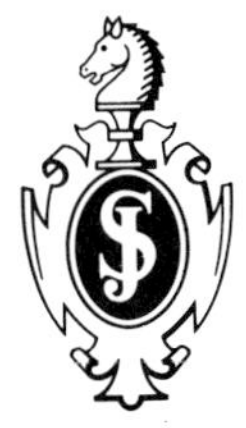

Springer-Verlag
New York Berlin Heidelberg
London Paris Tokyo

Ronald J. Tallarida, Ph.D.
Professor of Pharmacology, Department of Pharmacology, Temple University School of Medicine, Philadelphia, Pennsylvania 19140, USA

Robert B. Raffa, Ph.D.
Senior Scientist, Janssen Research Foundation, Spring House, Pennsylvania 19477; and Adjunct Assistant Professor, Department of Pharmacology, Temple University School of Medicine, Philadelphia, Pennsylvania 19140; and Adjunct Assistant Professor, Jefferson Medical College, Philadelphia, Pennsylvania 19107, USA

Paul McGonigle, Ph.D.
Assistant Professor, Department of Pharmacology, University of Pennsylvania School of Medicine, Philadelphia, Pennsylvania 19104, USA

Library of Congress Cataloging-in-Publication Data
Tallarida, Ronald J.
Principles in general pharmacology / Ronald J. Tallarida, Robert B. Raffa, Paul McGonigle.
p. cm. – (Springer series in pharmacologic science)
Bibliography: p.
Includes index.
ISBN 0-387-96602-1
1. Pharmacology. I. Raffa, Robert B. II. McGonigle, Paul. III. Title. IV. Series.
[DNLM: 1. Pharmacology. QV 4 T147p]
RM300.T317 1988
DNLM/DLC
for Library of Congress 86-12376

Typeset by Publishers Service, Bozeman, Montana.
Printed and bound by Arcata Graphics/Halliday, West Hanover, Massachusetts.
Printed in the United States of America.

9 8 7 6 5 4 3 2 1

ISBN 0-387-96602-1 Springer-Verlag New York Berlin Heidelberg
ISBN 3-540-96602-1 Springer-Verlag Berlin Heidelberg New York

To our children

Christopher, Diane, Karen, R.J., Valerie

Jonathan

Sean

Preface

This book deals with principles in general pharmacology—the key ideas that are applied to virtually all drug classes—and thus seems to us the proper subject matter with which to launch the *Springer Series in Pharmacologic Sciences*. The book is designed to meet the modern need for a better understanding of pharmacologic principles. It is an intermediate text directed mainly, but not only, to students who have completed a first course in pharmacology and who now need greater detail on concepts fundamental to understanding much of the research literature—especially the parts that are quantitative. Physicians having a special interest in pharmacology will also find much useful information here. The book integrates topics that we have included in several courses to health science students in graduate and professional schools in recent years. The "principles" are those key concepts that are applicable to a wide range of drug classes and include pharmacokinetics, drug biotransformation, receptor interaction, and the key ideas underlying the expression and interpretation of dose–response data. These concepts have their roots in the more basic sciences of physics and chemistry. Some readers may feel that we omitted concepts that might be considered "principles"; hence we have used the preposition "in," not "of," in the title of this book.

Because its individual chapters are essentially self-contained, the book can be used in a variety of courses. For example, Chapters 1, 2, and 4 are suitable for the "principles" sections of introductory courses in pharmacology of the kind given in most professional schools. Instructors teaching graduate pharmacology and pharmacy students will find that Chapters 1 to 5, 8, and 9 can form the basis of a one-semester course of 30–40 hours duration. The addition of Chapter 6 and 7, which present the fundamental physicochemical bases that underlie current thinking on chemical bonding and reaction kinetics, along with selected articles and other works cited from the literature, provide sufficient material for a two-semester graduate course.

We hope that this book, which combines the features of reference and text, will aid students and professionals alike in understanding drug actions. However, the literature in pharmacology, as in other scientific fields, is vast. Hence, we could not cite many excellent articles and books. We have instead carefully chosen those that best illustrate or extend the topics of this volume. We urge the student to read as many of these as possible, for no single book, however thick, is sufficient to teach this subject.

Series Preface

Pharmacology is both a basic and a clinical science. In contrast to other basic medical sciences, however, this discipline is bolstered by an active world-wide pharmaceutical industry that produces hundreds of new drugs each year. Further, researchers often find new uses for existing drugs – even old ones – while they are studying mechanisms of their action. Many compounds have become tools for further exploration of physiologic mechanisms. The result has been a dramatic and continuous proliferation of information about drugs and the various biologic systems on which they act.

This virtual explosion of knowledge presents a real challenge to students as well as to clinicians and researchers who must keep abreast of developments in their own and adjacent specialties. This challenge is further intensified when the new facts and mechanisms are related to completely new concepts necessary for their understanding. Many such concepts have been formulated from recent studies and thus were not taught until very recently in graduate and professional school courses. The experienced clinician or researcher who wants to keep up must have the new facts *and* the new mechanisms.

The *Springer Series in Pharmacologic Sciences* was conceived with these objectives in mind. The aim will be to produce volumes, each dealing with a particular therapeutic area or pharmacologic theme, that integrate the facts with the concepts needed to understand their underlying mechanisms. Physicians have long realized the importance of understanding mechanisms as a basis for rational drug therapy. The integration provided in these books also lends to each the flavor of a textbook, yet our intention is to give more recognition to the research literature than is usually found in student textbooks. This design helps to make each book rather self-contained, thus minimizing the need to consult many individual articles and reviews.

It is well known that drugs are categorized in a variety of ways, e.g., according to gross or intimate pharmacologic action, site of action, chemical structure, therapeutic use, etc. Accordingly, the books of this series will reflect this diversity of classification. In every book, however, the aim of the authors and editors is to sort, integrate, and interpret from among the large body of facts and conceptual ideas, and to provide a volume of modest size that is useful to large numbers of clinical and basic scientists and their students.

Some areas of pharmacology will surely advance more rapidly than others. Thus there will be a need to update with second editions in some areas. In this regard, this series has an advantage over the single, thick, comprehensive work. Our intention is to meet the needs for updated editions while continuing to expand the scope of the series with brand new titles.

Ronald J. Tallarida
Philadelphia, 1988

Contents

7 The Rate of Drug–Receptor Interactions

8 Pharmacodynamics: The Interaction of Drugs with Receptors

9 Radioligand Binding

1
General Principles: History and Overview

Introduction

Today there are drugs for treating virtually every ailment. Not all drug treatments are curative; in fact, most are only ameliorative. Yet, we are better equipped today than ever before in treating disease. For example, at the turn of this century more than 13% of all American children died before their first birthday. The fatal diseases were principally pneumonia, influenza, and tuberculosis.[3] The improvement in life expectancy during this century is, for the most part, largely due to advances in medicine, and an important component of that advance is the availability of new drugs. Most of the drugs used today have come from laboratory research. Only a few (e.g., digitalis and morphine) are products of ancient cultures, most of the others in the modern pharmacopeias having come from the synthetic chemistry laboratory.

It is interesting to note what the major classes of today's drugs are, based on use. Some indication of these classes and their relative rank is afforded by a sampling of prescription drugs in the United States, as shown in Table 1.1.

Though borrowing heavily from biochemistry, physiology, and even physics, pharmacology is today very much a science in its own right. It is a dynamic field, buoyed by advances in basic research that often apply to clinical situations. Its subject matter is now considered "core" in most medical school curricula, although this aspect of the education of the American physician is relatively recent. The first American professorship of pharmacology, awarded to John J. Abel, was established in 1891 at Michigan, but it was not until the mid-1930s, when chemotherapeutic drugs arrived, that pharmacology became deeply rooted as a separate discipline in the doctor's education.

Tracing the history of pharmacology, or even its significance in the formal education of physicians, is beyond the scope of this brief volume. Several excellent sources for historical information exist.[1,2] Even an historical tracing of pharmacologic principles will not be formally done, for such a task, with the space available, would result in something that is very incomplete. Yet, some minor historical perspective seems in order.

TABLE 1.1. Drug classification ranked according to pharmacologic action or therapeutic use.[a]

Rank	Drug group
1	Cardiovascular
2	Antibiotics
3	Analgesics
4	Antibacterials/antiseptics
5	Tranquilizers
6	Diuretics
7	Decongestants/expectorants
8	Antiarthritics
9	Antihistamines
10	Gastrointestinal preparations
11	Contraceptives

[a]Based on the number of different preparations within the category as determined from a sampling of new and refill prescriptions in US retail pharmacies. A particular drug may lie in more than one category. From Tallarida RJ: Most-Prescribed Drugs – 1985. Philadelphia, W.B. Saunders Co. 1985, pp. 219–230. Reprinted by permission.

Historical Perspective

In a general sense, "principles," those key points that apply to many drug groups, emerged in the first half of the 19th century when the active ingredients were isolated from natural preparations. Crude forms that had been used for ages became subject to quantitative analysis. With this quantitative precision it became possible to relate dose to response and thus instilled confidence in both the doctor and the patient. The London mathematician J.W. Trevan (1887–1955) would ultimately show in 1927 that the response to a fixed and precise dose in living material obeyed a normal distribution. The isolation of pure forms stimulated researchers to look for new compounds, or make alternatives to these natural products. The rise of chemistry aided in this effort. Products made at this time could now be screened for toxicity and effectiveness.

That a relation exists between the chemical structure of a compound and its biological activity was hypothesized by James Blake (1814–1893) and confirmed by his studies of inorganic salts. This work provided one of the earliest pieces of evidence for specific binding sites (receptors), for if the physiochemical composition of a drug influenced its activity, it was reasonable to suppose the existence of binding sites that specifically "recognized" the drug.

As chemistry advanced, the quest for new drugs and an understanding of their properties advanced. The accelerated pace led, for example, to a wide exploration for anesthetics and to the systematic work of Benjamin W. Richardson (1828–1896), who studied alcohols and hydrocarbons. Richardson discovered the importance of the number of carbon atoms in relation to the single-dose toxic effects of these compounds, the kind of study that now falls within molecular pharmacology. He also found and explored the dilation of blood vessels by amyl nitrate after Antoine Balard (1802–1876) made the compound and Thomas Brunton (1844–1916) reported its success in treating anginal pain. Brunton also noted the inotropic action of digitalis and its consequent diuretic action. Pharmacology was emerging as a science and textbooks on the subject appeared, such as that by Carl Ludwig (1816–1895): *Textbook of Pharmacology, Therapeutics and Materia Medica*, which was published in London in 1885.

Antagonistic drug action, a key concept in both theoretical pharmacology and modern therapeutics, was systematically studied by Thomas R. Fraser (1841–1920), who examined the antagonism between atropine and physostigmine. The latter compound, an alkaloid extract from the calabar bean, is today well known for its prominent parasympathetic effects.

Because the subject of pharmacokinetics is the movement of precise drug quantities throughout the body, pharmacokinetics could become a rigorous discipline only if methods of drug delivery could be made accurate. The first use of the hypodermic syringe by Alexander Wood (1817–1884) must therefore be regarded as a monumental advance in this branch of pharmacology, as well as in modern clinical medicine. The drug molecule must traverse many membranes (highly lipid structures) that divide the (largely aqueous) compartments of the organism. The studies of Hans H. Meyer (1853–1939) on the relative solubilities of compounds for fats and water, leading to the concept of the lipid/water partition coefficient, gave new insights that led to models patterned after the much studied diffusion of gases and studies of dilute solutions. Physical theories, along with chemical knowledge, therefore further permeated the discipline that is now known as pharmacokinetics. The physiochemical ideas provided a framework for the later precise studies of the biotransformation and elimination of drugs by Von Nencki (1847–1901), Von Mering (1849–1908), and Schmiedeberg (1838–1921).

Of course, the literature of the 20th century reveals an explosion in pharmacologic knowledge and much of the information has sharpened our definitions of key ideas or principles. The reader will become aware, while reading the chapters on quantitative pharmacology, that certain individuals are linked with certain ideas, so some additional sense of the history of the theoretical advances may emerge.

Principles

Just as the array of diseases is diverse, so, too, are the properties and actions of the drugs used to treat them. The results of laboratory research often seem at odds with clinical experience. Modell[4] has commented: "That a disparity should sometimes seem to exist generally arises through neglect of pertinent laboratory data or through improper interpretation or application." The point here is that, more often than not, properly evaluated laboratory findings are applicable to clinical situations, but the evaluation of laboratory data requires an understanding of some basic principles—the main subject of this book. The fundamental concepts broadly applicable to all drugs or to wide classes of drugs are the principles. Some readers will undoubtedly feel that we have overlooked some concept that might be considered a "principle." If so it is because our use here of the word is purposely narrow, including only those ideas that have their roots in the more fundamental sciences of chemistry and physics and the inevitable mathematical concepts that are required for their proper expression. The broader use of the term "principle" shall unfold in the accompanying volumes of this series in which individual systems and drugs affecting them are discussed.

Overview of Pharmacologic Principles*

In order to be effective a drug must be absorbed into the bloodstream and arrive at its locus of action on the target organ. In its movement the drug molecule must traverse various membranes and enter the capillaries. Only the smallest molecules can diffuse through the membranes pores; therefore larger molecules will pass by diffusion only if they are soluble in the membrane. Because membranes are mainly lipid, drug molecules that are lipid-soluble pass more readily than those that are not. Nonionized particles have greater lipid solubilities than do ionized molecules; thus, the degree of ionization of the drug molecules is an important factor in a drug's absorption. The lipid solubility of a drug is frequently expressed in terms of its lipid/water partition coefficient, a measure of the relative affinity of the drug for a lipid solvent and water at some specified temperature. Most drugs are absorbed by passive diffusion.

Besides passive diffusion, other mechanisms of transport exist. Some compounds of low solubility penetrate membranes more easily than can be accounted for by passive diffusion. The transport of some of these compounds is aided by carrier molecules. For compounds that move against a concentration gradient (actually an electrochemical gradient because of an accompanying difference in electric potential), energy is required and the transport is described as "active." In both active and carrier-mediated transport the drug must be in solution.

Drugs exist in a variety of different physical forms: aqueous solutions, suspensions, capsules, tablets, etc. The physical form is an important factor in the absorption of a drug by a particular route. For oral administration, the most common route, the degree and rate of absorption as a function of the physical form are generally greatest for oral solutions, then suspensions, capsules, tablets, and coated tablets, in that order. Tablets are frequently coated in order to prevent destruction of the drug by the acidic gastric juice.

---

*The balance of this chapter is from Tallarida RJ: Most-Prescribed Drugs—1985. Philadelphia, WB Saunders, 1985, pp 261–274. Reprinted by permission.

Ionization and Absorption

Because ions have low lipid solubility, and since many drugs are weak acids and bases that tend to form ions, it is useful to discuss the conditions that determine the drug's degree of ionization. Ionized molecules do not readily traverse the highly lipid cellular membranes. The degree of ionization of a drug molecule depends on the pH of the medium containing the drug and a property of the drug called "pK." The computation of the degree of ionization of both acidic and basic drugs uses the Henderson–Hasselbalch equations. The ionization constant (K) is often expressed as the negative (common) logarithm, or pK value: $\mathrm{p}K = -\log(K)$.

The degree of ionization depends on the pK of the drug and on the pH of the medium that contains the drug. For drugs that are weak acids, the ratio of nonionized to ionized concentrations is determined from the equation

$$\mathrm{pH} = \mathrm{p}K + \log_{10} \frac{(\text{ionized})}{(\text{nonionized})} \tag{1.1}$$

In contrast, drugs that are weak bases obey the equation

$$\mathrm{pH} = \mathrm{p}K + \log_{10} \frac{(\text{nonionized})}{(\text{ionized})} \tag{1.2}$$

As an example, consider acetylsalicylic acid, whose pK is approximately 3.3, in gastric juice of pH 3. The ratio of nonionized to ionized forms, computed from the Henderson–Hasselbalch equation, can be shown to be 1.99, that is, approximately twice as much is nonionized as is ionized, a situation that favors absorption. In contrast, diazepam, a weak base with pK of 3.3, has the ratio of approximately 2 of ionized to nonionized in the same gastric juice and, thus, exhibits, less absorption from the stomach. Of course, other factors besides ionization affect the absorption of drugs. These are outlined below and discussed in greater detail in Chapter 3 on pharmacokinetics.

Oral Administration

The most popular route of administration is the oral route, and drugs given this way must be absorbed from the stomach or the intestines. As previously discussed, the pH of the medium is one important factor in the absorptive process. The stomach juice is acidic, usually in the pH range 1 to 4, whereas in the duodeum the pH ranges from 5 to 6. The remainder of the intestine is neutral to slightly basic with a pH of about 8 in the lower ileum. These facts relate to ionization and its importance in absorption. Other factors, however, also affect absorption of orally administered rugs. (See Fick's law.) Because the intestines contain such a large absorptive area compared with that of the stomach, most of the absorption takes place in the small intestine. Solubility may depend on pH as well. A swallowed tablet must first disintegrate and then be dissolved if it is to enter the bloodstream. A drug that is not absorbed from the stomach must enter the intestine; hence, the rate of gastric emptying is important for such a drug. As previously noted, in some cases it is undesirable for the drug to be soluble in gastric juice, for example, when the drug would be destroyed by the gastric juice, or when the drug is irritating to the gastric lining. In such cases enteric-coated tablets are used, for these resist dissolution in the stomach. Gastric irritation can sometimes be avoided by taking the drug with food or milk.

Some preparations are designed to be released at a controlled rate by using different coatings, each destroyed at a different rate, thereby releasing the drug molecules at a controlled rate. Many widely prescribed drugs are formulated as sustained-release or controlled-release preparations.

Portal Circulation

The liver is the most important organ for drug metabolism. The drug metabolite or metabolites may or may not have activity, or they may have activities that are much less than that of the parent drug. A drug in the blood is carried to the liver, resulting in a decrease of the drug's concentration (in time) at a rate that depends on the hepatic blood flow and the chemical machinery of the liver. The latter consists of numerous enzymes contained in the endoplasmic reticulum of the liver. Drugs taken orally are particularly susceptible to this enzymatic activity, since drainage from the gastrointestinal system is into the portal circulation, a direct route to the liver (further discussed in Chapter 4). For example, nitroglycerin is rapidly degraded in the liver; accordingly, the oral route is not used. Instead, nitroglycerin is administered sublingually (and, more recently, transdermally). Drainage from the mouth is into the superior vena cava and not into the portal circulation. Of course, it is necessary that a drug given this way be highly potent (such as nitroglycerin) since the amount absorbed from this route is small.

Parenteral Administration

Although the oral route is the most common and the most convenient, it cannot always be used for reasons previously mentioned. In such cases parenteral administration may be used. The important parenteral routes are subcutaneous, intramuscular, and intravenous. The subcutaneous route is used, provided that the drug is not too irritating and that the volume is reasonably small. This route usually results in fairly constant absorption. The insulin preparations are good examples of drugs given subcutaneously.

Drugs administered via the intramuscular route are often in solutions in oil and are absorbed at a slow, steady rate. This route is not used when bleeding may be a problem, as in patients on anticoagulant drugs. Sometimes this route is also painful because of its irritating effect on muscle and other tissue.

In contrast to the subcutaneous and intramuscular routes, which are extravascular, the intravenous route delivers the precise amount to the blood and delivers the drug to the target sight(s) more rapidly than do the other common parenteral routes. Usually intravenous administration must be slow and carefully monitored. Drugs in oily vehicles should not be given this way. Also, drugs that directly affect blood components should not be given intravenously.

Other Routes of Administration

A number of other routes are used, and this information for any particular drug is provided by the manufacturer of the drug. Thus, inhalation is used for administering certain bronchial dilators (e.g., albuterol sulfate), topical for skin conditions (e.g., betamethasone), and rectal for controlling vomiting (e.g., prochlorperazine). Generally, only the routes recommended by the drug manufacturer should be used, and the dosages should also be in accord with these recommendations, since they are based on the known absorptive and elimination properties of the drug. These considerations are important even when drugs are given topically, that is, applied directly to the skin or to the mucous membranes of the vagina, colon, nasopharynx, etc. When these routes are used, there may be a tendency to apply too much of the drug. Absorption from mucous membranes is generally good, and absorption through the skin, though usually more difficult, should be relied on for drugs designed to be given that way. Principles of pharmacokinetics underly the dosage form and regimen (see Chapter 3).

Knowledge of these principles is especially important when normal mechanisms for either absorption, distribution, metabolism, or excretion are impaired as in certain disease states.

Drug Binding

Drug molecules may bind to sites other than the organ for which they are intended. These sites include blood proteins, fat, bone, skeletal muscle, etc. Protein binding is of special interest. A drug that is bound to protein will not usually be active; only the free (unbound) drug will act and only the free drug will be eliminated from the plasma. However, a drug that is protein-bound is not tied up permanently. If we denote the drug by *D* and the protein by *P* then the interaction may be written

$$\mathrm{D} + \mathrm{P} \rightleftharpoons \mathrm{D{-}P}$$

where D–P is the drug–protein complex. The reaction is reversible with a dissociation constant $K = (\mathrm{D}) \cdot (\mathrm{P})/(\mathrm{D{-}P})$. Many low-molecular-weight drugs bind to plasma albumin (molecular weight approximately 67,000) with high affinity (low K). The affinity ($1/K$) is related to the equilibrium concentrations of D, P, and D–P by the Scatchard equation given below:

$$\frac{(\mathrm{D{-}P})}{(\mathrm{D})} = -\frac{1}{K}(\mathrm{D{-}P}) + \frac{(\mathrm{P}_t)}{K} \tag{1.3}$$

The left-hand side is the ratio of bound to free concentration and is linear when plotted against (D–P). The vertical intercept is the ratio (P_t) to K, where (P_t) is the total protein concentration. The horizontal intercept gives P_t. Scatchard analysis is used to determine the degree of drug binding and the affinity of the drug for the protein (as well as in the study of receptor binding, discussed in Chapter 9). Besides rendering the drug inactive, and impeding its elimination from the plasma, protein binding is often the cause of adverse drug-drug interactions. When two drugs have affinity for the same protein-binding site, the drug with the higher affinity will be bound to a greater extent. When a patient is receiving both drugs simultaneously, the presence of the pair may significantly affect the free concentrations of each, requiring dosage adjustments of each. For example, anticoagulants such as warfarin bind strongly to plasma proteins, and it is this property that accounts for warfarin's interactions with many other drugs that also bind to protein.

When a drug is bound to protein, the complex dissociates as the free drug is eliminated by the kidney. This dissociation tends to maintain a fairly constant concentration of the free form of the drug. The protein fraction is therefore a depot for the drug. In some disease states, especially those of the liver, the dissociation constant may change (increase), thereby affecting (decreasing) the protein binding of the drug.

Drug Metabolism

The body contains numerous enzymes that act on foods, foreign bodies, and drugs. Many of these enzymes are located in the smooth endoplasmic reticulum of the liver. Four important kinds of chemical reactions involved in metabolizing drugs are oxidation, reduction, hydrolysis, and conjugation. (See Chapter 4 for a detailed discussion.) Regardless of which of these reactions metabolizes the drug, each represents a mechanism for deceasing the concentration of the drug. The metabolite(s) may or may not have activity similar to that of the parent compound. The organism, therefore, does not depend solely on excretion for ridding itself of drugs and other foreign substances. Indeed, metabolism of the drug is an important factor in its disappearance rate. Especially noteworthy is the heme protein known as *cytochrome P-450*, present in high concentration in liver microsomes, and responsible for hydroxylating (oxidizing) many lipid-soluble drugs. Some drugs (e.g., phenobarbital) cause an increase in the concentration of cytochrome P-450 so that many lipid-soluble drugs, in the presence of phenobarbital, have increased rates of metabolism. This kind of *enzyme induction* is an important mechanism of drug-drug interaction, often requiring dosage adjustment of one or both drugs. In contrast to enzyme induction, the presence of a second drug may inhibit the metabolism of a drug or food ingredient. Monoamine oxidase (MAO) inhibitors, for example, are frequently noted among the contraindications of many popular drugs as agents that can cause untoward effects when present concomitantly with these other drugs. (Chapter 4 provides a detailed discussion of drug metabolism.)

Excretion

Besides metabolism, an equally important process for the elimination of drugs is excretion. By far, the kidney is the most important organ of drug excretion. For many drugs elimination also involves other routes, such as those into bile, sweat, saliva, tears, and expired air. Drugs may also be excreted into breast milk, and, for this reason, virtually every drug package insert contains warnings about nursing while the mother is taking the drug. Yet, the kidney is the most important excretory organ, and several important principles emerge from a discussion of renal excretion.

Renal Excretion

The nephron is the functional unit of the kidney and is comprised of tubules and capillaries. The tubules, known as proximal, loop of Henle, and distal, contain materials outside the circulation and lead to the collecting duct, which is a conduit to the bladder. The capillary network makes up the glomerulus. Arterial blood enters the glomerular capillary network where the plasma and many of its solutes are filtered across these capillaries of the glomerulus. The filtration is selective and based on the molecular size of the solutes so that proteins and drugs bound to proteins do not enter the tubules. Accordingly, drugs that are highly protein bound are excreted slowly. As the filtrate passes through the tubules, the drug and other dissolved compounds may be reabsorbed, either actively or passively. (Reabsorption is favored if the drug is in the nonionized, lipid-soluble form.) Further, the drug or other solutes may be secreted from the capillary network into the tubules. If the drug or substance is not secreted or absorbed, then its only passage out is via glomerular filtration. The glomerular filtration rate (GFR), measured as milliliter per minute, is approximately 130 ml/min in healthy adults. If the glomerular filtration rate is reduced, as in some disease states, then the elimination of a drug that is normally excreted by filtration will be reduced. For this reason, drug dosages are adjusted in patients with impaired renal function, often quantitated by determination of the GFR.

Clearance

The amount of drug excreted per unit time, denoted by F, can be calculated for a drug that is not protein bound from the drug's plasma concentration, C_p, and the GFR (provided it is not reabsorbed or secreted)

$$F = C_p \cdot (\text{GFR}) \tag{1.4}$$

More commonly, the drug's clearance is calculated, that is, the volume of blood per minute that is cleared of the drug. In terms of the plasma concentration

C_p (mg/ml), the volume of urine excreted per minute V' (ml/min) and urine concentration of drug C_u (mg/ml), the clearance is

$$Cl = C_u \cdot V'/C_p \tag{1.5}$$

The mean values of C_u and C_p (over time) are used in equation (1.5). It is noteworthy that older patients (greater than 70 years) and neonates clear many drugs at a lower rate than the rest of the patient population.

Besides renal clearance there is hepatic clearance, which includes biliary excretion and hepatic metabolism. Total clearance involves both organs, the kidney and the liver.

Volume of Distribution

If a chemical is in solution, or if it is uniformly suspended in a liquid or gaseous medium, its concentration (C) is defined as total amount (I) per volume (V). Equivalently,

$$V = I/C \tag{1.6}$$

so that the volume is determined from I and C. If, however, the concentration is not uniform (perhaps because some of the chemical adheres to the inner wall of the container), then C is lowered and consequently the value of V computed from equation (1.6) will be larger than the true volume—a kind of virtual volume. It follows that if a drug binds to sites outside the plasma, the concentration of the latter will be lower than its value in the absence of binding. Consequently, routine use of equation (1.6) may lead to large value of V, perhaps even larger than the volume of the total body water. In pharmacology such a volume is called the *apparent volume of distribution*; its numerical value is an indicator of the degree of tissue binding (see also p. 40).

First-Order Elimination

Both excretion and metabolism contribute to the disappearance of a drug from the body. For most drugs the rate of elimination is proportional to the drug concentration in the body (or plasma). Stated differently, the drug concentration–time relation, viewed after absorption is complete ($t = 0$), is a decreasing exponential:

$$C = C_0 \cdot \exp(-kt)$$

where C is the concentration at any time, C_o is the concentration at $t = 0$, and k is the elimination rate constant. Exponential elimination, also called "first-order" elimination, is characterized by the half-life (t^*), which is related to k by the equation

$$t^* = \ln 2/k = 0.693/k \tag{1.7}$$

In *four half-lives*, 1/16 ($= 1/2^4$) remains. In practical terms, this amount is often small enough to be negligible. The relation between half-life, volume of distri-

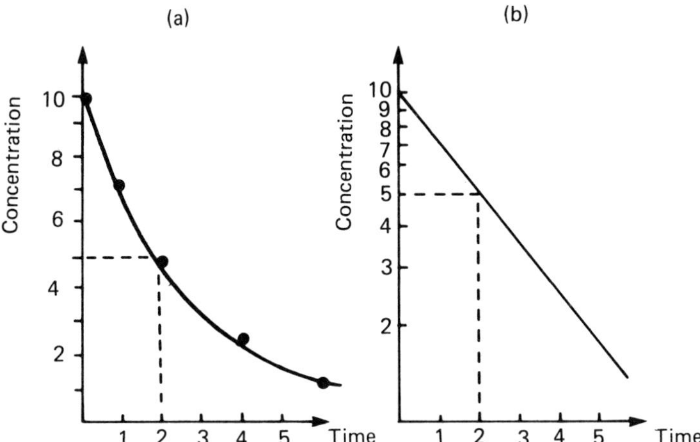

FIGURE 1.1. Exponential elimination. (a) Linear scales. (b) Semilogarithmic plot. The half-life is 2 (time units). (From Tallarida RJ: Most-Prescribed Drugs-1985. Philadelphia, WB Saunders Co., 1985, pp. 219–230. Reprinted by permission.)

bution, and clearance of a drug is discussed mathematically on p. 43. Suffice it to say here that a large value of the apparent volume of distribution, indicative of appreciable tissue binding, generally means a large half-life of elimination and low clearance.

Exponential elimination is illustrated in Figure 1.1 in two ways—with linear scales on both axes, and with a logarithmic ordinate and linear abscissa. In the latter the graph is theoretically linear. For many drugs, however, the elimination curve appears to contain two linear segments. The first segment demonstrates a rapid elimination from plasma to tissue-binding sites. The second is indicative of disappearance from plasma. The extrapolated concentration, shown as C_o' in Figure 1.2, is less than the actual concentration. The apparent volume of distribution is usually computed by dividing the amount of drug administered* by this lesser concentration C_o', and, as previously mentioned, this ratio may be larger than the real volume. For example, the apparent volume of distribution of digoxin is approximately 500 L, many times the value of total body water.

In contrast to first-order elimination, a few drugs are eliminated at a constant rate, a process called "zero order." When a drug obeys zero-order elimination, it is not meaningful to talk about its half-life.

Figure 1.3 illustrates graphs of plasma-time relations for a drug given by an absorptive route and by the intravenous route. Elimination is first order, and the ordinate scale is linear in both cases. Several points are noteworthy. First, absorption may not be complete so that the plasma concentration at peak will be less than the some concentration following use of the intravenous route. Even if

*Assuming complete and rapid absorption or intravenous administration.

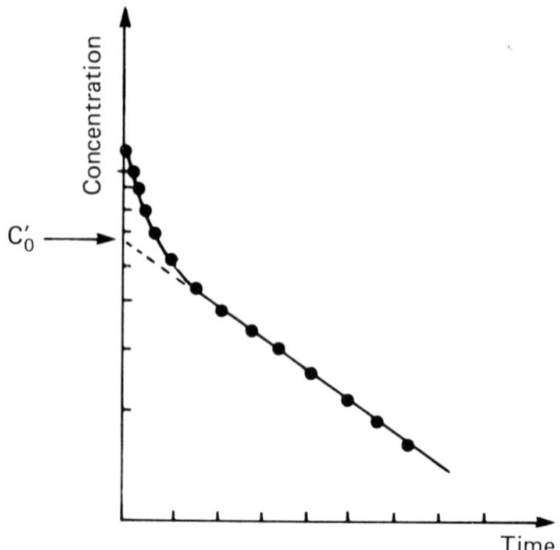

FIGURE 1.2. Bi-exponential decay of drug from plasma. The extrapolated value C_o' is used in computing the apparent volume of distribution of the drug. The ordinate is calibrated logarithmically. (From Tallarida RJ: Most-Prescribed Drugs-1985. Philadelphia, WB Saunders Co., 1985, pp. 219–230. Reprinted by permission.)

Even if absorption is complete, the peak concentrations will not be the same since the absorbed drug is partly eliminated even before its absorption is complete. Second, following complete absorption, the kinetic patterns are identical. Finally, there is a minimum concentration needed for effect (illustrated by the broken horizontal line) so that the onset and termination of effect occur at the times shown.

Repetitive Dosing

If a second dose is administered before the first has been eliminated, the concentration will build. If the elimination is first order, it may be shown that the buildup will be bounded, since the higher levels result in increased rates of elimination. In this context, "elimination" refers to removal by all routes and metabolic pathways. Figure 1.4 illustrates the concentration–time relation for dosing at regular time intervals T. The broken curve is the mean concentration and, as shown, it is bounded or approaches a plateau. The plateau concentration, denoted C, is given by the following equation (derived and discussed in detail on page 57).

$$C = \frac{1.44\, F \cdot D \cdot t^*}{T \cdot V}$$

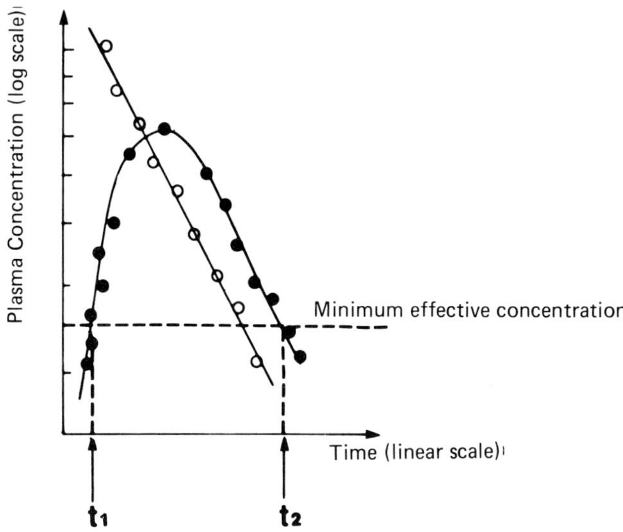

FIGURE 1.3. Plasma concentration following intravenous administration (○) and following administration via an absorptive route (●). Also shown are times of onset (t_1) and termination (t_2) of drug effect for the absorptive route. (From Tallarida RJ: Most-Prescribed Drugs-1985. Philadelphia, WB Saunders Co., 1985, pp. 219–230. Reprinted by permission.)

where D = dose
F = fraction absorbed
V = apparent volume of distribution
$t_{1/2}$ = elimination half-life
T = dosage interval

It may also be shown that the time to achieve 95% of this plateau is approximately 4.3 half-livcs (p. 54).

DOSE-EFFECT RELATION

The magnitude of a drug's effect often depends on the dose; that is, if a small dose D_1 produces an effect E_1, then a larger dose D_2 will generally produce a larger effect E_2. This correspondence between the dose and the effect constitutes a graded dose–response (dose–effect) relation for the particular drug and the particular effect observed. For small doses, below a certain threshold value, the organism may show no perceptible effect, whereas for doses above a certain value, the change in effect may be negligible. Between these two dosage extremes

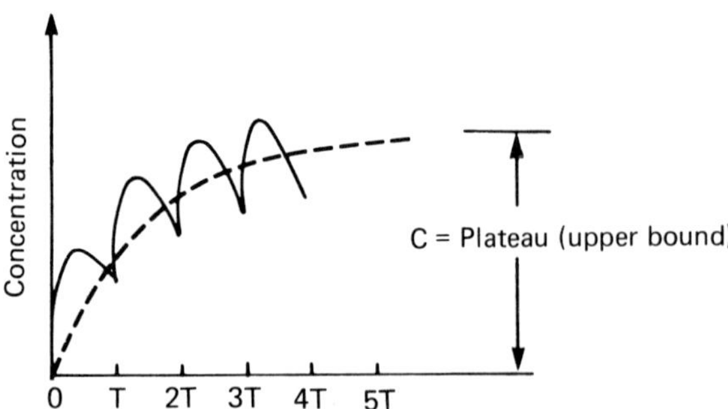

FIGURE 1.4. Repetitive dosing at time intervals T via an absorptive route. The broken curve is the mean concentration, which approaches an upper bound. (See text.) (From Tallarida RJ: Most-Prescribed Drugs-1985. Philadelphia, WB Saunders Co., 1985, pp. 219–230. Reprinted by permission.)

is the range in which there is a gradation of response. The graph of such a relation is shown in Figure 1.5 where a curve is shown connecting the individual (D_i, E_i) pairs. The upper limit of effect, E_{max}, is a measure of the drug's *efficacy.* A drug with efficacy is called an *agonist* and is said to possess *intrinsic activity.* (Intrinsic activity is discussed more fully in Chapter 8.)

The left-to-right position of the dose–response curve is an indicator of *potency*, or the dose needed to achieve a desired level of effect. Potency is often expressed as the dose needed to produce an effect that is 50% of the maximum, the so-called D_{50} dose. A small value of D_{50} suggests high potency, whereas a large D_{50} indicates low potency. An illustration of potency differences is provided in the comparison of the two popular antihypertensives chlorothiazide and hydrochlorothiazide. Both lower blood pressure to the same extent, but the former does so with higher dosage (e.g., 500 mg/day) requirements than the latter (e.g., 50 mg/day) in the typical patient with mild hypertension.

The steepness of a graded dose–response curve, measured by its slope, reveals the therapeutic dosage range. A steep curve means a narrow dose range. (A more thorough discussion of dose–response relations is given in Chapter 8).

ANTAGONISTS

In contrast to drugs that possess intrinsic activity, many useful therapeutic agents have little or no intrinsic activity. The importance of such agents, called antagonists, is that they inhibit or abolish the unwanted effects of other drugs, endogenous compounds, or toxic substances. Antihistamines are examples of antagonists; they antagonize the effects of histamine. Propranolol (Inderal®) antagonizes many effects of catecholamines, and hydralazine (Apresoline®) antagonizes pressor effects of vasoconstrictors on vascular smooth muscle. The mechanisms of antagonistic action vary. Some of these are explained in terms of the receptor theory of drug action.

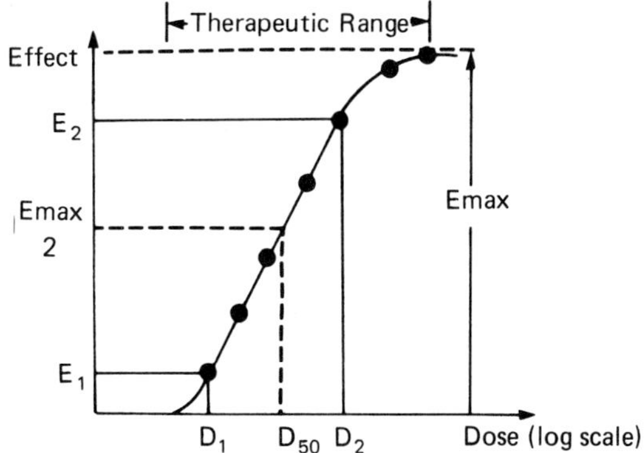

FIGURE 1.5. Graded dose-response curve. (From Tallarida RJ: Most-Prescribed Drugs-1985. Philadelphia, WB Saunders Co., 1985, pp. 219–230. Reprinted by permission.)

Receptors

Most drugs act by combining with specific binding sites or receptors on the cell membrane. If we denote the drug by D and the receptor by R, the reaction between drug and receptor is most simply viewed as a bimolecular reversible reaction resulting in the formation of a drug–receptor complex, DR:

$$D + R \frac{k_1}{k_2} DR$$

If the drug has intrinsic activity the DR complex stimulates the production of an effect (E). If the drug lacks intrinsic activity, the complex produces no direct effect of its own and is classified as an antagonist because it will inhibit the action of other drugs that act on R. Some drugs have activity somewhere between that of full agonist and antagonists; these are *partial agonists*.

The ratio, k_1/k_2 of forward and reverse rate constants in the above reaction is a measure of the *affinity*. If a drug has affinity for a specific receptor but lacks intrinsic activity it will antagonize other compounds or drugs that interact with this same receptor. An example of this pharmacologic antagonism is afforded by cimetidine (Tagamet®), which antagonizes histamine at the histamine H_2 receptor, or propranolol which antagonizes beta-adrenergic compounds. When an agonist's dose–response relation is determined in the presence of a fixed dose of a pharmacologic antagonist, the agonist's dose–response curve is shifted to the right, as in Figure 1.6 (curve 2). The same value of E_{max} may be attained, as shown, if the agonist dose is sufficiently large, in which case the antagonism is surmountable or reversible. This phenomenon is similar to that of competitive inhibition in enzyme–substrate reactions, and the term "competitive" is also used in characterizing pharmacologic phenomena of this kind. A more detailed discussion of receptors is given in Chapters 5 and 8 based on information from a quan-

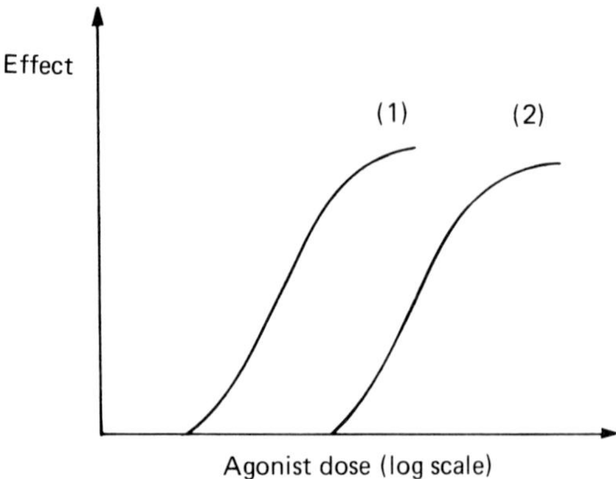

FIGURE 1.6. Competitive antagonism. Curve 1 is the dose-effect curve of the agonist alone. Curve 2 is the agonist dose-effect curve in the presence of a fixed dose of a reversible pharmacologic antagonist. (From Tallarida RJ: Most-Prescribed Drugs-1985. Philadelphia, WB Saunders Co., 1985, pp. 219–230. Reprinted by permission.)

titative analysis of dose–response relations and in Chapter 9, which discusses radiolabeled binding of ligands to receptors.

Other kinds of antagonism exist. For example, each drug may combine with its own specific receptor and each may have intrinsic activity, but the expressions of these at the effector organ produce opposite effects. We call this *physiologic* or *functional antagonism*. The effects of cholinergic and adrenergic compounds on organs having both kinds of receptors are typical of physiologic antagonism. Also, the previously mentioned example, hydralazine, which directly dilates vascular smooth muscle, is a physiologic antagonist of both endogenous and exogenous vasoconstrictors.

Knowing the mechanism of the antagonism may provide a rational basis for proper therapeutic usage. For example, propranolol is an effective antihypertensive with beta-adrenergic blocking action. Generalized beta blockade is undesirable, however, in patients with bronchial asthma, since bronchiolar smooth muscle contains beta receptors that mediate relaxation. Hence, beta blockade impedes the relaxating effects and is, therefore, contraindicated, since it may cause an adverse reaction in the asthmatic. Drugs with relatively cardioselective beta-blocking action have less effect on bronchioles and are therefore used (though with caution).

Adverse Drug Reactions

No useful drug produces just a single effect. Both desirable and undesirable additional effects occur as well. These adverse effects may be mild, serious, or very serious. Some adverse reactions result from the exaggerated, but otherwise normal, pharmacologic action of the drug. Other adverse reactions are unpredictable from knowledge of the drug's normal pharmacologic action and frequently are not detected in toxicologic screening. The ultimate adverse effect is death. Hence, for every drug there is a dose–response relation, determined from animal experimentation, in which death is the effect. The dose that kills 50% of the animals is termed the LD_{50}. The dose that produces the desired effect in 50% of the subjects is termed the ED_{50}. Obviously, it is desirable that the LD_{50} greatly exceed the ED_{50} in order to have a margin of safety. The therapeutic index, TI, is the ratio of LD_{50} to ED_{50} and is a guide to the drug's safety. Clearly, it is desirable that the TI be large. Unfortunately, this value may be small (e.g., digitalis glycosides have a small TI, approximately 2.5.)

Between these extremes of desirable effects and death there may be a continuum of undesirable, or adverse effects. The individual volumes in this series deal with particular systems and drug groups used in treating these and will provide information of the most important adverse reactions. (Additional information may be found among the various references below.) The total risk of a drug in the form of adverse reactions is dependent on both the severity of the adverse reaction and its incidence. The magnitude of the drug risk must be weighed against the severity of the condition being treated and alternative treatments available.

References

1. Holmstedt B, Liljestrand G (eds): *Readings in Pharmacology.* Oxford, Pergamon Press Ltd, 1963.
2. Leake CD: *An Historical Account of Pharmacology to the 20th Century.* Springfield, C Thomas, 1975.
3. Lowrance WW: *Of Acceptable Risk.* Los Altos, Wm Kaufmann Inc, 1976, p. 5.
4. Modell W: *Drugs of Choice–1979*–1981. St. Louis, Mosby, 1981, p. 3.
5. Tallarida RJ: *Most-Prescribed Drugs–1985.* Philadelphia, WB Saunders, 1985, pp 219–230.

Additional Readings

Davies DM: *Textbook of Adverse Drug Reactions.* New York, Oxford University Press, 1977.

Goldstein A, Aronow L, Kalman SM: *Principles of Drug Action: The Basis of Pharmacology,* ed 2. New York, John Wiley & Sons, 1974.

Karch FE, Smith CL, Kerzner B, et al: Adverse drug reactions–a matter of opinion. *Clin Pharmacol Ther* 1976; 19:489.

Reidenberg MM, Lowenthal DT: Adverse non-drug reactions. *N Engl J Med* 1968; 279:678.

Rowland M, Tozer TN: *Clinical Pharmacokinetics.* Philadelphia, Lea & Febiger, 1980.

Tallarida RJ, Jacob LS: *The Dose-Response Relation in Pharmacology,* New York, Springer-Verlag, 1979.

Tallarida RJ, Murray RB: *Manual of Pharmacologic Calculations* (with computer programs). New York, Springer-Verlag, 1981.

Tallarida RJ, Murray RB, Eiben C: A scale for assessing the severity of diseases and adverse drug reactions: Application to drug benefit and risk. *Clin Pharmacol Ther* 1979; 25:381.

2
Dose–Effect Relations

The terms drug "effect," "response," and "action" are often used synonymously to describe the same kind of event, namely, a change in the function or properties of a component of the organism. The change may be clinically observable or it may not be. It might be primarily chemical or physiologic in nature, or it might be some combination of these. At the level of the cell, drug action results in intimate events, such as contraction, secretion, or alteration in electrical properties. At the level of groups of cells, or organs, the action of a drug is due to an integration of the intimate events, resulting, thereby, in clinically observable effects. These effects include both desirable and undesirable consequences of drug administration.

Certain clinical effects of drugs are readily measurable; for example, changes in body temperature, heart rate, respiratory rate, blood pressure, pain tolerance, tumor size, blood clotting time, bacterial growth, etc. Other effects are less easily measured, such as changes in mood, anxiety state, and behavior. The last represent a challenge for the clinical pharmacologist who must quantitate drug effects in order to determine efficacy and toxicity, and for the physician who must assess the progress of a patient being treated with drugs.

Precise demonstration of drug effects in humans is further complicated by the placebo response, that is, the real change in function that accompanies the mere act of administering a substance with no known action in the amount given. More specifically, a placebo is a substance that exerts effects (at times), but these effects are independent of its chemical nature. To demonstrate that an experimental chemical or drug is efficacious in producing an effect, it is necessary to prove that the magnitude of the chemical's effect is significantly greater than that of a placebo given under the same conditions. Part of this proof involves an experimental design in which neither the recipient of the chemical nor the physician knows whether the substance is the chemical or the placebo (a double-blind study.)

In a double-blind study 72 obese patients were given a sustained-release capsule containing phenylpropanolamine (37.5 mg) and caffeine (140 mg) or a placebo. After six weeks the placebo group lost 2.07 pounds compared with a loss of 4.64 pounds in the drug group.[1]

Dose-Effect Graphs: Potency and Efficacy

Notwithstanding the problems of accurately measuring the real effect(s) of a drug, it is generally found that (1) all drug effects are limited or bounded, that is, there is a practical maximum effect (E_{max}) in the sense that further increases in dosage produce no discernible increase in effect; (2) zero dose produces zero effect; and (3) between these dosage extremes there is a gradation of responses. The effects come on in time, hence, practically, one uses the peak effect for each dose, yielding a time-independent dose–response curve. The shape of a typical dose–response curve, when plotted with conventional rectangular coordinates, is as shown in Figure 2.1. No widely accepted theory accounts for the shape of a graded dose–response curve; however, a rather simple theory of drug action (classical occupation theory) has proved valuable in this regard. Often the magnitude of the effect is plotted against the common logarithm of the dose (or concentration) since this procedure allows for a wide dosage range. The shape of a typical log dose–response curve is sigmoidal, as shown in Figure 2.2. Both graphs (linear or logarithmic) convey the same quantitative information; the difference in shape is merely due to the transformation of the horizontal scale.

Several features of the graded dose–response curve are useful in describing some of the terminology. As previously noted, the height, E_{max}, is a measure of intrinsic activity or efficacy, the innate ability of the drug to produce an effect. The left-to-right position is an indicator of the potency or quantity of drug needed to produce a given level of effect. One index of potency is the dose that yields a half-maximal effect (Figure 2.1). We denote this dose D_{50}. If a drug has a small value of D_{50} it is very potent, whereas a large value is indicative of low potency. The slope (steepness) gives an idea of the therapeutic range. A large value of slope indicates a narrow therapeutic range, whereas a small slope (shallow curve) is indicative of a wide therapeutic range. According

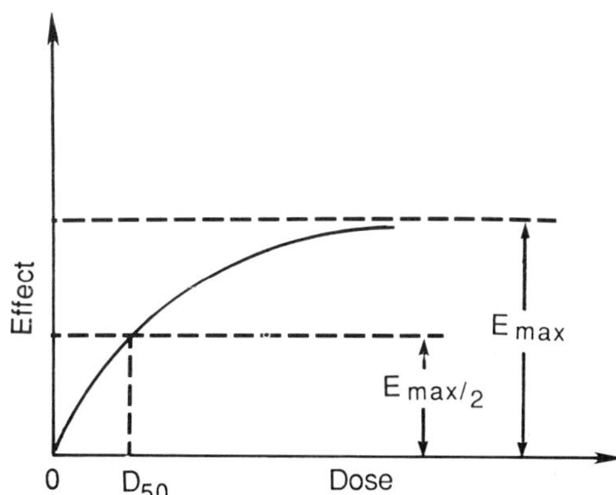

FIGURE 2.1. Graded dose–effect curve. D_{50} is the dose that produces a half maximal effect.

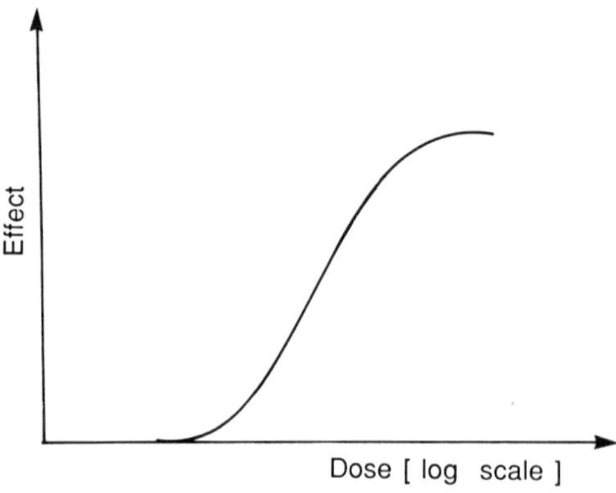

FIGURE 2.2. Effect vs dose plotted with a logarithmically calibrated scale for dose.

to the classical theory previously referred to, the slope of the log dose–response curve is 0.567.

It should be noted that the solid curves of Figures 2.1 and 2.2 are drawn from data derived from a sample of patients, and, hence, a point on the curve is a mean response for the dose indicated. Also noteworthy is that the effect at each dose is usually the peak, or steady-state effect, since the effect is a time-varying function as well.

Antagonists

Antagonists are substances that reduce or abolish the effects of an active drug or chemical. Several examples of antagonists were given previously (p. 14). The term "pharmacologic" antagonism has been used when the agonist and antagonist act on the same drug receptor. Most pharmacologic antagonists are of the reversible (also known as competitive) type, that is, the effect of the antagonist can be overcome with sufficiently high doses of the agonist. Accordingly, the dose–response curve of the agonist is merely shifted to the right, meaning that higher doses of the agonist are needed at any level of effect. As an example, Figure 2.3 illustrates the antagonism of morphine's antinociceptive action by naloxone. In contrast to the reversible antagonism of morphine and naloxone, consider the graph for the antagonism produced by phenoxybenzamine (Dibenzyline) on norepinephrine-induced contraction of vascular smooth muscle (Figure 2.4). In this case the full agonist effect is not achieved with this concentration of the antagonist, regardless how large the agonist concentration. Indeed, an even high dose of phenoxybenzamine would completely mask any norepinephrine action. This kind of irreversible antagonism, involving a single receptor, is called *noncompetitive* by analogy with the corresponding terminology in enzyme substrate studies.

Physiologic or functional antagonism refers to situations in which each compound acts on its own individual receptor but the effects of each are opposite.

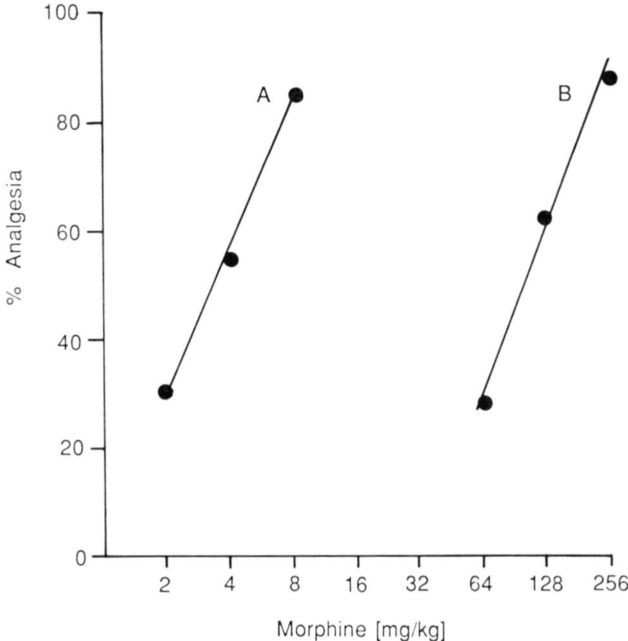

FIGURE 2.3. Dose-response curve for morphine (in rats). Curve A is in the absence of naloxone, whereas curve B is after administration of 0.10 mg/kg of naloxone. (Adapted from Tallarida RJ, Harakal C, Maslow J et al: The relationship between pharmacokinetics and pharmacodynamic action as applied to *in vivo* pA_2: Applications to the analgesic effect of morphine. J Pharmacol Exp Ther. 206:38. © by the American Society for Pharmacology and Experimental Therapeutics 1978.)

Indeed, the actions of acetylcholine and norepinephrine best exemplify this kind of antagonism. There is no general rule that can be applied to predict whether the antagonism can be overcome in this case. If it cannot be overcome, the pair of dose–response curves can very well resemble those for irreversible (noncompetitive) antagonism just discussed. The dose–response curves are not sufficient in themselves to classify the antagonism. Other information from experiments designed to determine whether one or two different receptors are involved is needed in such cases. A quantitative discussion of dose–response data and the effects of antagonists is presented in Chapter 8.

Quantal (All-or-None) Dose–Response Relations

In contrast to the graded dose–response relation previously discussed, there is another common method for expressing drug effects and doses needed to produce them. This method uses a particular end point or level of effect and determines

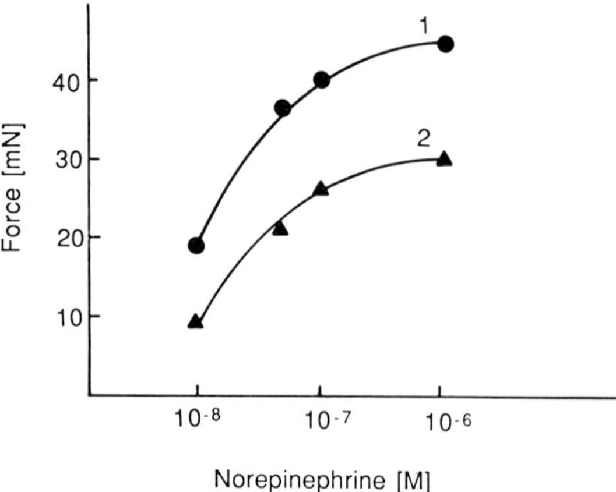

FIGURE 2.4. Curve 1 represents developed force in isolated strips of rabbit aorta as a function of norepinephrine concentration. Curve 2 illustrates the same experiment in the presence of a fixed dose of the noncompetitive antagonist phenoxybenzamine. (Adapted from Tallarida et al.[3])

among the population of subjects the relative number (or percentage) of those who respond at various dosages of the drug. For example, the end point might be the production of sleep (determined by some appropriate test) among a sample of subjects drawn from the population. A low dose is administered and the percentage responding is recorded and plotted. A higher dose, in turn, produces the effect in a greater percentage, and it includes all those who previously experienced the effect with the lower dose plus additional responders (a cumulative process), yielding another pair (dose, %), which is also plotted. The experiment is continued until eventually 100% respond. (At this dose, some of the early, most sensitive individuals may be experiencing toxic effects.) The plot of these data is shown in Figure 2.5, curve (a).

The dose that is effective in 50% of the subjects is termed ED_{50} and is a kind of potency index. The ultimate effect is death. Accordingly, there is a lethal curve, determined (obviously in animals) by plotting the percentage of animals that die at each dose. Clearly, the lethal curve, such as that in Figure 2.5 curve (b), should be far to the right of curve (a). The dose that is lethal in 50% of the animals is denoted LD_{50}, as shown in the figure. Commonly one quotes the ratio LD_{50}/ED_{50} or therapeutic index (TI). Large values of TI are clearly desirable. Unfortunately this index is rather low for some drugs; e.g., it is about 2.5 for digitalis glycosides, meaning that even a small excess (2.5 times normal) can be fatal in 50% of the population.

The sigmoidal-shaped curves of Figure 2.5 can be rectified by converting the percentages, plotted on the vertical axis, to "probits." The probit is related to the area under the normal distribution (discussed subsequently). The conversion from percentages to probits generally results in a linear plot when the probit

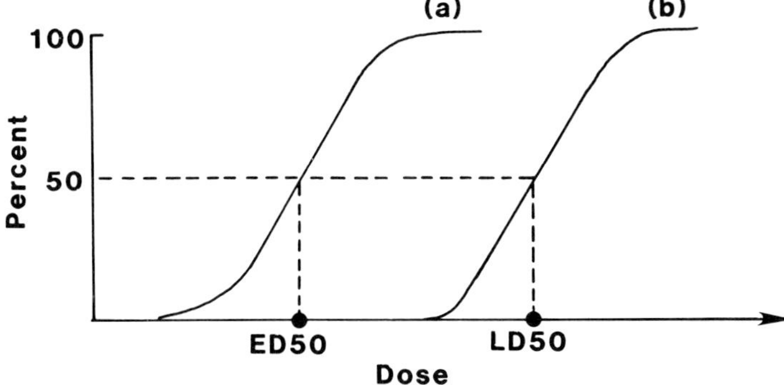

FIGURE 2.5. All-or-none (dose, percentage) curves for effect (curve a) and death (curve b), illustrating ED_{50} and LD_{50} doses.

(corresponding to each percentage) is plotted against log dose, as shown in Figure 2.6. Table A.3 gives the conversion from percentage to probit.

Although the probit transformation is most suited to the quantal dose–response curve just discussed, it is also convenient for the graded dose–response curves previously discussed. In the graded response there is a maximum. Hence, each response less than the maximum can be converted to a percentage of the maximum, a normalizing process. Then these percentages can be converted to probits

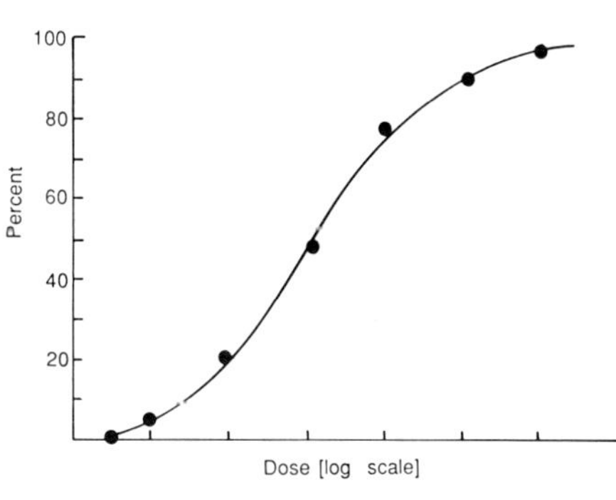

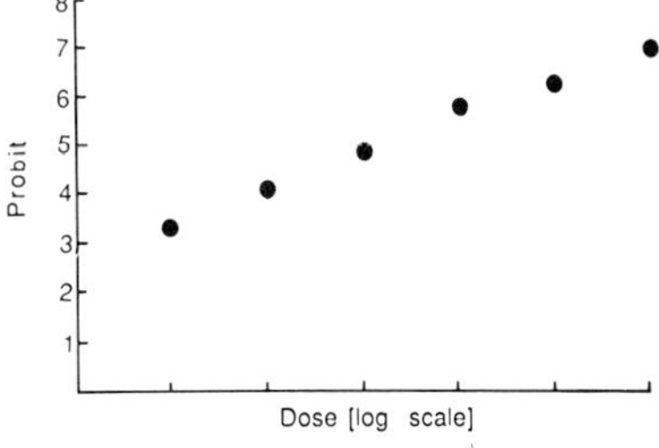

FIGURE 2.6. Top curve is a graph of percentage responding against dose. The bottom curve illustrates the conversion of percentages to probits for the same data.

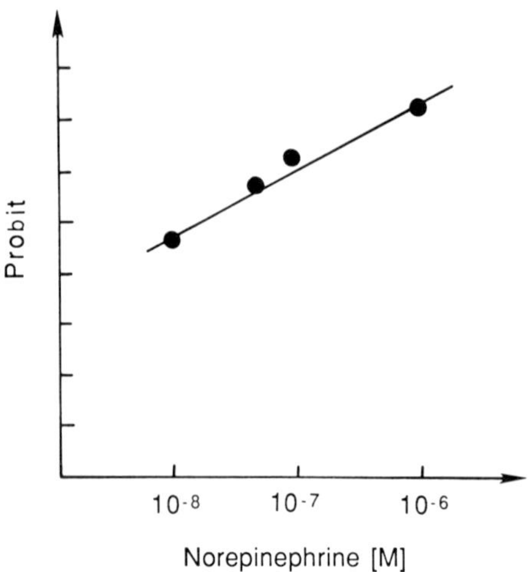

FIGURE 2.7. Probit transformation of graph (1) of Figure 2.4.

also, a conversion that may result in a linear plot against log dose. Although this technique may have no mechanistic basis, it may be useful as a curve-fitting device and is often used (see discussion below). As an example, consider the conversions of the graded responses of norepinephrine on contraction of vascular smooth-muscle strips illustrated in Figure 2.7.

PROBIT TRANSFORMATION

When the effect is expressed as a percentage of the maximum effect in a graded concentration–effect graph, or when the percentage of subjects showing an effect (all-or-none) to a dose or concentration is plotted against dose, it is common to convert the percentage to probability units or "probits." The probit is related to the percentage area under the normal distribution curve when the latter is shifted so that its center of symmetry is at $Z = 5$ rather than at $Z = 0$ (see Figure 2.8). Since one half (or 50%) of the area lies to the left of $Z = 5$, the probit corresponding to 50% is 5. Moving one Z unit to the right, that is, to a probit of 6, adds an additional 34%, or a total area of 84% of the area of the shifted normal curve. Moving one Z unit to the left, hence to a probit of 4, subtracts 34% so that only 16% of the area (50 − 34) is to the left of $Z = 4$. Thus, 16% corresponds to a probit of 4, 50% to a probit of 5, and 84% to a probit of 6. The advantage in converting percentages to probits, in either the graded or the quantal (all-or-none), is that the plot of probit (on the vertical scale) against log (concentration) displays a *linear* trend for many drug-effector systems. One may then either estimate the construction of the line that best fits the data or use regression techniques. A table of probits is given in Appendix Table A.

Regression analysis is commonly used in plotting and analyzing straight line data. Data points (x_i, y_i) may not be colinear, but yet display a linear trend suggesting that there is a straight line that can "best" describe the relation between the dependent (y) and independent (x) variables. The technique of finding the equation, $y = mx + b$, that best fits the data points uses the least–squares criterion and is well known, being now standard in textbooks of statistics. The procedure gives the slope m and vertical intercept b, as well as the standard errors of these. For the k points (x_i, y_i), $i = 1$ to k, the values of slope (m) and intercept (b) are given by

$$m = \frac{\Sigma\,(x_i - \bar{x})\,(y_i - \bar{y})}{\Sigma\,(x_i - \bar{x})^2} \tag{2.1}$$

and

$$b = \bar{y} - m\,\bar{x} \tag{2.2}$$

where $\bar{x}$ is the mean of the x_i and $\bar{y}$ is the mean of the y_i. In the analysis of dose-effect date the x_i are frequently values of log dose or log concentration since the distribution of log values gives a better fit to the observed distribution. A further discussion of the probit transformation, linear regression, and the errors in the estimates of m and b (including computer programs) is given by Tallarida and Murray.[5] (See also Busby and Tallarida[2].)

In the current context the y_i are probits corresponding to percent response and the x_i are values of log (concentration). In actual experiments generating concentration–effect data it is common to administer the same dose (concentration) to a sample of subjects and measure the effect in each.

Not all subjects will respond identically to the same dose; that is, to a given dose, x_i, (or log dose) there will be responses $y_{i1}, y_{i2}, \ldots y_{ik}$ in the k subjects. A common procedure is to "average" the responses ($\bar{y}_i$ = mean of y_{ij}) and use a single point $(x_i, \bar{y}_i)$ in the plot instead of the individual k points or effects corresponding to log dose x_i. It has been shown[2] that it is desirable to use *all* the points for each log dose, rather than to use the mean response, in that the confidence intervals of slope and intercept of the resulting regression line are smaller than if the mean response at each dose is used. Further aspects of regression analysis are covered in the discussion of Schild plots for competitive antagonists.

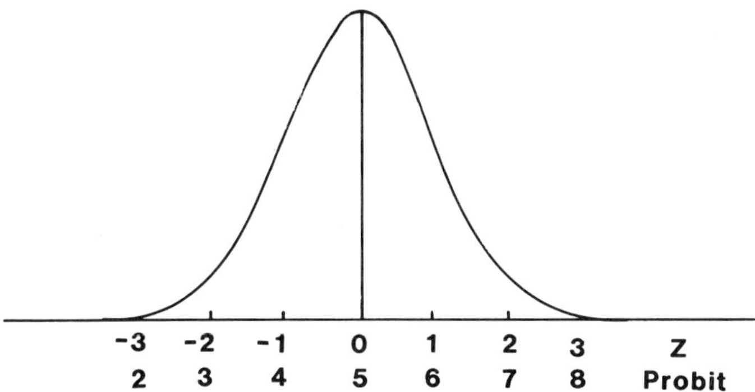

FIGURE 2.8. Percentage of the area under the standard normal curve corresponds to a value of the probit ($Z + 5$).

TABLE 2.1. Common drug-drug interactions

Drugs	Adverse effects
Allopurinol, and	
Anticoagulants, oral	Increased anticoagulant effect
Ampicillin, and	
Contraceptives, oral	Decreased contraceptive effect
Antacids, and	
Digoxin	Decreased digoxin effect
Indomethacin	Decreased indomethacin effect
Tetracyclines, oral	Decreased tetracycline effect
Anticoagulants, oral, and	
Allopurinol	Increased anticoagulant effect
Barbiturates	Decreased anticoagulant effect
Carbamazepine	Decreased anticoagulant effect
Cimetidine	Increased anticoagulant effect
Contraceptives, oral	Decreased anticoagulant effect
Hypoglycemics	Increased sulfonylurea hypoglycemia
Indomethacin	Increased risk of bleeding
Phenylbutazone	Increased anticoagulant effect
Phenytoin	Increased phenytoin toxicity (dicumarol)
Quinidine	Increased anticoagulant effect
Barbiturates, and	
Anticoagulants, oral	Decreased anticoagulant effect
Antidepressants, tricyclic	Decreased antidepressant effect
Beta-adrenergic blockers	Decreased beta blockade
Contraceptives, oral	Decreased contraceptive effect
Haloperidol	Decreased haloperidol effect
Phenothiazines	Decreased phenothiazine effect
Quinidine	Decreased quinidine effect
Benzodiazepines, and	
Cimetidine	Increased effect of chlordiazepoxide (Librium) and diazepam (Valium)
Carbamazepine, and	
Anticoagulants, oral	Decreased anticoagulant effect
Contraceptives, oral	Decreased contraceptive effect
Doxycycline	Decreased doxycycline effect
Propoxyphene	Increased carbamazepine effect
Cimetidine, and	
Anticoagulants, oral	Increased anticoagulant effect
Benzodiazepines	Increased effect of Librium and Valium
Theophylline	Increased theophylline toxicity
Clonidine, and	
Antidepressants, tricyclic	Decreased antihypertensive effects
Hypoglycemics, oral	Decreased signs of hypoglycemia
Propranolol	Paradoxical hypertension
Tolazoline	Decreased antihypertensive effect

TABLE 2.1. *Continued*

Drugs	Adverse effects
Contraceptives, oral, and	
Ampicillin	Decreased contraceptive effect
Anticoagulants, oral	Decreased anticoagulant effect
Barbiturates	Decreased contraceptive effect
Carbamazepine	Decreased contraceptive effect
Hypoglycemics, oral	Decreased hypoglycemia
Phenytoin	Decreased contraceptive effect
Tetracyclines	Decreased contraceptive effect
Corticosteroids, and	
Barbiturates	Decreased corticosteroid effect
Diuretics (except potassium-sparing)	Increased loss of potassium
Phenytoin	Decreased corticosteroid effect
Digoxin, and	
Diuretics (except potassium-sparing)	Increased digoxin toxicity
Kaolin-pectin	Decreased digoxin effect
Quinidine	Increased digoxin effect
Dipyridamole, and	
Aspirin	Increased effects on platelet function
Erythromycin, and	
Theophylline	Increased theophylline effect
Furosemide, and	
Digoxin	Increased digoxin toxicity
Indomethacin	Decreased antihypertensive and natriuretic effect
Phenytoin	Decreased diuresis
Propranolol	Increased beta-adrenergic blockade
Haloperidol, and	
Barbiturates	Decreased haloperidol effects
Methyldopa	Increased haloperidol toxicity
Phenytoin	Decreased haloperidol effects
Hypoglycemics, oral, and	
Clonidine	Decreased signs of hypoglycemia
Contraceptives	Decreased hypoglycemia
Dicumarol	Increased hypoglycemia
Methyldopa	Increased hypoglycemia (tolbutamide)
Phenylbutazone	Increased hypoglycemia
Propranolol	Prolonged hypoglycemia
Salicylates	Increased hypoglycemia
Sulfonamides	Increased hypoglycemia
Indomethacin, and	
Antacids, oral	Decreased indomethacin effect
Anticoagulants, oral	Increased bleeding risk
Beta-blockers	Decreased antihypertensive effect
Furosemide	Decreased antihypertensive effect
Thiazides	Decreased antihypertensive effect

TABLE 2.1. *Continued*

Drugs	Adverse effects
Iron, oral, and	
Tetracylines	Decreased tetracycline effect
Methyldopa, and	
Haloperidol	Increased haloperidol toxicity
Tolbutamide	
Naproxen, and	
Probenecid	Increased naproxen effects
Papaverine, and	
Levodopa	Decreased levodopa effect
Phenothiazines, and	
Barbiturates	Decreased phenothiazine effect
Phenytoin	Decreased mesoridazine effects
Propranolol	Increased effects of chlorpromazine and propranolol
Phenylbutazone, and	
Anticoagulants, oral	Increased anticoagulant effect
Hypoglycemics, oral	Increased sulfonylurea hypoglycemia
Phenytoin	Increased phenytoin toxicity
Phenytoin, and	
Antidepressants, trycyclic	Increased phenytoin toxicity (imipramine)
Chloramphenicol	Increased phenytoin toxicity
Contraceptives, oral	Decreased contraceptive effect
Corticosteroids	Decreased corticosteroid effect
Dicumarol	Increased phenytoin toxicity
Doxycycline	Decreased doxycycline effect
Furosemide	Decreased diuresis
Haloperidol	Decreased haloperidol effect
Levodopa	Decreased levodopa effect
Phenylbutazone	Increased phenytoin toxicity
Quinidine	Decreased quinidine effect
Propranolol, and	
Barbiturates	Decreased beta-blocker effect
Chlorpromazine	Increased effects of each
Clonidine	Paradoxical hypertension
Furosemide	Increased beta-adrenergic blockade
Hypoglycemics, oral	Prolonged hypoglycemia
Indomethacin	Decrease in antihypertensive effect
Theophylline	Increased theophylline effect
Quinidine, and	
Anticoagulants	Increased anticoagulant effect
Barbiturates	Decreased quinidine effect
Digoxin	Increased digoxin effect
Phenytoin	Decreased quinidine effect
Salicylates, and	
Anticoagulants, oral	Possible risk of increased bleeding
Dipyridamole	Increased effects on platelet function
Hypoglycemics	Increased hypoglycemia

TABLE 2.1. *Continued*

Drugs	Adverse effects
Spironolactone, and	
Potassium	Hyperkalemia
Sulfonamides, and	
Anticoagulants, oral	Increased anticoagulant effect
Hypoglycemics	Increased sulfonylurea hypoglycemia
Tetracyclines, and	
Antacids, oral	Decreased tetracycline effects
Barbiturates	Decreased doxycycline effect
Carbamazepine	Decreased doxycycline effect
Contraceptives, oral	Decreased contraceptive effect
Iron, oral	Decreased tetracyline effect
Phenytoin	Decreased doxycycline effect
Theophylline, and	
Cimetidine	Increased theophylline toxicity
Erythromycin	Increased theophylline effect
Propranolol	Increased theophylline effect
Thiazide diuretics, and	
Corticosteroids	Increased loss of potassium
Digitalis drugs	Increased digitalis toxicity
Indomethacin	Decreased antihypertensive and natriuretic effects
Salicylates	Increased CNS toxicity (acetazolamide)
Thyroid, and	
Anticoagulants, oral	Increased anticoagulant effect
Triamterene, and	
Potassium	Hyperkalemia

From Tallarida RJ: Most-Prescribed Drugs—1985. Philadelphia, WB Saunders Co., 1985, pp. 219–230. Reprinted by permission.

Additivity and Synergism

Whereas an antagonist reduces the effects of an active drug or other compound, there are substances that may enhance drug action. Mechanisms underlying augmented responses vary considerably. One substance may enhance the absorption of the other, or impede the excretion of the other, or have similar actions so that the combination is additive. In some cases the presence of one compound sensitizes the receptor to the combination of the second compound. These are just a few mechanisms. Combinations may have therapeutic advantages or disadvantages. Certainly the adverse effects, when summed, represent a total disadvantage. When the side effects are tolerable, many combination drugs are extremely effective. For example, combinations containing a diuretic and an antihypertensive drug are often indicated. Accordingly, pharmaceutical manufacturers frequently formulate drugs that are combinations. For example, Hydropres, a popular antihypertensive agent, is a combination of hydrochlorothiazide and reserpine. The presence of the diuretic (which also has antihypertensive action) allows a smaller dose of reserpine than would otherwise be needed to lower the blood pressure to the same degree.

Another rational combination is a vasodilator (e.g., hydralazine) and a beta-adrenergic blocker (e.g., propranolol or atenolol). The vasodilator may reflexly cause stimulation of sympathetic outflow that would excite the heart. Beta blockade affords a component of protection against this cardiac stimulation. Further, the combination of triamterene (which conserves potassium) and hydrochlorothiazide (which excretes potassium) is a particularly useful and popular formulation (Dyazide).

Some combinations are dangerous. For example, the combined effects of alcohol and drugs that are central nervous system depressants, such as barbiturates, are responsible for many accidental deaths.

Certain combinations produce effects (desirable or undesirable) that are greater than the sum of the effects of the individual components. This kind of synergism is often called *potentiation* in pharmacology.* The diuresis produced by the combination of a mercurial diuretic and ammonium chloride is often sighted as an example of potentiation. Several examples of drug–drug combinations—additive, antagonistic, and generally undesirable—are contained in Table 2.1. The drugs listed are among the most widely prescribed in the United States. (For a discussion of the modification of metabolism induced by concomitant drug administration, see Chapter 4.)

References

1. Altschuler S: *Int J Obesity* 1982; 6:549.
2. Busby RC, Tallarida RJ: On the analysis of straight line data in pharmacology and biochemistry. *J Theor Biol* 1981; 93:867.
3. Tallarida RJ, Sevy R, Harakal C, et al: The effect of preload on the dissociation constant of norepinephrine in isolated strips of rabbit thoracic aorta. *Arch Int Pharmacodyn Ther* 1974; 210:67.
4. Tallarida RJ, Harakal C, Maslow J, et al: The relationship between pharmacokinetics and pharmacodynamic action as applied to *in vivo* pA_2: Applications to the analgesic effect of morphine. *J Pharmacol Exp Ther* 1978; 206:38.
5. Tallarida RJ, Murray RB: *Manual of Pharmacologic Calculations with Computer Programs*, Second Edition. New York, Springer-Verlag, 1987.
6. Tallarida RJ: *Most Prescribed Drugs—1985*. Philadelphia, WB Saunders, 1985.
7. Tallarida RJ, Porreca F, Cowan A: Statistical analysis of drug-drug and site-site interactions with isobolograms. (Submitted as *Life Sciences* minireview, 1988).

*A detailed statistical treatment for distinguishing potentiation from simple additive or subadditive action is given by Tallarida et al.[7] (See also Chapter 8, "Drug Combinations: Isoboles.")

3 Pharmacokinetics

Pharmacokinetics is concerned with the kinetics or movement of compounds throughout the organism. For the most part, we are here concerned with the kinetics of drugs and endogenous compounds as well as their metabolites. The processes studied in pharmacokinetics include absorption, distribution, metabolism, and excretion of substances. Ideally we wish to know the amounts and concentrations of these substances as a function of time in various body compartments and in excreta. The term "compartment," for the present, refers to a space into which the drug distributes. For example, we shall speak of drug concentrations in blood, gut, and brain; however, in pharmacokinetics these compartments require further definition, as we shall show later. The time course of effect, not necessarily the same as the time course of concentration in the effector organ, is also considered by some to be part of pharmacokinetics.

Factors influencing the time course of concentration and effect include the chemical form of the drug, its physical state, its route of administration, as well as unknown factors. The study of pharmacokinetics requires measurement of the drug concentration in various body compartments or tissues, but usually such measurements are confined to blood, plasma, serum, and urine, since these compartments are the most conveniently reached.

Absorption

Drugs are administered by several different routes. These include oral, sublingual, buccal, intramuscular, subcutaneous, inhalation, rectal, vaginal, transdermal, intravenous, and intra-arterial. The last two routes are intravascular, whereas the others are extravascular and, therefore, require absorption into the blood. Of the various extravascular routes of administration, oral ingestion is the most common. We shall therefore discuss this route first and, in so doing, introduce pharmacokinetics as a quantitative branch of pharmacology. Many, but not all, of the pharmacokinetic concepts involved in oral administration will be applicable to other extravascular routes. Some factors that are important in assessing absorption from the oral route are the drug's solubility, the blood flow to the site of absorption, and the drug's degree of ionization.

The gastrointestinal epithelium contains small membrane pores and is composed largely of lipids so that passage across this membrane requires either that the drug molecule be lipid soluble or that it have an extremely small molecular diameter. For example, a water-soluble substance such as urea can pass through the narrow water-filled channels, whereas most drug molecules would be too large to pass through these channels. Therefore, the absorption of most drugs must be due to passage through the highly lipid membrane.

The epithelial cells of the small intestine transfer water and dissolved substances from the intestinal lumen to the interstitial fluid and, hence, to the blood. The rate of transfer of different substances is selective, and the transfer may be either active or passive. Active transport means movement against a concentration gradient (electrochemical gradient is discussed later) and requires energy, whereas a passive process does not require energy. Generally, the absorption of water and most solutes is greater in the duodenum and jejunum than in the stomach, ileum, and colon. Yet drugs taken orally must pass through the stomach; thus the rate of *gastric emptying* is a controlling step in the absorption. Further, while in the stomach the drug is in an acid environment; hence, if the drug molecule is acid unstable (e.g., penicillin, erythromycin) it will be destroyed before it can be effectively absorbed. The rate of gastric emptying is affected by many influences such as anxiety and stress, food, and the existence of other drugs. For most drugs the passage through membranes is by diffusion.

Diffusion

Passive diffusion through the intestinal membrane is usually described by a model identical to that governing the diffusion of gases. In this model, illustrated in Figure 3.1, the flux (amount per unit time) through area A is directly proportional to the concentration gradient

$$J = b \cdot dC/dx \tag{3.1}$$

in which J is the flux; dC/dx, the concentration gradient; and b, the constant of proportionality, which itself is the product of surface area A, partition coefficient K (discussed in a later section), and the diffusion coefficient D:

$$b = A \cdot K \cdot D \tag{3.2}$$

Equation (3.1) is generally referred to as Fick's first law of diffusion. An approximate form of this equation in terms of outer and inner concentration, C_o and C_i, is given by

$$J = A \cdot K \cdot D\,(C_o - C_i)/h \tag{3.3}$$

where h is the membrane thickness.

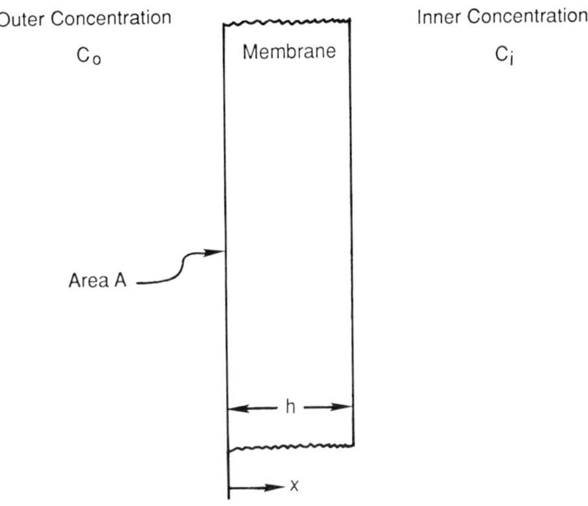

FIGURE 3.1. Flux, amount/time, through area A is proportional to the concentration gradient dc/dx. The latter is approximately $(C_o - C_i)/h$.

In equation (3.3) the concentration gradient dC/dx, which varies along the depth of the membrane, has been replaced by the term $(C_o - C_i)/h$ and permits the definition of the *permeability constant* P:

$$P = K \cdot D/h \tag{3.4}$$

The permeability constant is a characteristic of the drug and the membrane. From equations (3.3) and (3.4) the flux may be expressed as follows:

$$J - P \cdot A\,(C_o - C_i) \tag{3.5}$$

When all the drug is on the outside of the membrane, a time we call $t = 0$, $C_i = 0$, and the initial flux is proportional to the outer concentration. Experimentally, one may isolate the membrane, vary C_o, and measure the initial flux. If the relation is found to be linear, it is reasonable to suppose that the transport is taking place by passive diffusion, whereas nonlinearity indicates another mode of transport (see Figure 3.2). The experiment described measured *initial* flux. At times after $t = 0$, both C_o and C_i change and eventually become equal (provided that the molecule is electrically neutral), at which time the net flux would be zero, meaning that equilibrium has been attained. Equilibrium is not usually achieved in vivo, since blood flow to the region assures continuous absorption by removing the drug molecule that has penetrated the region. Drugs that are highly lipid soluble or otherwise able to penetrate the aqueous pores may rapidly reach equilibrium with blood so that the absorption rate becomes dependent on the blood flow to the region. Blood flow is therefore a potential rate-

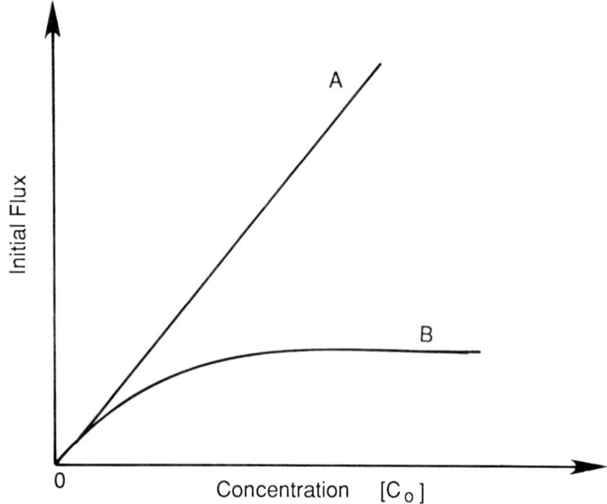

FIGURE 3.2. The initial flux (amount/time) is plotted as a function of drug concentration. Curve A suggests that the transport process is passive diffusion, whereas curve B demonstrates saturation, thereby suggesting a carrier-mediated transport process.

limiting factor in the absorption of a particular drug molecule. Another factor is the degree of ionization of the drug in the compartment from which absorption takes place. In general, the nonionized form is able to pass through most membranes whereas ionized molecules do not pass readily.

Since most drugs are either weak acids or bases and, therefore, ionizable, their degree of ionization in the compartment from which absorption occurs will greatly affect the amount of absorption. The relative concentrations of ionized and nonionized forms at equilibrium depend on the pK of the drug and the pH of the medium, according to the Henderson–Hasselbalch equation (discussed in Chapter 1). The pH along the gastrointestinal tract is variable (Table 3.1) and, therefore, drugs taken orally are most affected. The variation in pH is less in most other parts of the organism, and, indeed, the degree of ionization is of less consequence when the drug must cross capillaries as in parenteral routes such as subcutaneous and intramuscular.

Rate Constant for Absorption

The oral absorption of many drugs proceeds at a rate that is proportional to the amount (X) remaining to be absorbed, or $dX/dt = k_a X$. The absorption rate constant k_a may be related to the physical constants of the Fick's law as follows:

$$J = \mathrm{P} \cdot \mathrm{A}\,(C_o - C_i).$$

TABLE 3.1. Variation of pH along the gastrointestinal tract.

	pH
Stomach	1–3
Duodenum and jejunum	5–7
Ileum	7–8

The flux $J = dX/dt$. If C_o is greater than C_i, as is the case when C_i is the blood concentration, then $J = \text{PA}C_o = \text{PA}X/\text{V}$, where the outer concentration has been replaced by X/V, the amount per unit volume. Because P, A, and V are constants, the expression PA/V may be viewed as the proportionality constant k_a and, with adjustment of sign to account for outward movement, $dX/dt = -k_a X$. This form is convenient and will be referred to as a first-order process. Viewed from the gut, the drug is leaving so the sign is negative. Clearly, the rate entering the blood is $k_a X$.

Lipid–Water Partition Coefficient

The lipid–water partition coefficient K, a parameter of importance in the diffusion of the drug through the lipid membrane, is the ratio of concentrations of the drug at equilibrium in a lipid solvent (such as mineral oil) and water. Denoting the concentrations in lipid and aqueous phases by C_l and C_a, respectively, we have

$$K = C_l/C_a \tag{3.6}$$

In this definition it is assumed that the concentrations are those of the same species in both fluids, that is, the drug molecule does not undergo a physicochemical change in one of the two fluids. A number of different nonaqueous solvents have been used to measure K and to compare the values among a series of drugs to actual gastrointestinal absorption. The agreement has been generally good, but not perfect. The partition coefficient as used in pharmacology is often referred to as the *apparent* lipid–water partition coefficient, since the "true" coefficient is defined for ideal solutions of two immiscible liquids in which the solute does not change form and in which the concentration in either is low. As previously mentioned, polar drugs do not pass well across the lipid membrane. In terms of K, such drugs have low values compared with nonpolar drugs. Despite its limitations, the lipid–water partition coefficient is a reasonable indicator of a drug's absorption potential and also of drug storage in the body's fat. If a drug has appreciable storage in fat its release from this depository will extend its effective time in the body, a phenomenon well known for some drugs such as barbiturates. Further discussions of the partition coefficient will occur when we discuss volume of distribution and protein binding.

Transport Mechanisms

It is well known that some substances move against their concentration gradients. The movement of sodium is an example. Clearly this movement requires energy, in contrast to passive diffusion as just discussed. In one such active transport process the molecule attaches to a specific carrier, usually believed to be an enzyme located on the outer surface of the membrane. The molecule joins with the carrier and moves, as the complex, across the membrane, utilizing energy provided by the breakdown of adenosine triphosphate (ATP). Once inside the membrane, the drug molecule dissociates from the carrier and the latter moves back to the outer membrane. When the drug molecules exceed the number of carriers, the transport system becomes saturated. In contrast to passive diffusion in which the initial rate of transport is linearly related to the drug concentration at the absorptive site, in carrier-mediated transport such a relation is not linear but plateaus at sufficiently high drug concentrations (see Figure 3.2). This type of transport is also affected by substances (e.g., cyanide) that interfere with cell metabolism and by competing substances (such as other drugs) that also have affinity for the same carrier. Michaelis–Menten kinetics is often used to describe the interaction between drug molecules and carrier molecules, as well as to describe the effects of various kinds of competition.

Electrochemical Potential

Diffusion from a region of high concentration to a region of lower concentration results from the random motion of molecules. If these molecules possess an electrical charge, however, the movement across a membrane of a second molecule is influenced by the charge of the first. Each successive molecule that traverses the membrane must do more work than its predecessor. Accordingly, the potential energy, or capacity to do work, is due to both electrical and diffusion phenomena and is calculated from a function called the *electrochemical potential*. When a state of dynamic equilibrium is reached, the electrochemical potential is zero. At equilibrium the tendency to move because of the concentration difference is balanced by the repulsive force of the opposing electric field set up by the separation of like charges.

The spatial derivative of potential constitutes a potential gradient. If the potential is denoted by V and the spatial coordinate is denoted by s, then the electric potential gradient is dV/ds. When such a gradient exists, the transport of charged (drug) molecules requires energy and is termed "active."

The study of the absorption of vitamin B_{12} reveals the necessity of a carrier, *intrinsic factor*, produced in the stomach; yet the absorption is not against a gradient. This absorptive process is called *facilitated* transport, and although generally considered to be a subset of active transport, it does not proceed against a gradient. This mode of transport is not very common for drugs, yet it occurs in normal physiology, as exemplified by the transport of glucose into red blood cells.

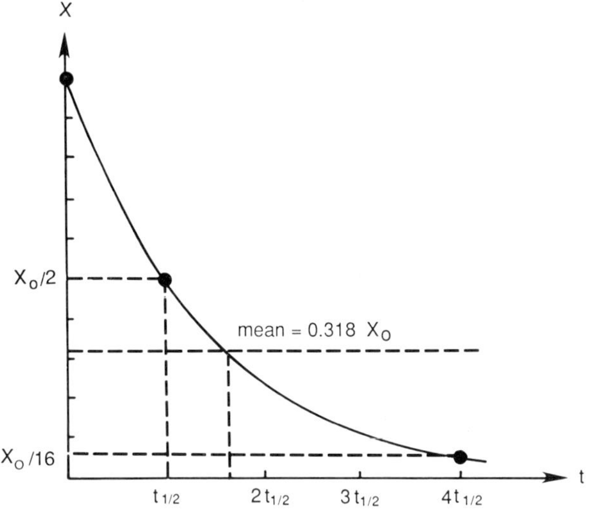

FIGURE 3.3. First-order elimination. At time $t = 4\ t_{1/2}$, one sixteenth of X_0 remains. The mean value over the interval 0 to 4.3 $t_{1/2}$ is 0.318 C_o *(see text)*. *Inset*: Plot on logarithmically calibrated ordinate showing fraction of X_o at integral multiples of the half-life.

Another kind of transport, called ion-pair transport, is believed to exist. Because some highly ionized compounds are absorbed in the physiologic pH range, and neither of the absorption mechanisms discussed provides an adequate explanation, it has been proposed that an ion of the opposite polarity may neutralize the compound, rendering it absorbable by passive diffusion. The opposite-polarity ions may exist naturally in the gastrointestinal tract. This mechanism may explain the observation that several quaternary ammonium compounds that are highly ionized in the gastrointestinal tract are apparently absorbed and produce systemic effects. Therefore, *the degree of ionization of a compound in the gut is not an infallible indicator of its ability to be absorbed.*

The Liver

The liver is the most important organ involved in the biotransformation of most drugs. The drug metabolites formed may be pharmacologically inactive, or far less active than the administered drug. In such cases hepatic extraction represents a pathway out of the circulation of the active drug. Hepatic extraction is especially important when drugs are administered orally, since the venous blood from the gastrointestinal tract drains into the portal vein and is delivered to the liver. For some common drugs, e.g., nitroglycerin, even a single pass through the liver results in appreciable degradation; hence, this agent is not usually given by the oral route. When the "first-pass effect" is not so appreciable, the oral route is used, but it would still require a larger dose than that used in parenteral administration. (Hepatic metabolism is discussed in Chapter 4.)

Drug Elimination

Much of the terminology and many concepts in pharmacokinetics arise from a *model* in which the body is regarded to be a single homogeneous compartment in which a drug distributes very rapidly. Thus we consider a compartment of volume V into which an amount X_0 of drug is introduced at the time $t = 0$. Further, the drug is to move out of this compartment and not return. We wish to describe mathematically the kinetics that might apply to this simplified situation, that is, the amount of drug that exists (remains) in the compartment as a function of time after $t = 0$. Several conceptual points are fundamental to an understanding of actual drug kinetics.

The simplest mathematical description is that in which the drug, in amount X_0, is distributed in a constant volume V and leaves at a constant rate b (amount per unit time). In this case, the amount X at time t is given by

$$X = X_0 - bt \tag{3.7}$$

Dividing each term by the constant volume V yields an expression for the *concentration* C remaining as a function of time:

$$C = C_0 - (b/V)t \tag{3.8}$$

where C_0 is the initial concentration. The time to complete passage is easily seen to be equal to X_0/b. The transport process described here is called "zero order" for reasons to be explained subsequently. Although mathematically the simplest case, the zero-order process is not the most common in pharmacokinetics. More commonly, the rate of movement of drug from one compartment to another is not constant but, instead, depends on the amount or the concentration of the drug in the compartment containing the drug. Using the common notation for the derivative, dX/dt, we can write $dX/dt = f(X)$, where $f(X)$ denotes, in a general way, a function of X. The function $f(X)$ may be a direct proportion, in which case

$$dX/dt = -k \cdot X \tag{3.9}$$

The constant of proportionality k is the *elimination rate constant*, or fraction per unit time, that leaves the compartment; thus, k has the unit of reciprocal time. The negative sign in equation (3.9) is necessary, since the derivative, or time rate of change, is negative because the drug is leaving the compartment. Equation (3.9) defines a transport process that is called *first order*, whereas if there were an integral power n on X, that is, $dX/dt = -kX^n$, the order would be n. (When $n = 0$ the process is zero order and since $X^0 = 1$, dX/dt is constant.) From equation (3.9)

$$X = X_0 \cdot \exp(-kt) \tag{3.10}$$

TABLE 3.2. Biologic half-life of selected drugs.*

Drug	Half-life
Acetaminophen	1–4 h
Desipramine	12–24 h
Diazepam	20–40 h
Digitoxin	5–8 d
Digoxin	0.7–2 d
Indomethacin	2–8 d
Meperidine	1.5–4 h
Phenobarbital	50–120 h
Propranolol	3–6 h

*Illustrates range among individuals. From Pribor et al.[2]

The graph of equation (3.10) is shown in Figure 3.3. Also shown is the *half-life* or time interval during which the concentration halves. From equation (3.10) the half-life is obtained by letting $X = X_0/2$ and solving for t (denoted, $t_{1/2}$):

$$\frac{1}{2} X_0 = X_0 \cdot \exp(-kt_{1/2})$$

$$t_{1/2} = \ln(2)/k \tag{3.11}$$

Equivalently,

$$k = \ln(2)/t_{1/2} \tag{3.12}$$

For computation, ln(2) is approximated by 0.693. Note that after four half-lives, only 1/16th (6.2%) of the drug remains and after 4.3 half-lives, 5% of the drug remains. When this analysis is applied to actual drugs that obey first-order elimination from a compartment, it is common to assume that after 4.3 half-lives the drug is gone. Half-lives of selected drugs are given in Table 3.2.

The mean value of concentration (or amount X) in an exponential elimination process may be found over an interval, 0 to T, by integrating the concentration function $C(t)$ between 0 and T and dividing the integral by T. Graphically, the integral is the area under the concentration–time curve (Figure 3.4). Because an exponential theoretically never reaches zero, it is necessary to define the interval 0 to T in some practical way. As previously noted, the practical value of T is 4.3 half-lives. Thus, for concentration $C = C_0 \exp(-kt)$, the integral between $t = 0$ and $t = T = 4.3\ t_{1/2}$ is

$$\textstyle\int_0^T C_0 \exp(-kt)\, dt = C_0/k \cdot [1 - \exp(-kT)].$$

For $T = 4.3$ half-lives, the term in brackets on the right-hand side is 0.95. Hence, the value of the integral is 0.95 C_0/k, and the mean is 0.95 C_0/kT. It is easily seen that $kT = -\ln(0.05) = 2.99$. Thus, the mean concentration is $(0.95\ C_0)/2.99$, or

$$C_{(\text{mean})} = 0.318\ C_0 \tag{3.13}$$

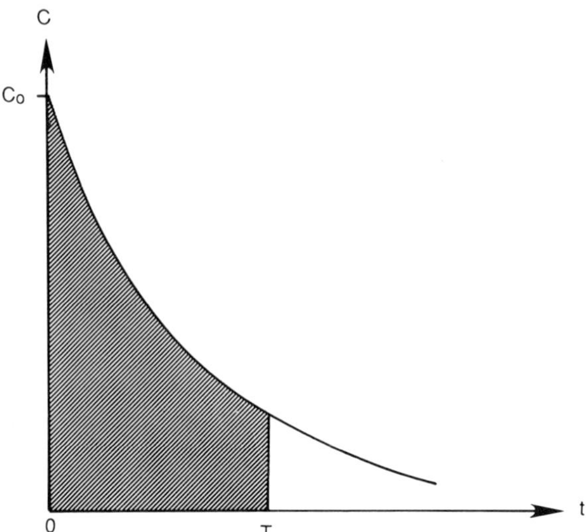

FIGURE 3.4. The mean value of a function (such as concentration, C) over the interval $t = 0$ to $t = T$ is the area shaded divided by the interval width T. For the exponential function that characterizes the elimination of many drugs, T is frequently 4.3 half-lives, the time to fall to 5% C_o.

For the elimination process discussed, the actual concentration attains its mean at time $t = 1.69$ half-lives (Figure 3.3). Note that in this figure the time axis is calibrated in units of half-life.*

Volume of Distribution

If a quantity X of a substance is distributed uniformly in a volume V, the concentration C at equilibrium is $C = X/V$, so that the volume $V = X/C$. The volume can thus be calculated from the concentration and the amount X. When drugs are administered to an organism, they will generally distribute to many body compartments. If, however, the entire amount were confined to a single compartment one could determine the volume of that compartment by sampling to determine the concentration and using the above equation. The plasma is an accessible fluid and, thus, the concentrations in plasma are readily determined. Because the drug will move from the plasma to other sites, the equilibrium concentration in plasma will be less than it would be if the drug remained in this compartment. Accordingly, the use of plasma concentration as C in the equation leads to a volume larger than the true plasma volume (Figure 3.5). This larger volume is thus an "apparent" volume of distribution.

*For future reference it may be of value to note that for arbitrary T, $e^{-kT} = (\frac{1}{2})^{T/t_{1/2}}$.

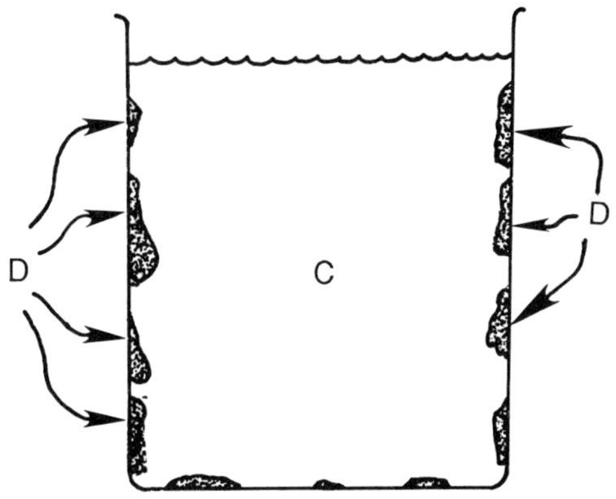

FIGURE 3.5. Binding of the drug D to the walls of the container results in a diminished concentration C. The apparent volume, determined by dividing the dose by C, is larger than the true volume.

Figure 3.6 is a graph of plasma concentration (log scale) against time following intravenous administration. The concentration declines in the plasma. The initial concentration $C(0)$, obtained by extrapolating data to zero time, is used in the calculation. The extrapolation is from the terminal segment of the decay curve. The initial rapid decline is due to movement of the drug to sites outside the plasma and, when such binding is appreciable, the extrapolated value $C(0)$ is very reduced so that the apparent volume of distribution is large. Clearly, the volume of distribution is an indicator of the degree of drug binding and, for a highly bound drug, will be a number larger than any true body volume. (Typical volumes in adults are 5 1, plasma; 15 1, extracellular fluid; 20 1, intracellular fluid.) Besides its use as an indicator of drug binding, the apparent volume of distribution is useful because it is a proportionality "constant" between the amount of drug in the body and the plasma concentration at any time. This value is therefore a characteristic of the drug, and the value is reasonably constant over the range of therapeutic concentrations.

Volume of distribution is most often computed from the total area under the plasma concentration–time curve $(\mathrm{AUC})_0^\infty$ and the elimination rate constant (k) of the terminal segment of the decay curve:

$$V = \frac{\text{amount absorbed}}{k\,(\mathrm{AUC})_0^\infty} \tag{3.14}$$

For intravenous administration the amount administered is, of course, used in equation (3.14) for amount absorbed. Equation (3.14) is actually a definition of the apparent volume of distribution. It is, therefore, independent of the mode of administration and the shape of the concentration–time curve. The motivation for the definition is, however, related to certain properties of exponential functions (as discussed below), and it is also shown that the above is equivalent to the previous formula $[V = X/C(0)]$ when drug elimination is exponential with a single elimination rate constant.

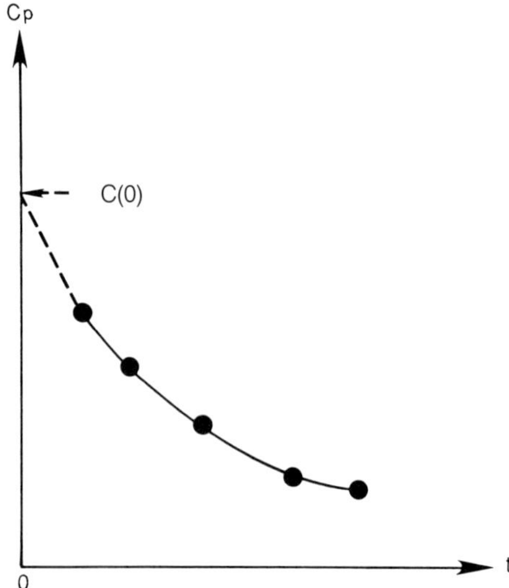

FIGURE 3.6. Initial plasma concentration, C_{p_o}, determined by extrapolating the smooth curve that best represents concentration-time data points.

A pure exponential decay of concentration is given by $C(0) \cdot \exp(-kt)$. The total area under the curve $(\text{AUC})_0^\infty$ is the integral $\int_0^\infty C(0) \cdot \exp(-kt)\, dt$. The value of the integral is $C(0)/k$. Thus, $C(0) = k(\text{AUC})_0^\infty$ so that V = amount absorbed/$C(0)$ becomes amount absorbed/$k(\text{AUC})_0^\infty$.

Clearance

Just as the amount of drug in the body is proportional to the plasma concentration (proportionality constant V), the total rate of removal (dX/dt) is also found to be proportional to the plasma concentration over the range of therapeutic concentrations. The proportionality constant is termed the clearance of the drug and is denoted Cl:

$$Cl = \frac{dX/dt}{C_p} \tag{3.15}$$

The clearance of a drug from a biological fluid, such as plasma, has the units of volume per time and may be viewed as fluid volume that is cleared of the drug in unit time. If the concentration used in equation (3.15) were that of blood, then the clearance would be the blood volume per unit time that is cleared. Clearance may be separated according to the organ or system that is responsible for elimination. For example, if renal excretion and hepatic metabolism are the only two modes of elimination, then

$$(dX/dt)_{\text{total}} = (dX/dt)_{\text{renal}} + (dX/dt)_{\text{hepatic}} \tag{3.16}$$

Division by C_p gives

$$Cl_{\text{total}} = Cl_{\text{renal}} + Cl_{\text{hepatic}} \tag{3.17}$$

so that clearances are additive.

Further insight into the concept of clearance and alternative methods for computing clearance follow from a *model* that views the body as a single compartment in which the amount of drug X is the product of concentration C and the apparent volume of distribution V. Thus, for first-order elimination

$$dX/dt = -k \cdot X = -k \cdot V \cdot C \tag{3.18}$$

Thus,

$$\frac{dX/dt}{C} = -k \cdot V \tag{3.19}$$

and clearance is given by

$$Cl = k \cdot V \tag{3.20}$$

or, from equation (3.14)

$$Cl = \frac{\text{amount absorbed}}{(\text{AUC})_0^\infty} \tag{3.21}$$

Equation (3.21) is often used in calculating the total body clearance of a drug. Since AUC is the total area ($t = 0$ to ∞), the amount absorbed is the amount eliminated. When the concentration–time curve is known only up to some time T, the clearance calculation may be made from the disposition of the drug. If the elimination (all routes) is denoted by A over the time interval 0 to T, then the average rate of removal is A/T and the average plasma concentration is $\frac{1}{T}\int_0^T C(t)dt$ so that clearance becomes

$$Cl = \frac{A}{\int_0^T C(t) \cdot dt} \tag{3.22}$$

If A in equation (3.22) is the total amount excreted into urine, then the clearance computed from it is the renal clearance. The largest possible value of renal clearance is the renal blood flow. Since $Cl = kV$ and $k = \ln(2)/t_{1/2}$, we get also the following relation:

$$Cl = \ln(2) \cdot V/t_{1/2} \tag{3.23}$$

Drug–Protein Binding

Many drugs bind to plasma proteins, mostly to the albumin fraction (see Table 3.3). This binding influences the distribution, excretion, metabolism, and interaction with the drug receptors. That is, the bound drug does not readily arrive at

TABLE 3.3. Protein binding of selected drugs.

Diazepam	96
Digitoxin	97
Digoxin	23
Glutethimide	50
Indomethacin	90
Lithium	0
Phenytoin	88
Procainamide	15
Propranolol	93
Quinidine sulfate	82
Tolbutamide	50–80
Trimethadione	0

From Pribor et al.[2]

its locus of action, nor is it filtered by the renal glomeruli. Differences in protein binding of a drug among humans and across species account, in part, for differences in a drug's action among people and in different species. The protein-bound drug is ultimately available, since the unbound drug is eliminated, thereby favoring dissociation of the drug molecule from its protein-binding site. Thus, protein binding, like binding to tissue, tends to maintain a fairly constant level of the free drug.

If we denote the protein by P, the drug by D, and the complex by PD, then it follows that

$$\frac{(\mathrm{PD})}{(\mathrm{P}_t)} = \frac{(\mathrm{D})}{K + (\mathrm{D})} \tag{3.24}$$

where (D) is the concentration of drug (assumed to greatly exceed the total protein concentration P_t) and K is the dissociation constant of the complex. The left-hand side of equation (3.24) is the fraction bound and, as seen, when plotted against (D), results in the familiar hyperbolic plot of Figure 3.7. Rearrangement of Equation (3.24) yields

$$\frac{(\mathrm{PD})}{(\mathrm{D})} = \frac{-1}{K}(\mathrm{PD}) + \frac{\mathrm{P}_t}{K}, \tag{3.25}$$

the Scatchard form. In this form a plot of the ratio (bound/free) against bound is linear, with slope $-1/K$ and vertical intercept $(\mathrm{P}_t)/K$, as shown in Figure 3.8. A further discussion of Scatchard plots is given in Chapter 9.

Protein Binding and Disease

Diseases, especially those of the liver and kidney, can affect the degree of protein binding of some drugs. For example, the popular drugs diazepam, morphine, and phenytoin are less extensively bound to proteins in states of impaired hepatic

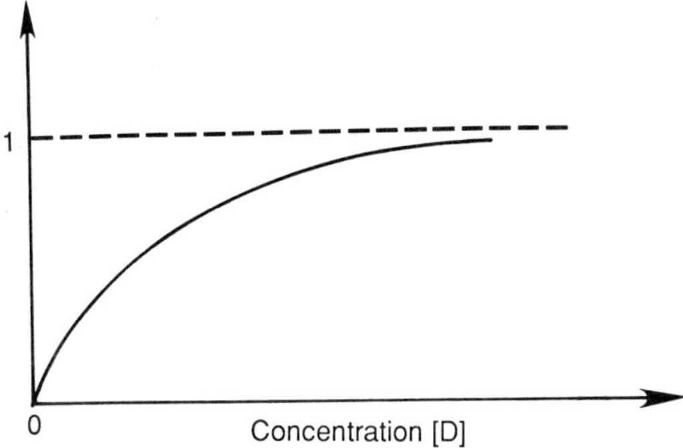

FIGURE 3.7. Drug–protein binding.

function; whereas barbiturates, digitalis, and furosemide display decreased protein binding in patients with certain kidney diseases. Patients having these diseases may require dosage adjustments of these drugs and others that are protein bound.

Renal Excretion

The kidney is the most important organ for excreting drugs and other substances in order to maintain a normal blood state. The functional unit of the kidney is the nephron. This unit consists of a combination of tubules and capillaries. The tubules are known as the "proximal," the "loop of Henle," and the "distal." This last tubule leads to the collecting duct. The capillary network of the nephron is the glomerulus. Arterial blood enters the glomerulus. Fluid and many plasma solutes are filtered across the capillary walls that comprise the glomerulus and

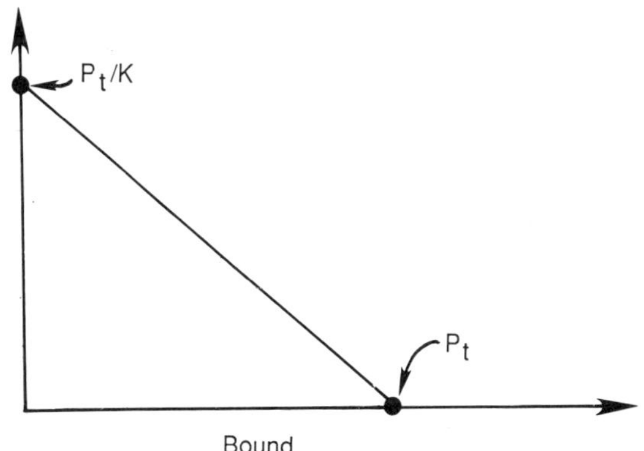

FIGURE 3.8. Scatchard plot.

enter the tubule portion of the nephron. This filtration is selective so that large molecular weight substances, such as proteins, do not normally enter the tubular region. Accordingly, drug molecules attached to plasma proteins will not usually be filtered so that the degree to which a drug is bound to protein will be an important determinant of its excretion rate. Further, a drug or other substance that is filtered may be reabsorbed during the passage of the filtrate through the proximal tubule, the loops, and the distal tubule before entrance to the collecting duct. This reabsorption can be either passive or active. Also, substances may be secreted from the peritubular capillaries into the kidney tubular network. Thus, the amount of a substance excreted will equal its amount filtered only if it is neither reabsorbed nor secreted. The extent of reabsorption or secretion depends on factors such as molecular size, lipid solubility, pK_a and the pH of the urine. Thus, if the urine pH is altered (as with other drugs), one can either facilitate or impede reabsorption and secretion. Inulin is a substance that is neither reabsorbed nor secreted, and its clearance (milliliter per minute) provides a measure of the glomerular filtration rate (GFR). In a normal adult this value is about 125 ml/min. Hence, the GFR is a physiologic "constant." For a non-protein-bound drug of plasma concentration C_p, the amount leaving per unit time, denoted by A, is therefore

$$A = C_p \cdot (\mathrm{GFR}) \tag{3.26}$$

It is noteworthy that those drugs that constrict renal arterioles will lower the GFR and may therefore lower the value of A.

Regardless of the particular mechanism of excretion, the renal clearance (Cl) of a drug may be determined from the definition [equation (3.15)] using the concentration of drug in plasma (C_p), the volume of urine excreted per minute (V'), and the concentration of drug in urine (C_u)

$$Cl = \mathrm{C}_u \cdot V'/C_p \tag{3.27}$$

Of course, at any given time the amount excreted is the product of drug concentration in urine and volume of urine. One may obtain a "corrected" clearance by using only the unbound concentration in equation (3.27). If we denote by f the fraction of drug bound to plasma proteins, then the free-drug concentration is $(1 - f) \cdot C_p$. Since C_u and C_p vary with time, their mean values over the collection time interval are used in the calculation with this equation. Alternatively, urine may be collected over some short time interval (e.g., one hour) and the amount of drug in the urine determined. This amount divided by the time interval is thus the numerator in equation (3.27). For the denominator C_p one uses the average concentration in plasma over the time interval. This average may be approximated as the plasma concentration at the midpoint of the interval. More precisely, the average is (for time interval T) $(1/T) \int_0^T C_p \cdot dt$. Thus, the renal clearance is the amount of drug in the urine divided by the area under the plasma–time curve over the interval 0 to T [see also equation (3.22)]. Many factors influence the clearance of the drug, including the chemical nature of the drug, the age and sex of the subject, the existence of pathology, etc. In the very young human (less than 6 months) and the old (greater than 70 years), clear-

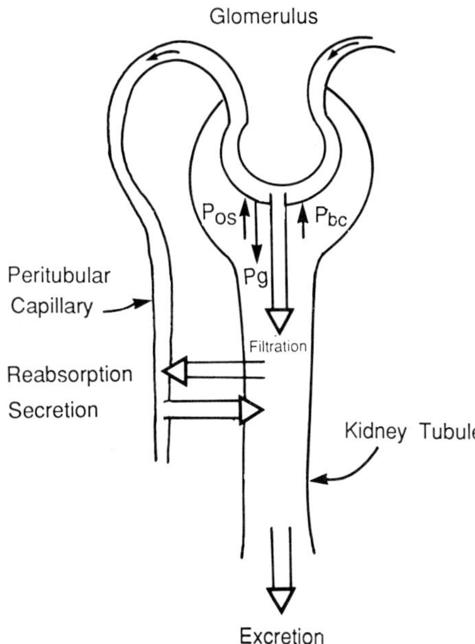

FIGURE 3.9. Glomerular filtration, reabsorption, and secretion as related to excretion. Typical pressures (mm Hg) are P_g = 50, Pos = 30, and P_{bc} = 10 mm Hg.

ances are generally lower. Also noteworthy is that throughout adulthood creatinine clearance (discussed below) diminishes at a rate of 1%/yr.

Glomerular Filtration

The capillary part of the nephron, as previously mentioned, is the glomerulus. Blood enters the glomerulus via the afferent arteriole and leaves via the efferent arteriole. In this movement fluid, dissolved solutes, and small molecules pass through the capillary walls and enter the lumen of the tubule, being driven by a net pressure difference. The fraction entering the lumen, the filtrate, normally contains little or no protein or other high molecular weight substances. The filtrate moves along the lumen of the proximal tubule, loop of Henle, and distal tubule. In this transit, molecules can be actively or passively reabsorbed into the blood. Also, molecules can pass from the peritubular capillaries to the tubule, a process called secretion. Accordingly, the excreted amount is the difference: excretion = (filtration + secretion) − (reabsorption)

As illustrated in Figure 3.9, filtration is driven by the relatively high hydrostatic pressure of the glomerular capillaries (P_g) and is opposed by the pressure in the capsule (P_{bc}) and the osmotic pressure (P_{os}) resulting from the impermeable proteins in the blood: $P_g - (P_{bc} + P_{os})$. Figure 3.9 also shows reabsorption and secretion.

The GFR, an index of renal function, is normally about 125 ml/min. Clinically it is determined from the clearance of creatinine, a natural product of muscle metabolism that is neither reabsorbed nor secreted. (See also the discussion of

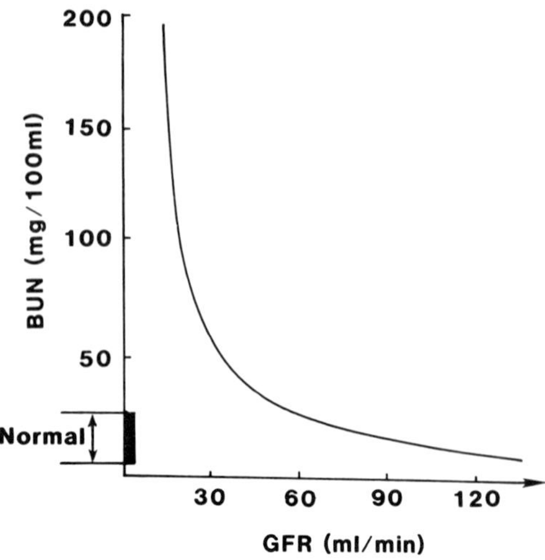

FIGURE 3.10. Estimation of GFR from value of blood urea nitrogen.

inulin, p. 46.) The GFR may also be estimated from the value of blood urea nitrogen (BUN), since these are related (Figure 3.10).

Rate Constants for Renal and Total Elimination

The appearance of the drug in urine allows the determination of *both* the rate constant for renal excretion (k_r) and the rate constant for total elimination (k_e) from a dose given as an intravenous bolus. The rate constant k_r is the proportionality constant between rate of appearance in urine dU/dt and the amount of drug in the body [dose $\cdot \exp(-k_e \cdot t)$]. Thus

$$dU/dt = k_r \cdot \text{dose} \cdot \exp(-k_e \cdot t). \tag{3.28}$$

Taking logarithms of both sides yields

$$\ln(dU/dt) = \ln(k_r \cdot \text{dose}) - k_e \cdot t \tag{3.29}$$

so that a plot of the logarithm of urinary excretion rate against time is linear with slope $= -k_e$ and intercept $= \ln(k_r \cdot \text{dose})$. In practice, $\ln(dU/dt)$ is plotted against midpoint time. The derivative is frequently approximated over the time interval $t_1 - t_2$ by the average rate of change $(U_2 - U_1)/(t_2 - t_1)$.

---

*Example**. A drug was given as an intravenous bolus (100 mg) and urine samples were collected at times t_i after administration. These samples yielded urine volumes and *unchanged* drug concentration as given in the table below. The table also contains the midpoint time of the collection interval (calculated from the collection times), the amount

*From Tallarida and Murray[4]

excreted during the collection interval (calculated from the data), the approximate values of dU/dt and the logarithms of these.

time (hr)	1	2	4	6	10	14
volume of urine (ml)	80	120	130	200	340	300
concentration (mg/L)	250	125	77	32.5	7.9	3.67
(calculated) midpoint time (hr)	0.5	1.5	3	5	8	12
(calculated) amount excreted (mg)	20	15	10	6.5	2.7	1.1
(calculated) dU/dt (mg/hr)	20	15	5	3.25	0.675	0.275
(calculated) $\ln(dU/dt)$	2.99	2.71	1.61	1.18	−0.39	−1.29

A linear regression of $\ln(dU/dt)$ against midpoint time gave slope = −0.385 and intercept = 3.06. Thus $k_e = 0.385$ and $\ln(k_r D) = 3.06$ so that $k_r = 0.213$. (It is noteworthy that the amount excreted as unchanged drug at the end of 14 hrs is approximately 55 mg, much less than the 100 mg administered. Hence, there is appreciable metabolism of this drug.

Urine pH and Clearance

As might be expected, urine pH can affect the reabsorption of drugs that are weak acids or weak bases. If the drug is a weak acid, an acidic urine will generally favor reabsorption and therefore reduce clearance of the drug. On the other hand, if the drug is a weak base, an alkaline urine will favor reabsorption and a lowering of drug clearance. Many factors can affect the pH of the urine; disease states, diet, and drugs are examples.

Hepatic Clearance

Hepatic clearance involves biliary excretion and hepatic metabolism. When these processes are first order, the rate constants are additive to that for renal excretion. A single rate constant for elimination, K_e, is the sum of these rate constants and will be used when applicable in describing the kinetics of drugs. (Drug metabolism is discussed in Chapter 4.)

Intravenous Dosing

When a dose D of a drug is administered as an intravenous bolus, it rapidly distributes throughout the blood or plasma. If the drug is not appreciably bound to tissues, the blood concentration–time relation will be a single exponential, as shown in Figure 3.11. Thus,

$$C = C_o \exp(-k_e \cdot t)$$

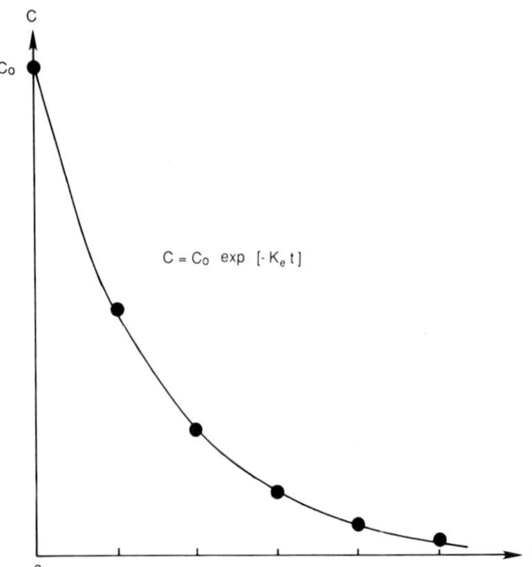

FIGURE 3.11. Blood concentration vs time, illustrating exponential decay.

where C_0 is the concentration immediately following administration, and k_e is the elimination rate constant (for all modes of elimination.) Taking logarithms,

$$\ln C = \ln C_o - k_e \cdot t.$$

Thus a plot of ln C against time is linear with vertical intercept ln C_o and slope $= -k_e$, as shown in Figure 3.12. As previously mentioned, for many drugs this logarithmic plot is not linear but, instead, may yield distinct linear segments, as in Figure 3.13. The rapid phase of elimination represents binding to tissues. For the biexponential decline illustrated, the concentration–time equation has the form

$$C = A \exp(-k_1 t) + B \exp(-k_2 t). \tag{3.30}$$

The constants A, B, k_1, and k_2 are determined from plasma concentration-time data and one of the several nonlinear curve-fitting computer programs that are in widespread use today. Estimates of these may be made with reasonable accuracy from a simple graphical procedure. For example, consider a case in which there is a rapid decline, that is, k_1 is much larger than k_2. Then $A \exp(-k_1 t)$ rapidly approaches 0 as t increases. Thus, after a sufficiently long time T, $C_p \approx B \exp(-k_2 t)$. It follows that a plot of ln C_p against time, *after time T*, is linear with slope $-k_2$ and vertical intercept ln B. With B and k_2 so determined, the value of $B \exp(-k_2 t)$ at each time may be computed and subtracted from C_p at that time:

$$C_p - B_e{}^{-k_2 t} = A\, e^{-k_1 t} \tag{3.31}$$

Taking logarithms of both sides yields

$$\ln(C_p - Be^{-k_2 t}) = \ln A - k_1 t \tag{3.32}$$

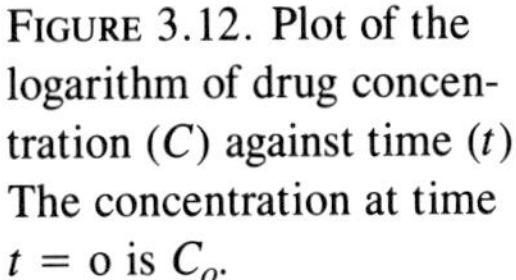

FIGURE 3.12. Plot of the logarithm of drug concentration (C) against time (t). The concentration at time t = o is C_o.

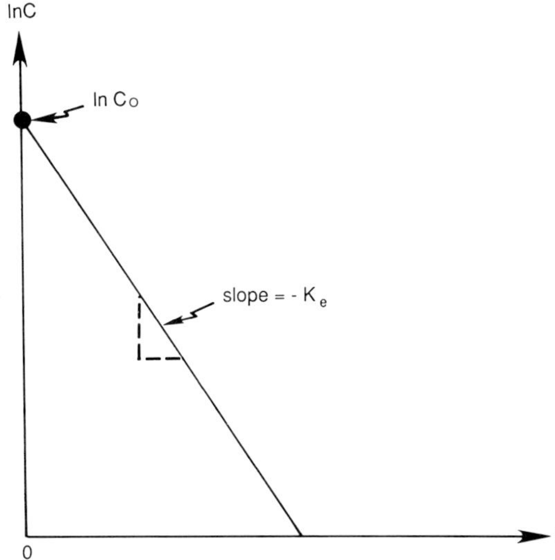

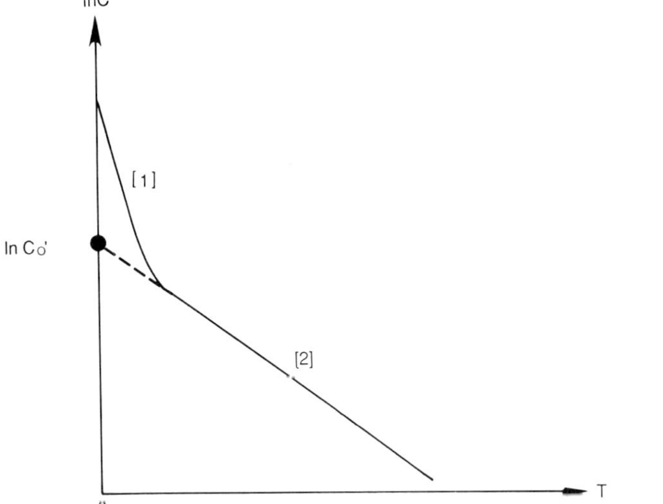

FIGURE 3.13. Graph of ln (plasma concentration) against time, illustrating binding to tissues [phase (1)] and elimination from plasma [phase (2)]. The quantity C_o' is obtained by extrapolation of phase (2) to time zero.

an equation also linear in t, with slope $-k_1$ and intercept ln A. It is convenient to use semilog graph paper when using this procedure. The half-life is obtained from the graph. Then the rate constant (either k_1 or k_2) is computed as 0.693/half-life. Also, the intercepts B and A are read directly from the vertical (logarithmically calibrated axis) instead of ln A or ln B.

Besides biexponential concentration–time relations, such as equation (3.30), triexponential curves are not uncommon. An example is afforded from the narcotic analgesic fentanyl, often used as an anesthetic supplement, especially in procedures of short duration. In a study of dogs[1] receiving intravenous injections of this narcotic (10 μg/kg), the plasma concentration at time t (minutes) after injection gave the following equation (based on mean values in four different animals):

$$C_p = 8.4 \exp(-0.340t) + 2.4 \exp(-0.0277t) + 0.60 \exp(-0.00385t)$$

The slow elimination (indicated by the rate constant 0.00385) is believed to be due to extensive uptake of the drug by body tissues. When this rate constant was used in the calculation of the apparent volume of distribution [according to equation (3.23)], the value obtained was $V_d = 10.2$ L/kg. It is noteworthy that the real volume per kilogram of the dog is approximately 1 L/kg, thereby indicating the large concentration of this narcotic in tissues.

Repeated Intravenous Injections

In this section we consider the kinetics of a drug administered repeatedly at time intervals T and in the same dose D. Further, the drug elimination is *first order*, with a single rate constant of elimination K_e. After time T, the amount in the blood is $D \cdot \exp(-K_e \cdot T)$. For convenience, we denote the constant $\exp(-K_e \cdot T)$ by f:

$$f = \exp(-K_e \cdot T) \tag{3.33}$$

The constant f is the fraction of the dose that remains after time T. (Regardless of the amount of drug at any time, after a time T, the same fraction f of that amount remains in the circulation.) Thus, at a time T, after administration of the first dose D, the amount remaining is $f \cdot D$. At this time a second dose D is administered so that the amount in the blood is now $D + f \cdot D = D(1 + f)$. After an additional time interval T, the amount remaining in blood is $f \cdot D(1 + f)$. Now a third dose is administered, instantly bringing the amount to $D + f \cdot D(1 + f) = D(1 + f + f^2)$. Continuing, after n doses [total time $= (n - 1)$T] the amount is $D(1 + f + f^{n-1})$. The expression in parenthesis is a geometric progression and has the sum S:

$$S = (1 - f^n)/(1 - f) \tag{3.34}$$

Thus, the amount after the nth dose is

$$\text{Amount}_{n+} = D(1 - f^n)/(1 - f) \tag{3.35}$$

Because f is a fraction less than one, as n increases, f^n tends to zero, so that the peaks approach an upper bound U given by

$$U = D/(1 - f). \tag{3.36}$$

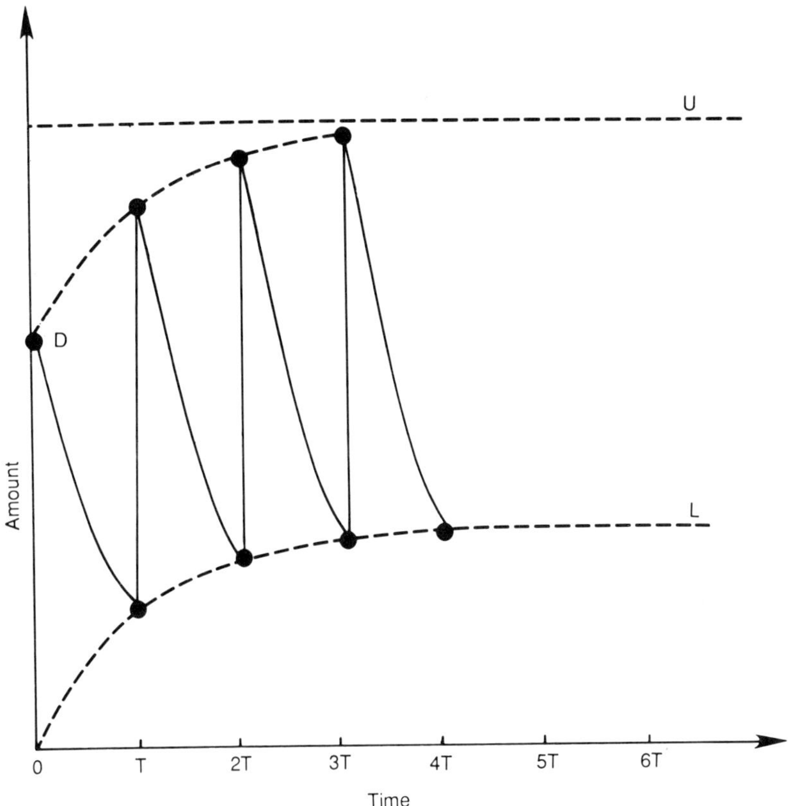

FIGURE 3.14. Repeated intravenous dosing in amount D, with first-order elimination. The amount of drug in the body varies between upper (U) and (L) lower bounds (see text).

The lower bound L is

$$L = f \cdot D/(1 - f).$$

Therefore, the blood levels do not increase boundlessly but stay within the amounts L and U (see Figure 3.14). It may also be shown that the mean amount X is computed from

$$X = D \cdot (-1/\ln f). \tag{3.38}$$

Example. A drug with elimination half-life of 2 hours is administered intravenously every four hours in amount 100 mg. The upper and lower bounds and the mean are to be determined. Since $t_{1/2} = 2$ hours, after four hours the fraction remaining is $f = ¼$. Thus $U =$

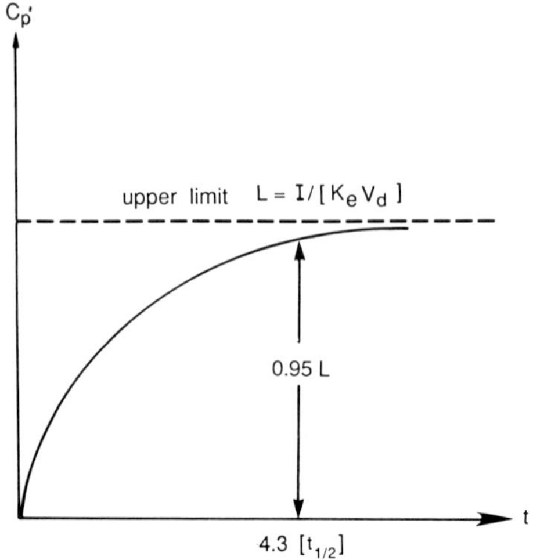

FIGURE 3.15. Constant intravenous infusion at rate I, for a drug with elimination rate constant K_e and volume of distribution V_d, results in the plasma concentration-time relation shown. The upper limit is practically attained (95%) in 4.3 half-lives.

$100/(1 - \frac{1}{4}) = 133$ mg, whereas $L = \frac{1}{4} \cdot (133) = 33$ approximately. The mean is $X = (100) \cdot [-1/\ln(\frac{1}{4})] = 72$ mg.

Intravenous Infusion

If a drug is infused intravenously at a constant rate I, has an apparent volume of distribution V, and is eliminated according to a first-order process with elimination rate constant K_e, the plasma concentration C_p follows from the differential equation

$$dC_p/dt = I/V - K_eC_p \tag{3.39}$$

The solution of equation (3.39) gives C_p as a function of time:

$$C_p = (I/K_e \cdot V)\,[1 - \exp(-K_e\,t)] \tag{3.40}$$

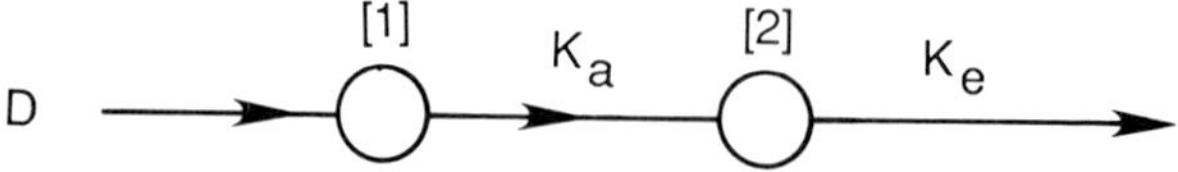

FIGURE 3.16. Dose D is rapidly administered into compartment (1) from which it is absorbed (rate constant k_a) into compartment (2) with volume of distribution V_d and elimination rate constant k_e (see equation 3.43).

From equation (3.40) it is evident that the concentration approaches the value $I/(k_e \cdot V_d) = I/clearance$. In terms of half-life the limiting concentration is approximately $1.44 \cdot I \cdot t_{1/2}/V$. Of course, this limiting value is never actually attained; however, as previously noted, after a time equal to $4.3t_{1/2}$, the concentration is 95% of the limiting value, as illustrated in Figure 3.15.

Example. A drug with elimination half-life of 6 hours is infused at the rate 120 mg/h and rapidly distributes into total body water (so that V may be taken to be 40 L). Thus, the limiting concentration is computed: (1.44)(120)(6)/(40) = 25.9 mg/L.

The constant intravenous infusion may be viewed as a zero-order process of absorption with first-order elimination. From the infusion rate and the limiting concentration, one may determine the drug's clearance. Also, when the clearance is known (and constant), one can determine the infusion rate in order to achieve a desired steady-state level or limiting value: $I = (Cl) \cdot$ (concentration). It should also be noted that intermittent intravenous (IV) dosing in amounts D every T hours (IV bolus) may be reasonably approximated as a constant infusion in which $D/T = I$, so that the mean level (I/Cl) is approximately $D/T \cdot Cl$.

$$\bar{C}_{\text{IV}} = \frac{D}{(T)(Cl)} \tag{3.41}$$

[This is equivalent to $D/V \ln f$ given in equations (3.38) when the latter is divided by V.]

Absorption and Elimination

Drugs administered from an extravascular route (e.g., oral) must be absorbed into the blood in order to be effective. As the drug appears in the blood it is also eliminated, and therefore the blood concentration is a time-varying function. The nature of this function depends on the dose and the kinetics governing the absorptive and elimination processes. Commonly, both absorption and elimination are first order, each therefore characterized by a rate constant. We shall denote these as K_a and K_e, for absorption and elimination, respectively. Figure 3.16 illustrates the process. Compartment 1 denotes the originating compartment (e.g., the gut) and compartment 2 denotes the blood. We wish to determine the plasma concentration as a function of time after dosing. If the amount (e.g., mg) administered is denoted by D and the absorption rate constant is denoted by K_a, then for first-order absorption, the amount absorbed per unit time is $K_a \cdot D(t)$, where $D(t)$ is the amount of drug at the absorptive site as a function of time and is given by $D \cdot \exp(-K_a \cdot t)$, so that the *rate of absorption* is $K_a \cdot D \cdot \exp(-K_a \cdot t)$. The amount absorbed distributes into a volume V and, thus, the rate of increase of plasma concentration is $K_a \cdot D \cdot \exp(-K_a \cdot t)/V$. The rate of decrease of

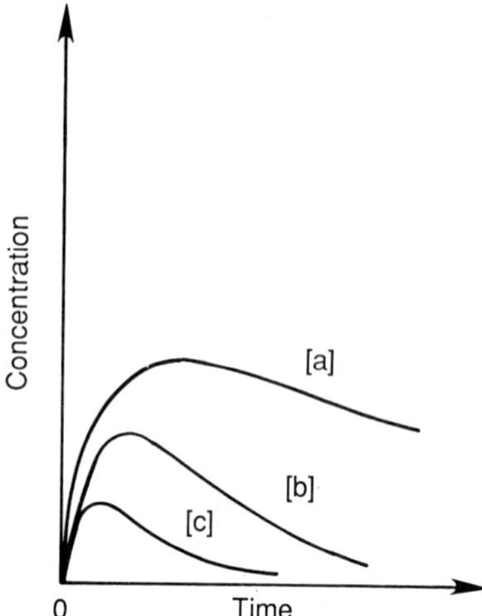

FIGURE 3.17. Blood concentration vs time following administration at time $t = 0$ via and absorptive route, illustrating the relative value k_e/k_a on the peak concentration and the time-to-peak. The relative value k_e/k_a for curves (a), (b), and (c) are 0.1, 0.5, and 2.0, respectively. Note that as the ratio of elimination to absorption increases, both the peak and the time to peak decrease.

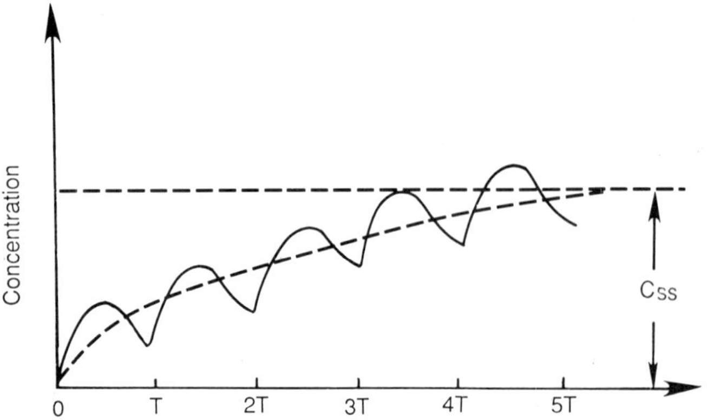

FIGURE 3.18. Blood concentration-time curve for repeated dosing at time intervals T via an absorptive route. The mean concentration (broken curve) approaches the steady-state value C_{ss} (see text).

plasma concentration is $K_e \cdot C_2$. Therefore, the net rate of change of concentration, dC_2/dt, is

$$dC_2/dt = K_aD \cdot \exp(-K_a \cdot t)/V - K_e \cdot C_2 \tag{3.42}$$

The solution of the differential equation given in equation (3.42) is

$$C_2 = \frac{K_aD}{V \cdot (K_e - K_a)} [\exp(-K_at) - \exp(-K_et)]. \tag{3.43}$$

Representative graphs of this equation are shown in Figure 3.17.

In absorptive processes the entire dose D may not be absorbed. Say only a fraction F_1 is absorbed from the gastrointestinal tract. Further, suppose that the liver removes a fraction during the first pass, leaving only F_2 for absorption, then the largest amount ever absorbed is $F_1 \cdot F_2 \cdot D$, and this term is used in equation (3.43) instead of D. If clearance is determined by monitoring the plasma concentration after this absorptive process we get [see equation (3.21)]:

$$Cl = F_1 \cdot F_2 \cdot D/\int C_2(t) \cdot dt \tag{3.44}$$

where the integral is the area under the plasma concentration–time curve. In determinations of clearance in this way the value is that due to renal and extrarenal (e.g., hepatic) pathways out of the blood.

Extravascular Multiple Dosing

In contrast to the sharp peaks in the concentration–time curve that typify intermittent intravenous dosing, the curves for multiple dosing with an extravascular route are illustrated in Figure 3.18. A mathematical analysis leading to the equations describing these curves is given at the end of this section. Here we present a frequently used approximate analysis. In this approximation we use the results of the previously derived equation for the plasma level attained with constant intravenous infusion at a rate $= I$ [see equation (3.40)]. In other words, a dose D, given at time intervals $= T$, is equal to a dosing rate D/T, and this rate is used for I in equation (3.40). Also, instead of the entire dose D being absorbed, we allow for fractional absorption, with the fraction being denoted by F. Thus, the mean concentration* is given by either of the formulas

$$C_{\text{mean}} = F \cdot D/T \cdot k_e \cdot V = F \cdot D/T \cdot Cl \tag{3.45}$$

or

$$C_{\text{mean}} = \frac{1.44\, F \cdot D \cdot t_{1/2}}{T \cdot V} \tag{3.46}$$

where Cl is the clearance.

*$\text{Exp}(-k_et) \sim 0$ after sufficiently long time in equation (3.40).

Example. An oral form of theophylline, which is completely and rapidly absorbed, is administered as a daily dose of 900 mg to an adult of mass 70 kg. Given that the clearance is 0.045 L/h/kg, the mean blood level is computed from equation (3.45):

$$C_{\text{mean}} = \frac{(1)(900)}{(24)(0.045 \times 70)} = 11.9 \text{ mg/L}.$$

A more precise analysis is based on the two-compartment model shown in Figure 3.16, where α and k denote rate constants for absorption and elimination, respectively, and F, V, and D have the same meaning as in the above discussion. For the first time interval, $t = 0$ to $t = T$, we have concentration $C(t)$ given by

$$C(t) = \frac{\alpha FD}{V(K - \alpha)} [e^{-\alpha t} - e^{-kt}] \tag{3.47}$$

At $t = T$, the concentration is $C(T)$, since the second dose has not yet been given. For convenience, we denote $C(T)$ by A and e^{-kT} by g in the following: For subsequent intervals

$$C(T + t) = C(t) + A \cdot e^{-kt}$$

$$C(2T + t) = C(t) + A(1 + g) \cdot e^{-kt}$$

$$C(3T + t) = C(t) + A(1 + g + g^2) \cdot e^{-kt}$$

$$\vdots$$

$$C(nT + t) = C(t) + A \cdot (1 + g + g^2 + \ldots + g^{n-1}) \cdot e^{-kt}. \tag{3.48}$$

The term in parentheses is a progression with sum $= (1 - g^n)/(1 - g)$. Hence, after sufficient time (or doses) this sum approaches the limit $1/(1 - g)$ and thus

$$C(nT + t) = C(t) + \frac{A}{1 - g} \cdot e^{-kt} \tag{3.49}$$

The time (nT) to attain 95% of this limit is $-\ln(.05)/k$, which, in terms of half-life, is approximately $4.3 \cdot t_{1/2}$. (In equations (3.48) and (3.49), $0 \le t \le T$.)

We now express the mean value by integrating over a time interval (for convenience, 0 to T) and dividing by T:

$$\bar{C} = \frac{1}{T}\left[\int_0^T C(t)dt + \int_0^T \frac{A}{1 - g} e^{-kt}dt\right]$$

$$= \frac{\alpha DF}{V(k - \alpha)} \cdot \frac{1}{T} \; \frac{1}{\alpha}(1 - e^{-\alpha T}) - \frac{1}{k}(1 - e^{-kT}) + \frac{A}{Tk} \tag{3.50}$$

For $\alpha > k$, the usual case, the above simplifies to approximately

$$\bar{C} = \frac{FD}{VTk}(1 - e^{-\alpha T}) = \frac{1.44\,FD\,t_{1/2}}{TV}(1 - e^{-\alpha T}) \tag{3.51}$$

When $e^{-\alpha T}$ is small compared with one, the above reduces to equation (3.46).

Time Course of Effect and Drug Receptor Concentration

Thus far we have discussed drug absorption, distribution, and elimination. The drug effect (or effects), however, may show a time course different from the plasma concentration of the drug. In other words, there may be a lag because of the transduction process between the drug-activated receptor and the expression of that complex, or the intensity of effect may be temporally unrelated to the complex concentration. It seems reasonable to assume that the intimate effects are more likely to be related to the plasma concentration than the more distal effects. Nevertheless, there is no a priori reason to make such an assumption in any specific case; instead, each drug–receptor–effector system must be examined. The cautions expressed here are especially applicable when experiments are conducted in vivo, because in such experiments the effect studied may be very far removed from the drug–receptor complex. In one study[3] the disappearance of the narcotic antagonist naloxone was examined based on the rate of decay of its antagonism of morphine, with good agreement found between the pharmacokinetic and pharmacodynamic properties. Yet, it should be recognized that such agreement may not hold for other drugs and effector systems. We shall see (Chapter 8) however, that certain experiments conducted in vivo may be designed to yield useful pharmacodynamic parameters, such as the apparent affinity of the drug for the receptor.

References

1. Murphy MR, Olson WA, Hug CC: Pharmacokinetics of ^{3}H-Fentanyl in the dog anesthetized with enflurane. *Anesthesiology* 1979; 50:13.
2. Pribor HC, Morrell G, and Scherr GH: *Drug Monitoring and Pharmacokinetic Data*, Pathotox Publishers, Inc. Park Forest South, Illinois, 1980, p. 168. See also MS P 089,090.
3. Tallarida RJ, Harakal C, Maslow J, et al: The relationship between pharmacokinetics and pharmacodynamic action as applied to *in vivo* pA_2: application to the analgesic effect of morphine. *J Pharmacol Exp Ther* 1978; 206:38.
4. Tallarida RJ, and Murray RB. *Manual of Pharmacologic Calculation with computer programs*. Springer Verlag 1987, New York p. 104. (2nd ed.)

Additional Readings

Gibaldi M: *Biopharmaceutics and Clinical Pharmacokinetics*, ed 2, Philadelphia, Lea & Febiger, 1977.

Notari RE: *Biopharmaceutics and Clinical Pharmacokinetics*, ed 3, New York, Marcel Dekker, 1980.

Ritschel WA: *Handbook of Basic Pharmacokinetics*, ed. 2, Hamilton IL, Drug Intelligence Publications Inc, 1980.

Rowland M, Tozer TN: *Clinical Pharmacokinetics, Concepts and Applications*. Philadelphia, Lea & Febiger, 1980.

Wagner JG: *Biopharmaceutics and Relevant Pharmacokinetics*. Hamilton IL, Drug Intelligence Publications Inc, 1971.

Wartak J: *Drug Dosage and Administration*. Baltimore, University Park Press, 1983.

4
Drug Metabolism (Biotransformation)

General Principles

When a drug molecule is introduced into a living organism or tissue, it is immersed in a highly reactive biological mixture in which thousands of chemical reactions are simultaneously proceeding in complex, but organized, patterns. These reactions operate in a coordinated manner within cells to conserve certain endogenous compounds and nutrients and to eliminate potentially harmful foreign material. A drug molecule will very likely be affected by one or more of the many chemical reactions occurring in a cell.

When cellular reactions alter the chemical structure of a drug, the drug is said to be "biotransformed" or "metabolized." The activity and fate of biotransformed drug molecules depend to a great extent on the compatibility of the metabolites with the chemical reactions in the cell and how closely the metabolites resemble endogenous chemicals.

In the normal, healthy individual, nutrients and endogenous compounds are largely conserved. For example, the renal reabsorption of many electrolytes is 90% or greater. In contrast, exogenous compounds (xenobiotics) are generally eliminated from the body. In humans, renal excretion is the major route of elimination of most drugs and foreign compounds. Other routes of elimination include urine, feces, sweat, exhaled air, saliva, semen, breast milk, and many others.

Drugs are excreted either unchanged or as metabolites. Most drugs are excreted in both forms, although exceptions exist. One exception is nitrous oxide, which is almost totally eliminated as unchanged drug. Most of it leaves the body in the expired gas; the rest leaves through the skin and other surfaces. Metabolites account for only a small fraction of the excreted nitrous oxide.

In most other cases, drugs are biotransformed to metabolites whose chemical structures closely resemble those of the original drug, but that are modified in specific ways. The relative contributions of metabolism and excretion to the elimination of a particular drug depend on many factors, especially the chemical nature of the drug and the degree of drug binding to tissues.

Most drugs are metabolized through the same chemical pathways responsible for the metabolism of nutrients and endogenous compounds. In this sense, there are no specialized reactions for inactivating drugs.[29] Drug metabolism (biotransformation) reactions are superimposed upon, and occur concurrently with, normal intermediary metabolism.[4] The extent to which a drug is metabolized depends on the degree to which its chemical structure forms a proper substrate for metabolizing enzymes.

Drugs are metabolized to compounds that have, as a general rule, two characteristics that affect their efficacy and duration of action. First, metabolites are often biologically less active than the parent compound. Because the shape of a drug molecule is critical to its affinity and efficacy, it can be inactivated by even minor changes in its chemical structure. Second, drug metabolites are generally more water soluble than the parent compound, thereby enhancing excretion via the kidney. But there are exceptions to these general rules. Drug metabolites are not always biologically inactive. Metabolites can be equally active (or toxic[25]) or more active (or toxic) than the original compound. Examples of each of these types of biotransformation are shown in Table 4.1. Likewise, metabolites are not always more water soluble than the original drug. Some sulfonamids are metabolized to less water-soluble metabolites that can precipitate in renal tubules in sufficient quantity to produce nephrotoxicity.

Any biological process that modifies the concentration of drug near its receptors also modifies the drug effect. Several processes that affect drug concentration near receptors have already been discussed (see Chapter 3). Another factor, considered here, is drug metabolism. The concentration of a drug near its receptor at any given time is the difference between drug influx (via administration and distribution) and drug efflux (via metabolism and excretion).

As previously noted, drugs must overcome several barriers in moving from the site of administration to the site of action (biophase). Thus, for a drug to be effective, it not only must possess affinity for its receptor and have intrinsic activity, but it must also possess the chemical properties that allow it to traverse membranes to reach the biophase. Many of these barriers are primarily lipid in nature (e.g., the gastrointestinal tract and the blood-brain barrier). A drug must also travel through polar media, such as blood, to reach its site of action. Therefore, a balance must be struck between lipid solubility and water solubility. Weak organic acids and weak organic bases ideally satisfy these criteria. Weak organic acids and bases can exist in both ionized (water soluble) and nonionized (lipid soluble) forms. The extent of dissociation into ions is determined primarily by the biological environment of the drug molecule. The ionized and nonionized forms of weak acids and bases are always in equilibrium. Therefore, a portion of these drugs is always in a form that is soluble in its immediate surroundings.

As is discussed subsequently, the metabolic fate of compounds is partly determined by whether the material is water soluble or lipid soluble. Drugs that are weak acids or bases, and thus soluble in both media, can be metabolized through multiple routes.

TABLE 4.1. Examples of biotransformation of drugs to less active, equally active, and more active metabolites.

To A Less Active Metabolite

1. Morphine to Morphine glucuronide

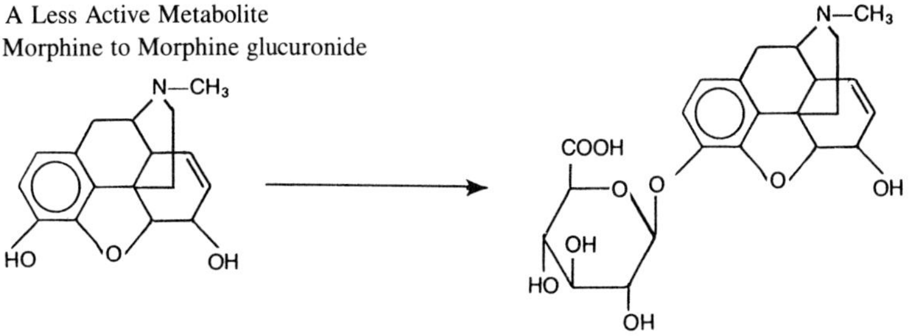

2. Norepinephrine to (3-methoxy-4-hydroxymandelic Acid (VMA)

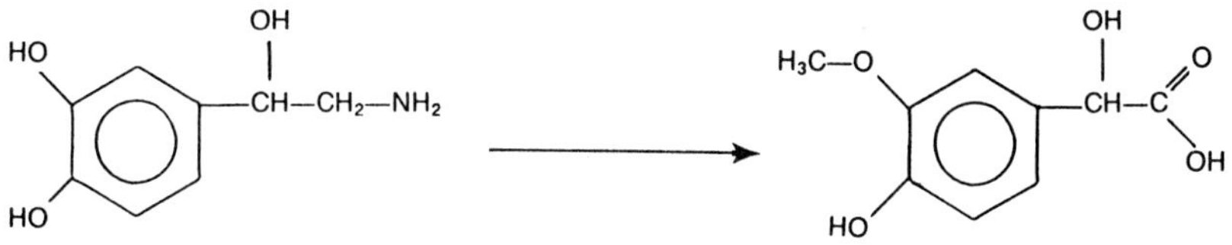

To An Equally Active Metabolite

Aspirin to Salicylic Acid

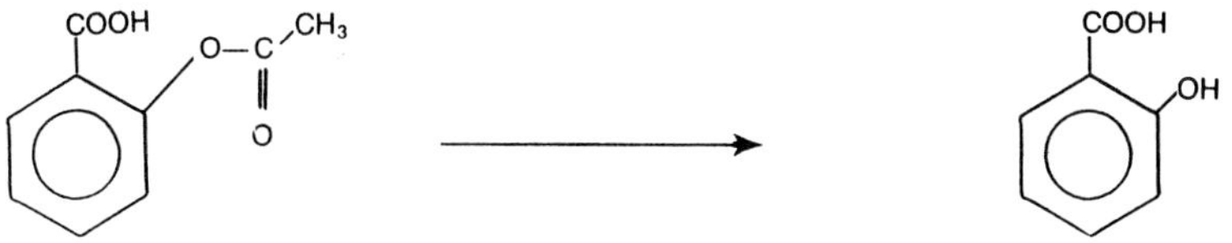

To A More Active Metabolite

1. Imipramine to Desipramine

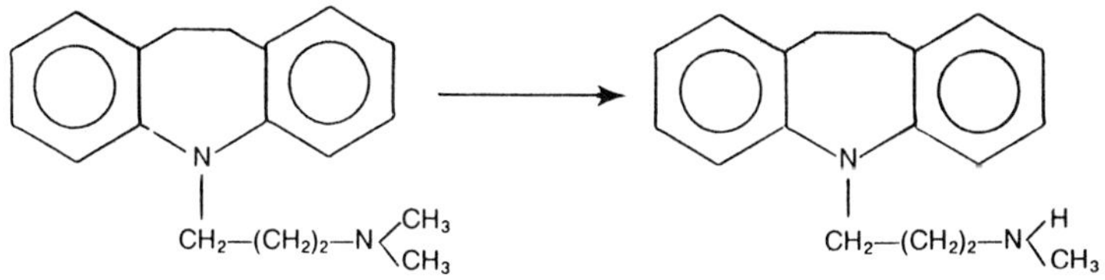

2. Chloral Hydrate to Trichloroethanol

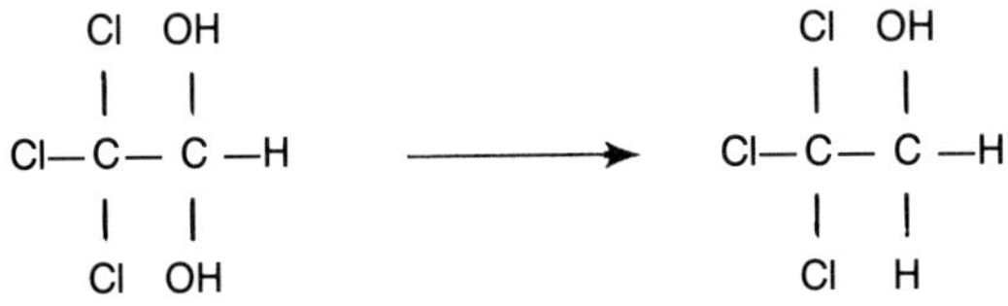

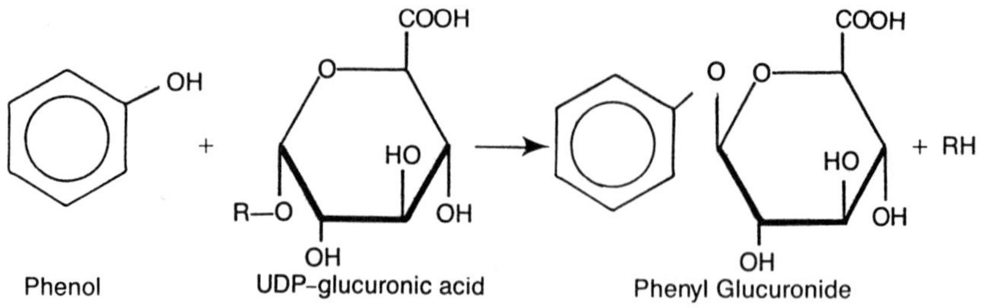

FIGURE 4.1. Example of a biotransformation reaction in which a large, bulky chemical group is attached to a comparatively small molecule (phenol). This addition disrupts the topology of the original molecule, rendering it less capable of stereospecific interaction with a receptor.

CLASSIFICATION OF DRUG METABOLISM REACTIONS

As a general rule, drugs are inactivated in the body by two mechanisms: (1) modification or removal of a critical portion of their chemical structure (e.g., by addition or loss of a reactive atom or side group), and (2) attachment of a large, bulky chemical group (Figure 4.1). Either alteration disrupts the shape and/or the properties of the drug molecule in such a way as to impede access to, or activation of, its receptor. Drug biotransformation reactions can be classified on the basis of which of these two mechanisms is involved. The first type (chemical modification) is termed *phase I*, or *nonsynthetic*. The second (attachment of an encumbering ligand) is termed *phase II*, or *synthetic*. Each type can be further divided on the basis of cellular location (e.g., microsomal versus nonmicrosomal) or the chemistry (e.g., oxidation, reduction, or hydrolysis). A drug molecule is not limited to only one mechanism of inactivation. Many drugs contain several functional groups, so it is not uncommon for multiple metabolites to be produced from a single drug precursor.

Drugs that are chemically related to endogenous compounds are usually suitable substrates for the same enzymes that metabolize their endogenous counterparts. Drugs possessing "foreign" chemical structures are normally metabolized by relatively nonspecific enzymes. Drug molecules that are substrates for more than one type of metabolizing enzyme can be biotransformed by a combination of mechanisms proceeding either in parallel or in series.

A general scheme of the more common routes of drug metabolism is shown in Figure 4.2. Details of each of these pathways are presented subsequently.

Any particular drug can be metabolized by one or more routes of biotransformation. The drug molecule can be biotransformed in either synthetic or nonsynthetic type reactions and can be excreted in this form. Additionally, the product(s) of the initial biotransformation reaction can undergo further biotransformation in subsequent phase I or phase II reactions. Commonly, a drug is metabolized by multiple routes simultaneously or sequentially. The full spectrum

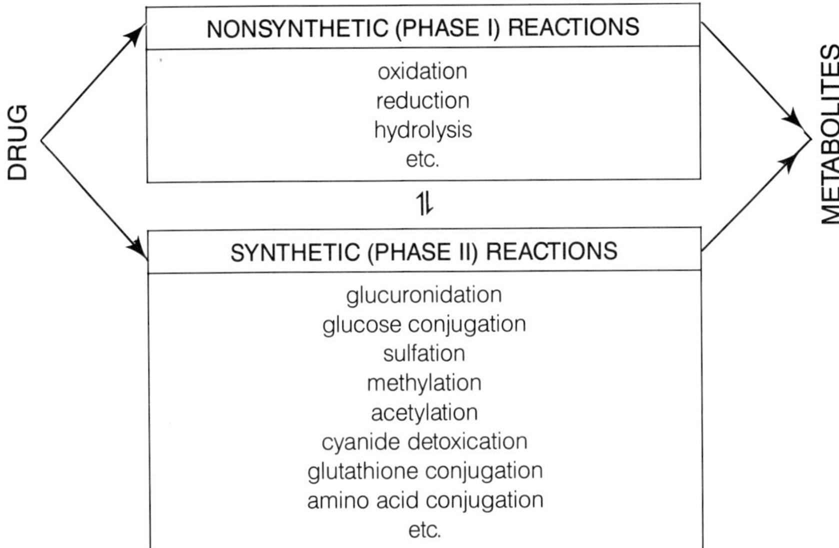

FIGURE 4.2. The most common pathways of drug metabolism (biotransformation). A particular drug may be metabolized via a single pathway or by multiple pathways, either simultaneously or sequentially (represented by arrow). Complete metabolism typically involves initial chemical modification in a phase I reaction, followed by conjugation in a phase II reaction.

of excreted metabolites of a drug represents the various products of these multiple routes of metabolism.

Diazepam (Valium) is an example of a drug biotransformed through multiple metabolic pathways (see Figure 4.3). The parent molecule can be *N*-dealkylated to *N*-desmethyldiazepam (the major route) or 3-hydroxylated to temazepam. Both of these reactions are nonsynthetic (phase I) types. Each of the intermediate metabolites (nordiazepam and temazepam) can be modified further in phase I reactions, yielding the same product—oxazepam. Oxazepam, and temazepam to a lesser extent, undergoes synthetic conjugation (phase II) reactions yielding glucuronidated metabolites. Each step in this pathway converts the parent compound to a less active and more water-soluble product.

Anatomical Sites of Biotransformation

Gross Anatomy

The site at which the biotransformation of a drug occurs is determined, to a large extent, by two major factors. The first is the pathway that the drug takes through the body from its site of administration to its sites of action and excretion. Since

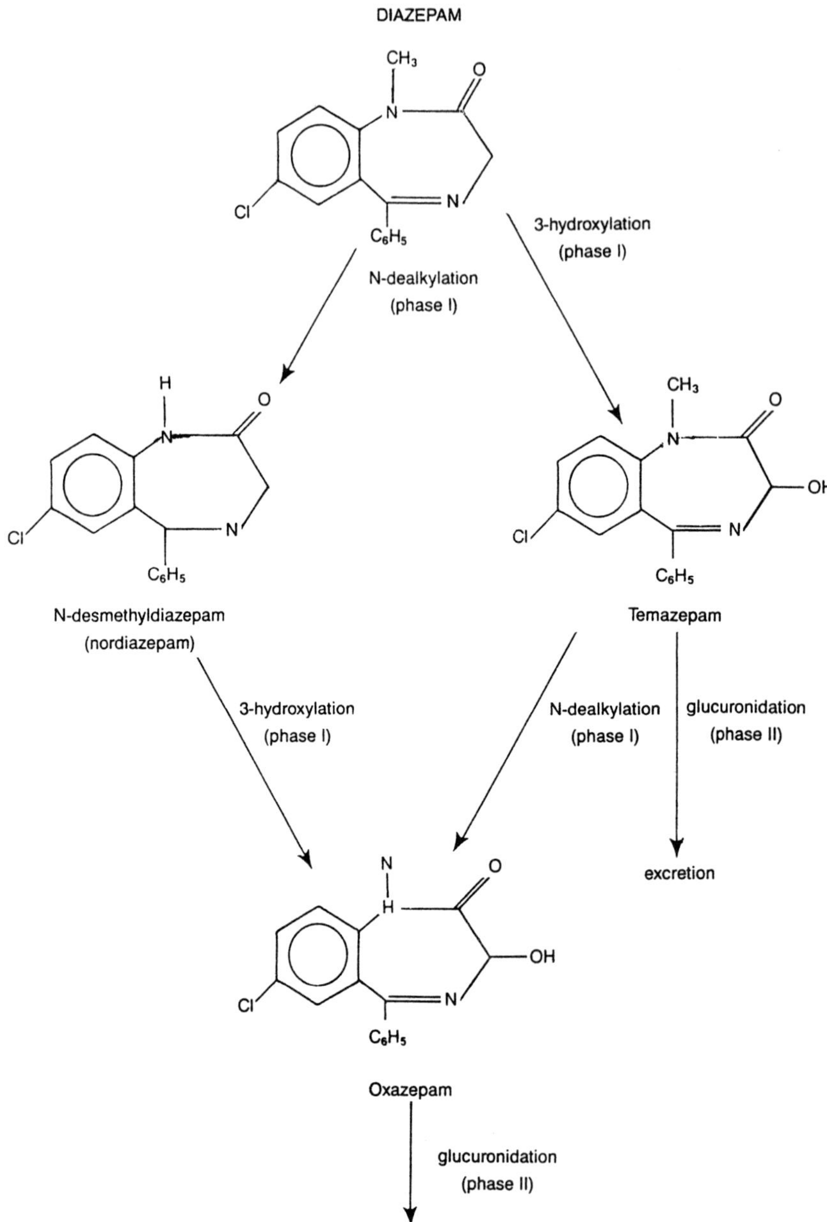

FIGURE 4.3. The multiple routes of diazepam (Valium) metabolism. The drug undergoes a series of phase I reactions (dealkylation and hydroxylation) that yield products that are then glucuronidated. All of these compounds can appear in the urine.

most cells of the body possess the capacity to biotransform most drugs to some extent, the actual sites of their biotransformation are determined by the distribution of the drug in the body. Second, some organs, especially the liver, possess cellular mechanisms ideally suited for metabolic activity and also possess the necessary enzymes in large quantities. In humans the liver has both the proper anatomical location and the specialized enzyme systems, a combination that makes it the major site of biotransformation of many drugs.

The anatomical location of the liver in the circulatory system establishes a specialized route for blood transport known as the "portal system." Drugs taken orally enter the liver, via the portal system, before entering into the general circulation (Figure 4.4). The portal system originates with the collective veins that exit from the organs involved in digestion such as the abdominal part of the digestive tract, the gallbladder, the pancreas, and the spleen. These veins then empty into the large portal vein, which carries the blood to the liver. In the liver, the portal system divides into an extensive network of venules. Blood from these venules then passes into capillary-like sinusoids, which provide a large surface area for exchange between the blood and the hepatic cells. From these sinusoids the blood collects into the hepatic vein, which empties directly into the inferior vena cava.

The liver eliminates a large portion of orally administered drugs before they enter into the general systemic circulation. The term "first-pass effect" is often used to describe this phenomenon. The term "presystemic elimination" is also used to emphasize that the liver continues to participate in drug biotransformation even after the first pass of drug. The term presystemic elimination is also sometimes preferred over first-pass effect because it includes other organs (such as the lung) through which blood also passes prior to entering the general circulation. Norepinephrine, for example, undergoes major inactivation during its passage through the lungs, whereas epinephrine does not. Thus, presystemic elimination can be a significant determinant of drug bioavailability and may account for the large differences in bioavailability of otherwise similar drugs.

Enzymes capable of biotransforming drugs are present in several tissues (e.g., liver, kidney, plasma, lung, intestine, and skin), but those present in the liver occur in high concentrations and are active in this function. They account for a large proportion of the total biotransformation of a drug. The subcellular sites of drug metabolism include the soluble, mitochondrial, and microsomal fractions of liver cells.

Microsomes

Although the term "microsome" is used in studies involving subcellular fractionation and in describing mechanisms of drug metabolism, it is noteworthy that there are no microsomes in the same sense that there are mitochondria, Golgi bodies, cell nuclei, or other components of the intact cells. Instead, "microsomes" describes a particular portion of cellular material that is isolated during

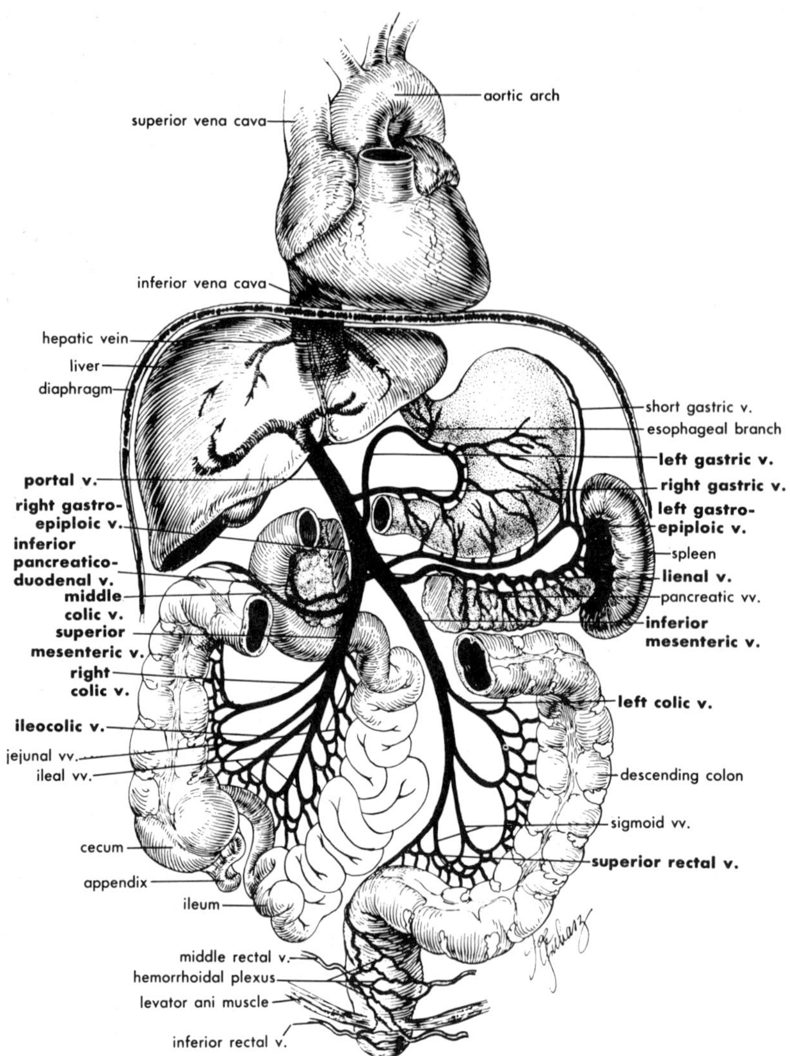

FIGURE 4.4. Anatomy of the portal system. Veins from the stomach, spleen, pancreas, gallbladder, and intestines empty into the portal vein, which conveys blood to the liver. In the liver, blood flow is directed into many small venules, passed through hepatic sinusoids, and collected into the hepatic vein. Blood from the hepatic vein empties directly into the inferior vena cava. (From Crouch, JE: *Functional Human Anatomy,* ed 2. Philadelphia, Lca & Febigen, 1972, p 329.

cell fractionation (usually by ultracentrifugation) and does not refer to discrete organelles having independent existence in the intact living cell. Hence, the term is an operational one denoting the cellular components that describe the pellet formed when tissue is centrifuged under specified conditions, usually for about 1 or 2 hours at approximately 100,000 *g* following prior elimination of heavier particles at 10,000 *g* (Figure 4.5). Viewed in the electron microscope, some of the material collected under these conditions appears to have aggregated in micelles and these micelles are sometimes called "microsomes." Of course, different centrifugation conditions result in different compositions of the pellets obtained. Even at 100,000 *g* for 1 or 2 hours, the pellet is a mixture of fragmented membrane pieces and a variety of cellular components. Thus, microsomes are a collection of intact and fragmented cellular membranes and organelles, the true nature of which depends on the conditions under which they are collected. The microsomal fraction derived from liver cells is particularly rich in drug-metabolizing enzymes that catalyze many important biotransformation reactions in humans.

The microsomal fraction contains enzymes that are active in various aspects of the biotransformation of endogenous compounds. For example, the microsomes:

1. Contain acyl-coenzyme A (CoA) synthetase (which catalyses the first step of fatty acid transformation and the synthesis of lipids);
2. Synthesize polyunsaturated fatty acids (important in cholesterol transport by plasma lipoproteins, in membrane structure, and as precursors of prostaglandins);
3. Are involved in the biosynthesis of ethanolamine plasmogens (the major constituent of myelin in the brain);
4. Metabolize endogenous ligands (such as steroid hormones);
5. Contribute to the biosynthesis of cholesterol, the formation of bile acids, carbohydrate metabolism, and glycoprotein synthesis.

The microsomal fraction of liver cells is obtained by first placing liver tissue in a buffered solution of carefully controlled ionic strength and pH. The tissue is then mildly homogenized in this solution. If the outer cell membrane has been broken, and the internal organelles have not been disrupted, the homogenate consists of cell fragments, including pieces of outer membrane and intact organelles. These individual cell components are then separated on the basis of such physical characteristics as size, shape, or density. Such a separation is most often accomplished using the ultracentrifuge.

In an ultracentrifuge, tubes containing the homogenate are rotated at a constant angular velocity ω, (radians/time), thereby producing a radial acceleration $L\omega^2$, where L is the distance from the center. Because individual particles are moving in a viscous medium and, hence, experiencing a retarding force proportional to their velocity, the equation for particle velocity is applicable:

$$v = \frac{m\,g}{K}\left(1 - e^{-\frac{k}{m}t}\right),$$

where K is the proportionality constant between retarding force and velocity, m is the particle mass, and t is the time. The large angular velocity (ω) results in large gravitational force g as mentioned above. Since the exponential term above → 0, the limiting velocity is $m\,g/K$. Hence, the more massive particles have the highest velocity, thereby effecting a

---

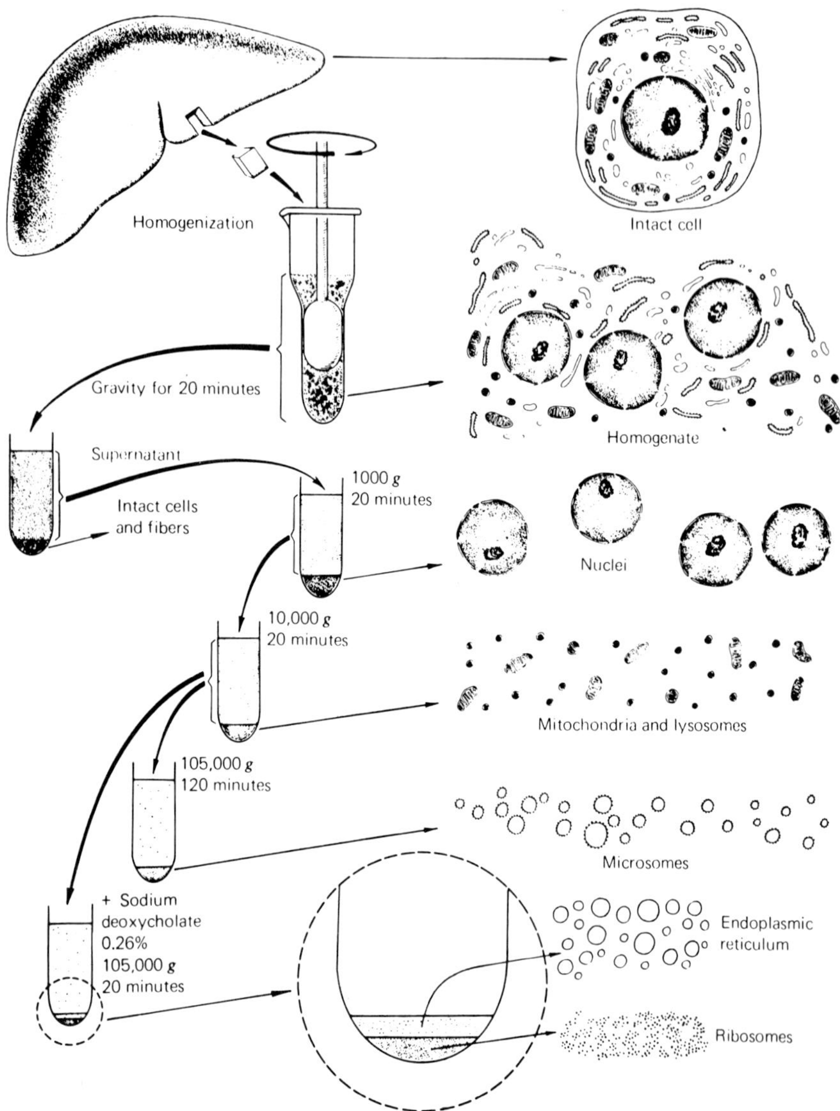

FIGURE 4.5. Isolation of hepatic cell constituents by differential centrifugation. After each step, the pellet is removed from the bottom of the tube and the supernatant of the tube is centrifuged again at higher speeds. The pellet at each stage consists of the cellular organelles shown at the right. Centrifugal force is expressed as a multiple of g, the force of gravity. From Bloom, W, and Fawcett, DW: *A Textbook of Histology,* ed. Philadelphia, WB Saunders, 1968. Reprinted with permission.

separation (since g is approximately the same for all the particles) depending on the square of angular velocity ω.

All particles ultimately settle to the bottom of the centrifuge tube, but they do not all settle at the same rate. The rate at which a particle of given mass will settle to the bottom of a centrifuge tube is a function of the size (mass) and angular velocity (squared) of the particle. This fact is exploited in the process of differential (also called fractional) centrifugation (see Figure 4.5).

Closer analysis of the microsomal fraction has revealed that it is composed primarily of vesicles or micelles of fragmented plasma membrane elements and of the endoplasmic reticulum of the liver cells. The microsomes are lipoprotein in nature, the major constituent of which is phosphatidyl choline. The proteins have enzymatic activities that can be modified by the lipids. Both have structural functions and influence membrane permeability.

Smooth Endoplasmic Reticulum

Endoplasmic reticulum, a collective term used to describe the lipoprotein complex and interconnecting network of tubular and vesicular structures present in the cytoplasm of cells (Figure 4.6), provides channels for conducting fluid to various parts of the cell.[12] Substances formed in one part of the cell can be transported to other parts of the cell via the endoplasmic reticulum.

The microscopic appearance of the endoplasmic reticulum suggests classification into two forms: rough endoplasmic reticulum (RER) and smooth endoplasmic reticulum (SER). The RER is characterized by a large number of small granular particles (ribosomes) attached to its surface, whereas the SER is devoid of such attachments. This difference in structure extends to differences in function. The ribosomes are believed to be responsible for protein synthesis and are not thought to play a significant role in drug metabolism. The agranular SER, in contrast, has functions more directly relevant to drug action. The SER contains a high concentration of drug-metabolizing enzymes and is a site of active drug biotransformation. The drug-metabolizing enzymes of the SER are collectively termed "microsomal enzymes."

The microsomal enzymes, as a group, have several properties that circumscribe their drug-metabolizing capabilities and limitations. First, they tend to be selective for lipid-soluble compounds.[16] Primarily lipid-soluble drugs (or the nonionized forms of weak organic acids and bases) are acceptable substrates for these enzymes. Microsomal enzymes metabolize substances of widely different chemical composition, but only if these substrates are at least partly lipid soluble. Second, the metabolized product is generally less lipid soluble and more water soluble (hydrophilic) than the original compound.

Nonlipid-soluble (water soluble) drugs are metabolized by the same route as endogenous water-soluble compounds, i.e., oxygenases, peroxidases, dehydrogenases, and other enzymes that act on water-soluble substrates. These soluble enzymes are dispersed throughout the cytoplasm of liver cells and other tissues of the body.

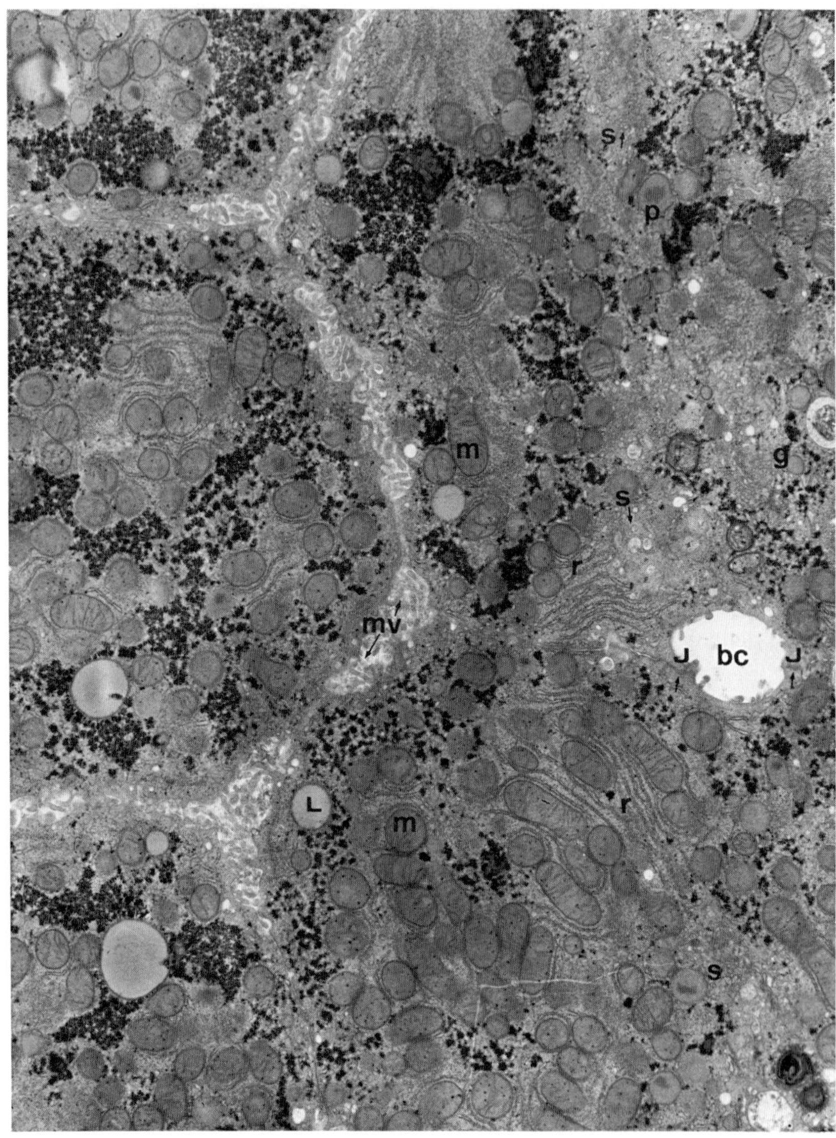

FIGURE 4.6. Photomicrograph of a rat liver cell. The rough endoplasmic reticulum (RER) is indicated by r, the smooth endoplasmic reticulum (SER) is indicated by s. Courtesy of Drs. G.D.V. Van Rossum and M. Mariani, Temple University, Philadelphia, PA.

Biotransformation Reactions

NONSYNTHETIC (PHASE I) REACTIONS

Biotransformations in which the drug molecule is altered in some way other than by covalent bonding to an endogenous compound are classified as nonsynthetic or phase I reactions. These reactions involve the modification of an essential portion of the drug molecule or the removal of a critical chemical group. Typical nonsynthetic reactions are oxidations, reductions, and hydrolyses. They may occur in the microsomes or at nonmicrosomal sites (Table 4.2). Most oxidation reactions are catalyzed by microsomal enzymes, whereas reduction and hydrolysis reactions are catalyzed by both microsomal and nonmicrosomal enzymes.

Oxidations

It is convenient to group together the biotransformation reactions in which one or more oxygen atoms become incorporated into the drug molecule. Several enzymatic systems capable of catalyzing the insertion of oxygen into drug molecules have been discovered, and together these systems account for the production of a great percentage of drug metabolites. The products of these reactions are either excreted unchanged or form the precursors for synthetic-type reactions. These enzymatic systems are also active in the metabolism of normal nutritional and endogenous substances. Hence, they provide a biochemical interface between drug metabolism and intermediary metabolism.

Insertion of O_2

Specific enzymes known as dioxygenases or oxygen transferases are capable of catalyzing the insertion of both atoms of an O_2 molecule into a suitable drug molecule. Tryptophan, for example, is metabolized by this type of reaction. Proof that both atoms of the O_2 molecule are introduced into the substrate molecule can be demonstrated using radiolabeled oxygen tracers.

When both atoms of the oxygen molecule are combined with adjacent hydrogen atoms, adjacent -OH groups are formed. Quite often, the dihydroxylated compound is unstable and induces sufficient strain on the -C-C- bond between the -OH groups to break it:

H H / —A—A— (ring) + O_2 → HO OH / —A—A— (ring) → HO OH / —A A— (open chain)

Such a sequence of events illustrates one mechanism by which cyclic drug molecules can be biotransformed to nonring metabolites.

TABLE 4.2. Classification of nonsynthetic (phase I) drug biotransformation reactions.*

	Examples
A. Microsomal	
1. Oxidation	
a. Addition of OH group	
(i) alkyl chain hydroxylation	Ketamine, meperidine, methohexital, pentobarbital, phenylbutazone, thiopental
$R{-}CH_2{-}R' \rightarrow R{-}CH(OH){-}R'$	
(ii) Ring hydroxylation	Acetanilid, fentanyl, hexobarbital, lidocaine, phenobarbital, propranolol, quinine
$R{-}C_6H_5 \rightarrow R{-}C_6H_4{-}OH$	
(iii) *N*-hydroxylation	Aniline, normeperidine
$RR'N{-}H \rightarrow RR'N{-}OH$	
$C_6H_5{-}NH_2 \rightarrow C_6H_5{-}NH(OH)$	
b. Addition of O atom	
(i) Epioxidation	Aldrin, hepatochlor, phenytoin
$R{-}CH_2{-}CH_2{-}R' \rightarrow$ R—CH—CH—R' (epoxide, O bridging the two C)	
$R{-}CH{=}CH{-}R' \rightarrow$ R—CH—CH—R' (epoxide, O bridging the two C)	
(ii) *N*-oxidation	Chlorpromazine, meperidine, morphine, nicotinamide, tetracycline, trimethylamine
$RR'R''N \rightarrow RR'R''N{=}O$	

TABLE 4.2. *Continued.*

	Examples
(iii) *S*-oxidation $R{-}S{-}R' \rightarrow R{-}S(=O){-}R'$	Chlorpromazine and other phenothiazines
c. Replacement of atom with an OH group or O atom	
(i) Halogens (dehalogenation) $R{-}C(H)(X){-}X \rightarrow R{-}C(=O){-}OH$ $C_6H_5{-}X \rightarrow C_6H_5{-}OH$	Enflurane, halothane, methoxyflurane, *p*-fluoroaniline
(ii) Sulfur (desulfuration) $R{-}SH \rightarrow R{-}OH$ $(R)(R')C{=}S \rightarrow (R)(R')C{=}O$ $(R{-}O)(R'{-}O)(R''{-}O)P{=}S \rightarrow (R{-}O)(R'{-}O)(R''{-}O)P{=}O$	Thiopental, other thiobarbs
(iii) NH_2 (oxidative deamination) 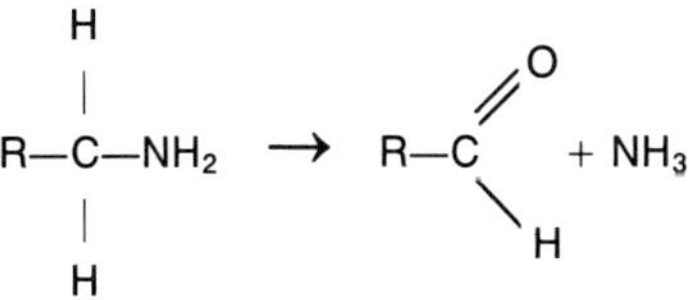	Amphetamine, epinephrine, other α-methylated amines
d. Removal of alkyl group	
(i) *N*-dealkylation $R{-}N(CH_3)_2 \rightarrow R{-}N(CH_3)H$ $(R)(R')N{-}CH_3 \rightarrow (R)(R')N{-}H$	Aminopyrine, atropine, codeine, diazepam, fentanyl, imipramine, ketamine, lidocaine, mephobarbital, morphine

TABLE 4.2. *Continued.*

	Examples
(ii) *O*-dealkylation	Acetapheneditin, codeine, pancuronium, phenacetin
$R{-}O{-}CH_3 \rightarrow R{-}OH$	
$C_6H_5{-}O{-}CH_3 \rightarrow C_6H_5{-}OH$	
(iii) *S*-dealkylation	Methylmercaptan, *S*-methylapteine
$R{-}S{-}CH_3 \rightarrow R{-}SH$	
(iv) Methalloalkane	Tetraethyllead
$Pb(C_2H_5)_4 \rightarrow Pb(C_2H_5)_3$	
2. Reductions	
a. Addition of H atoms (azo reductions), azobenzene, prontosil	
$R{-}N{=}N{-}R' \rightarrow R{-}NH_2 + R'{-}NH_2$	
b. Replacement of an atom by H atom	Chloramphenicol, dantrolene, nitrazepam, nitrobenzene
(i) Oxygen (nitro reduction)	
$R{-}NO_2 \rightarrow R{-}NH_2$	
(ii) Halogen (reductive dehalogenation)	Carbon tetrachloride, DDT, halothane, methoxyflurane
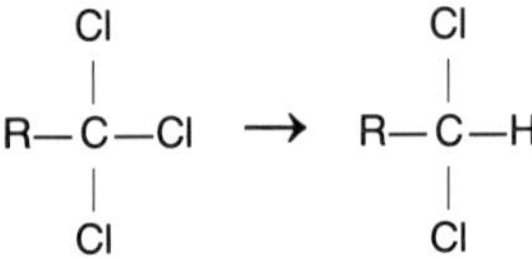	
3. Hydrolysis	
a. Ester (deesterification)	Acetycholine, carbachol, cocaine, meperidine, pancuronium, procaine, succinylcholine
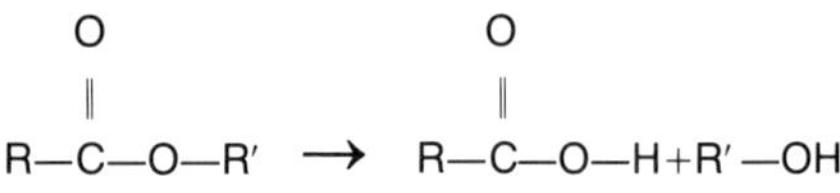	
b. Amide	Fentanyl, lidocaine, nicotinamide, procainamide
$R{-}C({=}O){-}NH{-}R' \rightarrow R{-}C({=}O){-}OH + R'{-}NH_2$	

References 8, 11, 14, 17, 20, 23, 24.

Insertion of an Oxygen Atom

Many enzyme systems can insert one atom of an O_2 molecule into a drug molecule that provides the proper substrate. In most of these reactions, the other oxygen atom of the O_2 molecule is combined with endogenous hydrogen to produce a water molecule. One such group of enzymes is collectively called *monooxygenases* or *hydroxylases*, terms that describe their role in inserting a single oxygen atom into a drug molecule (usually forming an -OH group). These same enzymes are also known as *mixed-function oxidases*, a term that emphasizes their dual role in catalyzing the reactions of both atoms of the oxygen molecule – one inserted into the drug molecule and the other reduced to water.

The general scheme of biotransformation via the mixed-function oxidases is represented by the chemical reaction:

$$AH + XH_2 + O_2 \rightarrow A(OH) + H_2O + X,$$

where AH is the drug molecule and XH_2 is the source of hydrogen atoms needed to reduce oxygen to water.

A supply of hydrogen (i.e., electrons or reducing equivalents) is necessary for this type of reaction. Ample amounts of hydrogen are usually available from the same two sources that supply adenosine triphosphate (ATP) production via oxidative phosphorylation. In the cytosol of cells, reducing equivalents are available from glycogen stores. Interestingly, particularly high levels of glycogen are present in the liver. The other major source of reducing equivalents is located within the mitochondria. Electrons are transported from inside the mitochondria to the cytoplasm (and then to the organelles comprising the microsomal fraction). This transport is mediated by various "shuttles." One such transport mechanism, the malate-aspartate shuttle, is particularly active in liver tissue.

Cytochrome P-450 System

The microsomal fraction of tissue (especially liver) contains specialized electron transport systems and enzymes associated with the endoplasmic reticulum. These systems, which have been extensively studied, participate in the biotransformations of a large number of drugs. They generally involve enzymes that are more complex than the monooxygenases and dioxygenases.

One of the most important of these systems involves a specialized electron carrier, cytochrome P-450. Cytochrome P-450 (P for "pigment")

"... refers to a group of heme proteins that are apparently unique in having a sulfur atom ligated to the iron and that form carbon monoxide complexes that have a major absorption band at an unusually long wavelength (approximately 450 nm)."[31]

This heme protein participates in what is thought to be the initial step of the chain of reactions leading to drug biotransformation via the microsomal metabolizing enzymes.[10] In this step, cytochrome P-450 combines with a drug molecule, probably through hydrophobic bonding (since lipophilic drugs are the primary substrates). The reaction then proceeds through a sequence of steps,

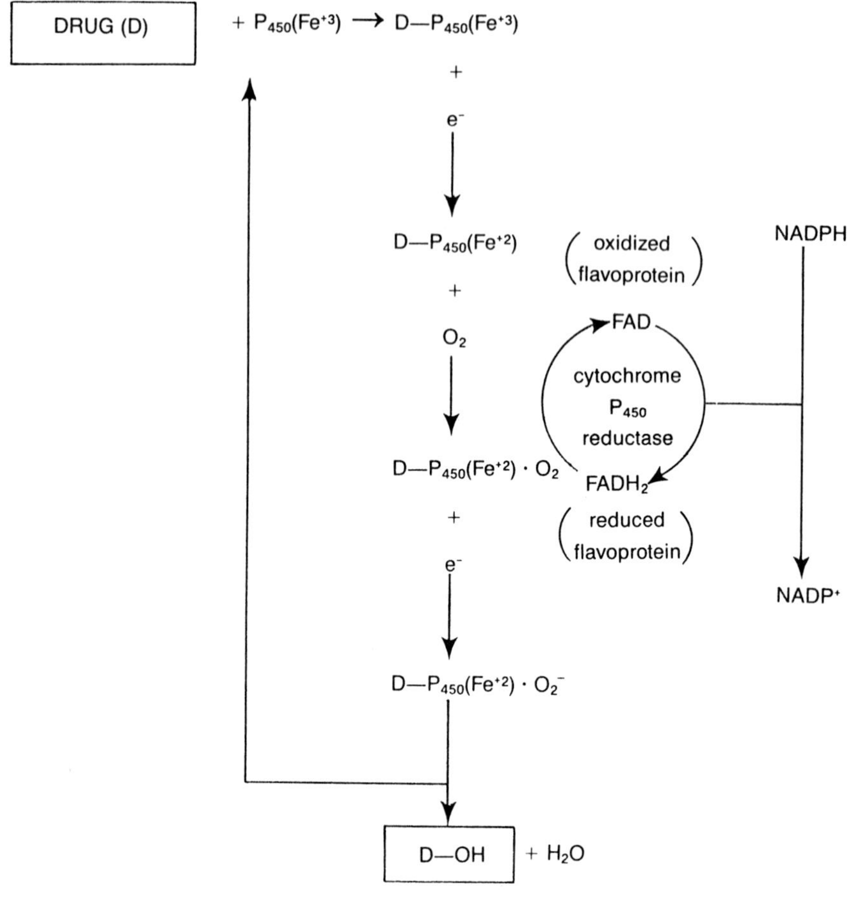

FIGURE 4.7. Series of steps postulated to mediate drug biotransformation via microsomal mixed-function oxygenase system involving cytochrome P_{450}.

with the result that one atom of molecular oxygen is inserted into the drug molecule and the other oxygen atom is reduced to water. For the reaction to proceed to completion, two electrons are required. Both of these are believed to be supplied by cellular sources such as the reduced form of nicotinamide-adenine dinucleotide phosphate (NADPH) (Figure 4.7) or the reduced form of nicotinamide-adenine dinucleotide (NADH).

The overall reaction scheme can be summarized by the representative equation:

$$\text{DRUG-H} + O_2 + \text{NAD(P)H} + H^+ \xrightarrow{X} \text{DRUG-OH} + H_2O + \text{NAD(P)}^+$$

where X represents cytochrome P-450, other electron transferring proteins, and various enzymes. When NADPH is the source of reducing equivalents, the heme protein is primarily cytochrome P-450 and the flavoprotein is NADPH cytochrome *c* reductase. When NADH is the source of reducing equivalents, the heme protein is primarily cytochrome b_5 and the flavoprotein is NADH cytochrome b_5 reductase.

Cytochrome P-450 is ubiquitous in the animal kingdom, but in any individual organism it is localized in specific tissue compartments. It is particularly abundant in hepatic microsomes, thereby accounting, in part, for the prominent role of the liver in drug metabolism. It is also present in low concentrations in the adrenal cortex and in other tissues. However, extrahepatic cytochrome P-450 systems differ in several important ways from the hepatic system. In the adrenal cortex, for example, they appear to be localized predominantly to the mitochondria and mediate the hydroxylation of steroids, but not of many drugs.

Recent research has revealed that cytochrome P_{450} in liver microsomes (sometimes designated P-450LM) is actually a composite of several distinct forms (isoenzymes) with overlapping substrate specificity.[31] Monoclonal antibodies to each isoenzyme are being produced.[15] The cytochrome P-450LM isoenzymes catalyse the hydroxylation of both endogenous compounds (e.g., steroids, fatty acids, squalene, prostaglandins, and some amino acids) and exogenous compounds (e.g., drugs such as phenobarbital, morphine, codeine, and amphetamine and toxic compounds such as petroleum products, insecticides, and carcinogens).[31] The specific reactions in which they participate include *N*-oxidation, sulfoxidation, epoxidation, *N*-, *S*-, *O*- dealkylation, peroxidation, deamination, desulfuration, and dehalogenation.

Reductions and Hydrolyses

Metabolic reduction and hydrolysis reactions are catalyzed by microsomal and nonmicrosomal enzymes in the liver and other tissues. In humans these reactions are less common routes of drug biotransformation than are oxidation reactions. Nevertheless, they play important roles in the metabolism of some drugs.

Nitrogen atoms are a common target of reducing agents (nitro and azo reduction), particularly of microsomal enzymes and intestinal flora. Other reduction reactions replace halogen atoms (e.g., Cl^-, Br^-, and F^- in halothane, methoxyflurane, and other volatile anesthetics) with hydrogen atoms. In these cases, the freed halogen ions are probably responsible for the toxic actions of these drugs. In a similar reaction, chloral hydrate (an aldehyde) undergoes aldehyde reduction (nonmicrosomal) in the presence of alcohol dehydrogenase (the most important nonmicrosomal enzyme that catalyzes reduction reactions) to trichloroethanol, a metabolite that is a stronger hypnotic than is the parent drug.

A familiar example of a hydrolysis reaction is the breakdown of acetylcholine by acetylcholinesterase. As in this example, hydrolysis reactions often result in cleavage of the substrate molecule with concomitant reduction of its biological activity. High concentrations of esterases (and other hydrolytic enzymes) are present in the plasma and contribute to the metabolism of several drugs (e.g., succinylcholine).

Synthetic (Phase II) Reactions—Conjugations

Biotransformations in which the metabolite is formed by the addition of some chemical moiety to the drug molecule are known as synthetic or phase II reactions. The term "synthetic" distinguishes this kind of reaction from that in which the drug molecule is altered by means other than the attachment of an endogenous ligand—such as oxidations, reductions, and hydrolyses. The term phase II refers to the fact that many drugs are metabolized in two sequential steps: (1) a nonsynthetic (phase I) type, and (2) a synthetic (phase II) type.

Conjugation reactions comprise the majority of synthetic biotransformations in humans. Although there is not total agreement on any single definition of conjugation, one definition has recently been proposed that is broad enough to engender widespread agreement.[6] According to this definition, conjugations are: "A group of synthetic reactions in which a foreign compound or metabolite thereof is covalently linked with an endogenous molecule or grouping to give a characteristic product known as a conjugate." The fact that the conjugation linkage involves a covalent chemical bond suggests that the linkage is essentially irreversible.

Conjugation reactions can occur in both the microsomal and the nonmicrosomal fractions of several tissues. Glucuronidation reactions are catalyzed by microsomal enzymes; all other conjugations are catalyzed by nonmicrosomal enzymes. Many conjugation reactions involve a specific transferase enzyme, a high-energy (often nucleotide) intermediate, and are often the final metabolic step in the overall pathway leading to drug detoxification and excretion. Conjugates are the major excretory products of the majority of drugs (and other xenobiotics).

The conjugated metabolites of a drug may differ from the parent compound in several important respects. Compared with the nonconjugated molecule, conjugated metabolites are more water soluble, more ionized (i.e., they are stronger acids), and are less likely to pass through membranes. Further, they have less intrinsic activity and are more readily excreted by the kidney.

Several authors[6,8,22] have conveniently summarized the major conjugation reactions occurring in humans, along with the conjugating agent and the functional group involved. Although there are more than two dozen different conjugation reactions, only eight are often encountered. Of these, glucuronidation is the most prevalent in humans. A summary of the information concerning these eight common conjugation reactions is presented in Table 4.3.

As is the case with other drug-metabolizing reactions, conjugation reactions can transform drugs to either less active, equally active, or more active compounds. The rate and extent of these reactions may be influenced by certain genetic and environmental influences, discussed later in the chapter.

In most conjugation reactions (1) the endogenous ligand is brought into the vicinity of, and attaches to, the drug molecule, and (2) the endogenous ligand is in abundant supply (and therefore minor losses are not vital to normal cell function). However, it has recently been discovered that some drug molecules cova-

TABLE 4.3. Summary of the eight most common types of conjugation reactions involved in drug metabolism in humans.[6] The major target groups and selected conjugate names are included.[6,8,22]

Reaction	Conjugating agent	Major target	Examples
1. Glucuronidation	UDP*glucuronic acid	-OH -COOH $-NH_2$ >NH -SH >CH	Disulfiram, bilirubin, chloral hydrate, chloramphenicol, codeine, fentanyl, lorazepam, morphine, nalorphine, naloxone, oxazepam, phenacetin, propranolol, sulfonamides
2. Glucose	UDP-glucose	-OH -COOH -SH >NH	
3. Sulfation	PAPS†	-OH $-NH_2$ -SH	Aromatic amines, catechols, fentanyl, lorazepam, morphine, phenols
4. Methylation	SAM‡	™OH $-NH_2$ <NH -SH	Dimercaprol, epinephrine, histamine, morphine, nicotinamide, norcodeine, norepinephine, serotonin, tryptamine
5. Acetylation	Acetyl CoA	-OH $-NH_2$ $-SO_2$, NH_2	Aniline, histamine, isoniazide, procainamide, sulfanilamide, sulfonamides
6. Cyanide Detoxification	Sulfane sulfur	-CN-	Dietary sources
7. Glutathione conjugation	Gluthatione	Arene oxide epoxide alkyl and aryl halides	Naphthalene, Acetaminophen
8. Amino acid conjugation	Glycine Glutamate (Ornithine) (Taurine)	Ar-COOH	

*UDP = uridine diphosphate
†PAPS = 3′-phospho-adenosine-5′-phosphosulfate
‡SAM = S-adenosylmethionine

lently bind to cell components that are not normally involved with drug detoxification or biotransformation reactions. When a drug binds to tissue macromolecules such as proteins, lipids, and nucleic acids (particularly -OH of serine, -SH of cysteine, and -NH of histidine), the binding, in contrast to most conjugations, promotes the retention of the drug and delays its excretion. Most conjugations of this kind also produce irreversible changes in the macromolecules to which the drug attaches, potentially leading to harmful consequences. Conjugation reactions permanently remove the conjugating agent (covalently bound to the drug molecule) from participation in normal cell function. Although such reactions are not usually detrimental to the cell, some pools of endogenous ligands are relatively limited (e.g., sulfate, sulfane sulfur, and methyl groups) and may be rapidly depleted by participation in extensive conjugation reactions. Loss of excessive amounts of these components can be harmful to the cell.

Glucuronidation

Glucuronidation is the most common conjugation reaction in humans, a fact due, at least in part, to the availability of large quantities of glucose in the body. Glucose is the precursor of the ligand (glucuronic acid) that is covalently linked to drug molecules during this type of biotransformation reaction. Glucuronidation is almost always a detoxification reaction. The products of these reactions are usually biologically inactive and highly water soluble. Many drugs are excreted as conjugated metabolites.

The enzymes needed to catalyze conjugation reactions are concentrated mainly in the liver but occur in other tissues including the brain. The major subcellular location of these enzymes is in the microsomal fraction of cells, but some of these enzymes are located in the supernatant (cytosol) fraction.

The conjugating agent in glucuronidation reactions, namely glucuronic acid, was first isolated by Schmiedeberg and Meyer in 1879. Convinced that the conjugating agent was a direct derivative of glucose and that its structure was intermediate between gluconic acid and saccharic acid, they arbitrarily named the compound glucuronic acid.[9]

Glucuronidation of drug molecules occurs in several sequential steps that, at the present time, are thought to include the following reactions:

[a] Glucose + ATP $\xrightarrow[\textit{hexokinase}]{}$ Glucose-6-phosphate + adenosine diphosphate (ADP)

[b] Glucose-6-phosphate $\xrightarrow[\textit{phosphoglucomutase}]{}$ Glucose-1-phosphate

[c] Glucose-1-phosphate + Uridine triphosphate (UTP) $\xrightarrow[\textit{UDP-glucose-pyrophosphorylase}]{}$ Uridine 5′-diphosphate (UDP)-glucose + pyrophosphate

[d] UDP-glucose + 2 NAD^+ + H_2O $\xrightarrow[\textit{UDPG-dehydrogenase}]{}$ UDP-glucuronic acid + 2 NADH + 2 H^+

[e] DRUG-XH + UDP-glucuronic acid $\xrightarrow[\textit{glucuronyl transferase}]{}$ DRUG-X-glucuronic acid + UDP

DRUG-XH $\longrightarrow$ DRUG-X-glucuronic acid (net drug biotransformation)

In this scheme, X is $-O-$, $-\overset{\overset{\displaystyle O}{\|}}{C}-O-$, $-NH-$, or $-S-$ and represents the functional group of alcohols, phenols, aromatic, and aliphatic carboxylic acids, amines (especially aromatic), and compounds containing sulfhydryl groups. Drugs containing these groups are prime substrates for glucuronidation. Morphine, for example, is metabolized to morphine glucuronide in a conjugation reaction:

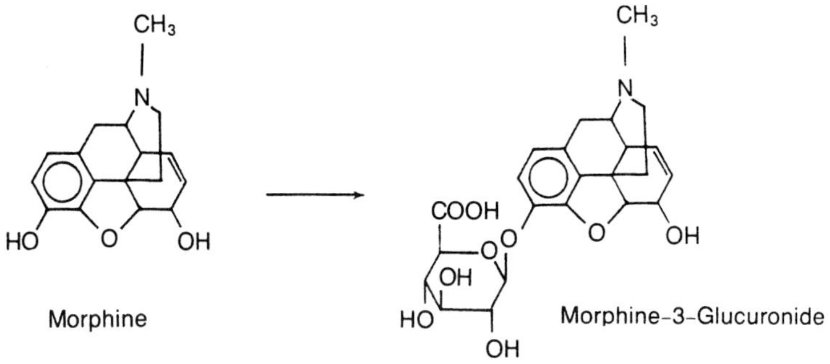

Morphine → Morphine-3-Glucuronide

The sites of glucuronidation mirror the distribution of the relevant enzymes. Glucuronyl transferase, the enzyme responsible for the actual conjugation reaction (step [e] in this scheme), is a microsomal enzyme present mainly in the liver, but also in the kidney, gastrointestinal tract, skin, and other tissue. Uridine diphosphate glucose (UDPG)-dehydrogenase is present predominantly in the supernatant fraction.

β-Glucuronidase can catalyze the breakdown of many glucuronides. This enzyme is present in most animal tissues (concentrated in lysosomes) and can delay the excretion of drugs. Glucuronidate metabolites of drugs that pass into the gastrointestinal tract with the bile (e.g., morphine glucuronide) can be broken down by intestinal or bacterial β-glucuronidase. The portion of drug that is liberated by such a mechanism can be reabsorbed, establishing an enterohepatic circulation that may prolong the action of the drug.

There are at least two features of the glucuronidation pathway that deserve special comment. The first is that steps [a] through [c] are not unique to drug biotransformation reactions. They are the same reactions (and enzymes) involved in the biosynthesis of glycogen from glucose. It is not until step [d] that the two pathways diverge. UDP-dehydrogenase catalyzes the formation of UDP-glucuronic acid for conjugation with drug molecules, whereas glycogen synthetase catalyzes the addition of a free glucose molecule to an existing glycogen chain. The significance of this common pathway in drug metabolism and intermediary metabolism is that it represents another point of potential interaction. Communication between the two pathways at these points probably accounts, in part, for the known influence of such factors as nutrition and hormones on drug metabolism.

Glucose Conjugation

In some cases, UDP-glucose is the conjugating agent, not glucuronic acid as in glucuronidation. This pathway is less common than glucuronidation, especially in humans.

Sulfate Conjugation

Phenols, aromatic amines, and some alcohols are the principal substrates for sulfate conjugation reactions. For example, phenol is metabolized to phenylsulfate by sulfate conjugation.

Methylation

Various phenols, aromatic amines, and sulfhydryl-containing drugs are the prime substrates for this type of reaction. These conjugations are also quite common in the intermediary metabolism of endogenous compounds. The methyl group is donated by *S*-adenosylmethionine (SAM), which is formed from ATP and the amino acid methionine.

Acetylation–Amide Synthesis

Acetylation is thought to occur predominantly in the reticuloendothelial cells (rather than parenchymal cells) of the liver, lung, spleen, etc. An interesting feature of acetylation conjugations is that they are active in neonates, in contrast to glucuronidation. Examples of acetylation-amide synthetic reactions are:

[a] Benzoic Acid

$$C_6H_5\text{-}COOH + CH_2NH_2COOH \xrightarrow[\text{CoA-SH}]{} C_6H_5\text{-}C(=O)\text{—NH—}CH_2\text{—COOH}$$

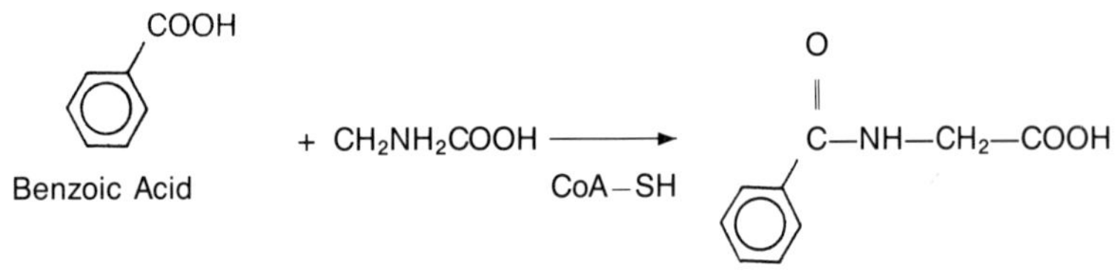

[b]

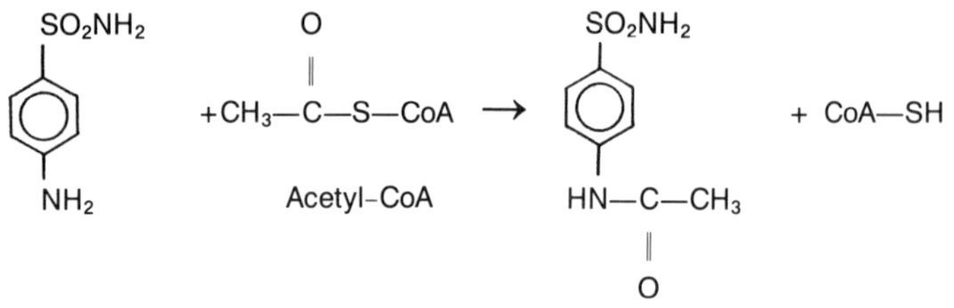

$$H_2N\text{-}C_6H_4\text{-}SO_2NH_2 + \underset{\text{Acetyl-CoA}}{CH_3\text{—}C(=O)\text{—S—CoA}} \rightarrow CH_3\text{—}C(=O)\text{—HN-}C_6H_4\text{-}SO_2NH_2 + \text{CoA—SH}$$

Cyanide Detoxication

This reaction primarily constitutes a line of defense against the toxicity that would result from dietary sources of cyanide.

Glutathione Conjugation

Arene oxides, epoxides, and alkyl and aryl halides can be metabolized via glutathione conjugation. Although this reaction is a relatively minor route of drug

$$\text{Glutamate} + \text{Cysteine} \xrightarrow{\text{ATP}} \text{Intermediate}$$

$$\text{Intermediate} + \text{Glycine} \xrightarrow{\text{ATP}} \text{Glutathione}$$

```
          COOH
           |
      H2N—CH
           |
          CH2
           |                 Glutamine
          CH2
           |
          C=O
           |
          HN
           |
  HS—CH2—CH                  Cysteine
           |
          C=O
           |
          HN
           |
          CH2                Glycine
           |
          COOH
```

Glutathione

metabolism in humans (because of the lack of significant amounts of glutathione-*S*-transferase, the enzyme that catalyses this conjugation reaction), it can be important in some circumstances, for example in the metabolism of acetaminophen.

Glutathione is thought to play a protective role in acetaminophen metabolism by inactivating a toxic intermediate.[26] Most (about 90%) of acetaminophen is metabolized by glucuronidation or sulfate conjugation reactions, but a small percentage is thought to be *N*-hydroxylated to a toxic compound that covalently binds to proteins and enzymes of hepatic cells, potentially producing hepatic cell damage or necrosis. Normally, sufficient glutathione is present (about 5 nmol in most tissue) to inactivate this intermediate compound through glutathione conjugation. In acute acetaminophen overdose, however, glutathione stores are depleted and liver tissue damage may occur.

Amino Acid Conjugation

One of the mechanisms by which benzoic acid is biotransformed is through conjugation to glycine, a fact of historical interest because benzoic acid was the first compound whose metabolic fate in the body was rigorously investigated (in 1824). In general, carboxylic acids are the major substrate for amino acid conjugation reactions, the conjugating agent most often being glycine or glutamate (in humans) and ornithine or taurine (in animals).

Factors Affecting Drug Metabolism

Many factors are known to alter the rate or the extent of drug biotransformation reactions. Because most drugs are metabolized by multiple routes, many of these factors shift the major drug-metabolizing activity from one pathway to another. The impact of these factors on the total metabolism of a particular drug depends on the number of metabolic pathways affected and the degree that they are altered.

Several factors that influence drug metabolism have been recognized and an extensive bibliography now exists.* Brief summaries of certain well-known factors that affect drug metabolism follow:

Age. The ability to metabolize drugs is a function of age. The sophisticated system of drug-metabolizing enzymes matures concurrently with other developing systems and is relatively underdeveloped in the fetus and the neonate.[27] In these situations drug actions are prolonged, usually more pronounced, and often toxic. Additionally, the incompletely formed blood-brain barrier at this stage of development permits passage of drugs into the central nervous system more readily than in older children and adults. Similar situations occur in the elderly. Age-related responses to drugs have been well documented. Barbiturates are sometimes excitatory in children, and amphetamine is sometimes a depressant for this age group.

Body Temperature. The rate of drug biotransformation reactions, as well as all other chemical reactions, is a function of temperature. (The "rule of thumb" in chemistry is that the rate of a chemical reaction changes by a factor of 2 for every 10°C change in temperature.) The direction of this change (increase or decrease in rate with an increase in temperature) depends on both the drug and the reaction.

Chemical Nature of Drug. Lipid-soluble drugs tend to be good substrates for microsomal enzymes; water-soluble drugs tend to be metabolized in the mitochondrial and cytosolic fractions of cells. The chemical nature of a drug also determines whether it can be oxidized, reduced, conjugated, or biotransformed in some other way.

The chemical nature of drugs can be modified in subtle ways to decrease their metabolism. Investigations of this kind have been prompted by the obvious realization that toxic metabolites limit the application of otherwise useful drugs. Such is the case for some volatile anesthetics, e.g., methoxyflurane, in which the inorganic fluoride produced during biotransformation reactions is responsible for the nephrotoxicity associated with this drug. Attempts to decrease the production of toxic metabolites by volatile anesthetics and other drugs have included the incorporation of deuterium atoms into the chemical structures of these drugs. Bonds involving deuterium are slightly stronger than those involving simple

*References 1–3, 5, 7, 13, 18–20, 28.

hydrogen. As a result, deuterium bonds are more resistant to chemical attack than are hydrogen bonds and deuterated drugs are metabolized at a slower rate than their nondeuterated counterparts. Such a chemical modification does not alter the anesthesia induced by these agents, but it may change their toxic potential. For drugs that are eliminated principally by sequential metabolism, deuteration decreases the rate, but not necessarily the pathway of metabolism. In such cases, toxicity is not greatly attenuated and may even be enhanced. Likewise, for drugs with multiple pathways of biotransformation, deuteration may merely shift the major route of metabolism from one pathway to another. Such shifts could actually increase the level of toxic metabolites produced by these compounds. In special cases such as volatile anesthetics, where alternative routes of elimination are available (such as the lungs), decreasing the rate of metabolism is advantageous because more drug is then available for elimination by these other routes. Unfortunately, to date, the potential of such an approach has not reached fruition in the development of many therapeutic agents with significant advantages over currently used drugs.

Circadian Rhythm. The extent to which circadian rhythms may affect drug metabolism has not been as extensively investigated as some of the other factors. However, the influence of this factor on drug response has been reported.

Diet and Nutrition. A decrease in dietary intake often results in a decrease in metabolic activity owing to depressed enzyme activity or lack of energy sources. A diet deficient in calcium will also have the same effect. Drugs that are conjugated to amino acids require a sufficient dietary source (protein) for this route of metabolism. The presence of protein in the diet or its absence (vegetarianism) can also affect pH enough to alter drug metabolism. It is well known that dietary intake of monoamine oxidase (MAO) inhibitors can dramatically alter responsiveness to monoamine drugs.

Disease. Drug metabolism can be directly affected by disease (e.g., in hepatic, renal, or respiratory system dysfunction) or indirectly by affecting the transport of drugs to their normal sites of metabolism (e.g., decreased hepatic perfusion in cardiovascular disease).

Dose. The metabolism of a drug via a particular pathway (e.g., conjugation) depends on the availability of the enzymes that catalyze the relevant biotransformation reactions and of the substrates of these enzymes. Normally, the enzymes and substrates are present in sufficient quantities in the liver and other tissues to metabolize relatively large quantities of drug. However, these enzymes can be saturated by high doses of drug, in which case the excess drug either remains unmetabolized (with possible toxic manifestations) or is biotransformed by alternative reactions, if available. In either case, the extent and rate of metabolism can be greatly affected. As previously noted, such a situation occurs in acute acetaminophen poisoning. A minor pathway of acetaminophen metabolism involves N-hydroxylation, via the cytochrome P-450 microsomal enzyme system, to a metabolite that is toxic, but that is normally rapidly further biotransformed via glutathione conjugation to a nontoxic end product:

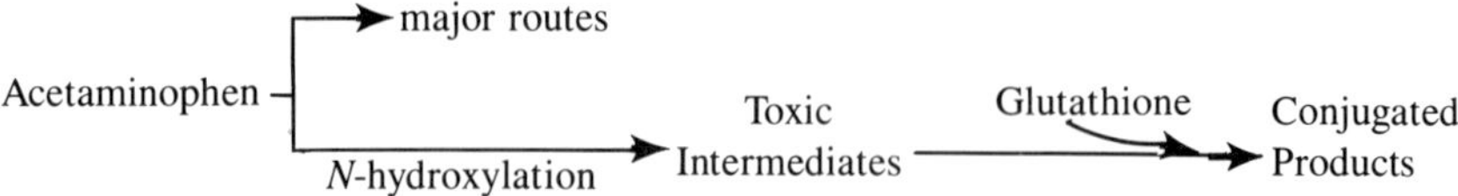

In acute acetaminophen poisoning, glutathione stores can be depleted, eliminating this route of detoxification. As a result, toxic intermediates can build up in sufficient quantities to cause hepatic damage.

Acetaminophen
N-hydroxylation
Toxic
Intermediates
covalent binding to
hepatic macromolecules
Hepatic
Damage

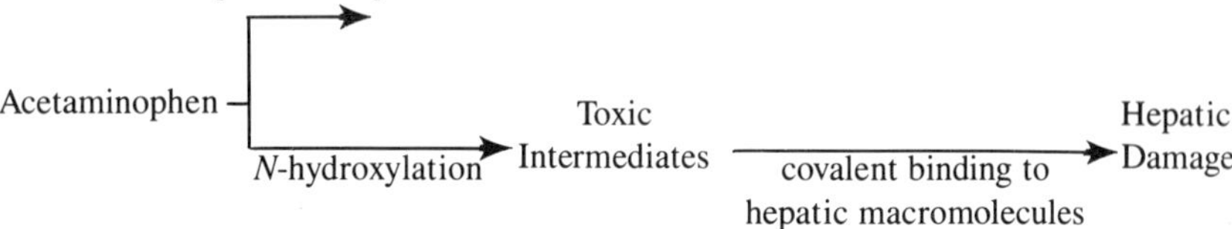

Drugs. The metabolism of a drug can be significantly modified by chronic administration of the drug or by coadministration of another drug. This modification can be manifested as either an increase or decrease in metabolic rate, depending on the drugs involved, and can result in an increase or a decrease in drug action and toxicity. Numerous examples of compounds that increase metabolic rate are known (e.g., alcohol, anticonvulsants, antipyretics, barbiturates, chloroform, central nervous system (CNS) stimulants, food additives, insecticides, muscle relaxants, nitrous oxide, polychlorinated biphenyls, steroids, and tranquilizers) and result in a more rapid metabolism of drugs. The increased metabolism is reflected in a lowered concentration of drug in the blood. Mechanistically, this increased metabolism can be due to two modifications in drug-metabolizing enzymes: increased enzyme activity, or increased enzyme quantity. The latter appears to be the more common mechanism of drugs that stimulate the microsomal enzyme system. Evidence for this includes electron micrographs suggesting an increase in smooth endoplasmic reticulum, biochemical data indicating an increased synthesis (or "induction" of drug-metabolizing enzymes), the inability to duplicate the phenomena in vitro, and the fact that inhibition of nucleic acid and protein synthesis prevents enzyme induction. Two types of microsomal enzyme induction have been described. The first, typified by phenobarbital, involves increased synthesis of several enzymes, including cytochrome P-450 and cytochrome P-450 reductase, and affects the metabolism of a wide variety of drugs. The second type, seen with polycyclic hydrocarbons, appears to involve fewer hepatic enzymes and to alter the metabolism of fewer drugs. The oxidative microsomal enzymes are the ones most commonly induced by drugs, but enzymes involved in glucuronidation can also be induced by a limited number of compounds such as benzpyrene and 3-methylcholanthrene. The site of enzyme induction is not limited to the liver, but occurs in other organs involved in the biotransformation of drugs. The induction is usually reversible, i.e., enzyme activity returns to normal levels following the cessation of the inducing agent. Induction of more prolonged duration can also be produced (e.g., by some dioxins).

Drug-metabolizing enzymes can be inhibited, as well as induced, by drugs and environmental chemicals. There are fewer examples of inhibition than of induction and there are qualitative differences as well. Induction usually involves increased synthesis of enzymes, whereas inhibition normally involves competition between substrates for available enzymes. Usually, drug-metabolizing enzymes are abundantly available and inhibition is not pronounced. But, drugs and experimental compounds that significantly inhibit the microsomal enzyme system are known. As in induction, alteration of these enzymes not only affects the metabolism of drugs, but also the metabolism of endogenous substances, an aspect of the phenomenon that perhaps needs additional attention.

Recently, an interaction between cigarette smoking and drug metabolism has been reported. Cigarette smoking appears to stimulate hepatic drug-metabolizing enzymes, resulting in reduced blood levels (and, hence, effectiveness) of affected drugs. The enzyme induction is of the type characteristic of polycyclic hydrocarbons (discussed above) and is probably caused by the presence of such chemicals in tobacco smoke. A list of some drugs suspected to be affected includes benzodiazepines, heparin, insulin, oral contraceptives, pentazocine, phenothiazines, propoxyphene, propranolol, and tricyclic antidepressants.

Gender (Hormones). Reviews of the literature regarding sex-related differences in drug metabolism reveal extensive evidence for differences in the rate that adult male and female rats biotransform drugs. These differences have been reported for hexobarbital, meperidine, methadone, morphine, pentobarbital, picrotoxin, strychnine, and other compounds. Female rats metabolize these compounds slower than do male rats, explaining the more pronounced and prolonged action of these compounds on the adult female rat. Investigation into the cause of this difference suggests that cytochrome P-450 in male rats has a greater capacity to bind with substrates. This would explain the observed differences in the rate of metabolism of drugs biotransformed via this route. In general, sex-related differences in the activities of hepatic microsomal enzymes are observed only in rats more than 50 days old (corresponding to sexual maturation). No significant differences in enzymatic activities are observed in younger rats.

Differences in the amount or activity of drug-metabolizing enzymes may be only one component of the observed sex-related differences in drug metabolism. Another component may be the effect of androgenic hormones, because castration of adult male rats appears to eliminate the sex-related differences in those situations where it has been observed.

Although sex-related differences in drug metabolism by the hepatic microsomal system are easily demonstrated in rats, these differences are less apparent in other species. No obvious sex-related differences in drug metabolism have been noted for mice, guinea pigs, hamsters, rabbits, dogs, or monkeys. Indeed, species differences can be used to ascertain whether sex-related differences in drug responsiveness are related to metabolism or to some other cause. If a drug produces a sex-dependent response in rats, but not in mice, the sex-related effects are probably explained by differences in metabolism. If both species show a sex-dependent response to a drug, the cause is less obviously attributable to metabolism.

Genetics. (1) Some individuals display a supersensitivity to the skeletal muscle relaxant succinylcholine and related compounds. This enhanced sensitivity is manifested as prolonged apnea, which can be attributed to subnormal rates of biotransformation of the drug. Succinylcholine is normally rapidly inactivated by plasma cholinesterase. However, individuals with low levels of the enzyme in their plasma are susceptible to otherwise nontoxic doses of the drug. Some variants have overactive plasma cholinesterase activity, making these individuals resistant to succinylcholine. (2) A major route of metabolism of the drug isoniazid (INH), which is used in tuberculosis, is through a conjugation reaction using acetyl-CoA as the substrate and yielding acetyl-INH. This conjugation reaction is catalyzed by *N*-acetyltransferase in the liver. Certain individuals ("slow acetylators") have subnormal quantities of this enzyme and, hence, metabolize INH at a slower rate than do the rest of the population. Other drugs biotransformed by *N*-acetyltransferase include sulfamethazine and hydralazine. (3) Genetics also appears to play a role in the metabolism of phenacetin, dilantin, primaquine, and warfarin.

Route of Administration. Drugs administered orally pass through the liver prior to entering the systemic circulation (first-pass effect). This attenuates the action of drugs that are inactivated by biotransformation in the liver and enhances the action of drugs that are biotransformed to active metabolites. Drugs administered intravenously enter the systemic circulation directly. Hence, hepatic drug concentration can vary considerably with the route of administration. If hepatic enzymes become saturated by one mode of administration, drug metabolism can be significantly altered.

Species. Marked species (and strain) differences in drug metabolism are known. These differences can be qualitative or quantitative and can alter drug metabolism by producing changes in rates or changes in fates. Aquatic animals, for example, lack a hepatic microsomal system and cannot metabolize compounds via any of the pathways associated with that system. Other examples exist. Cats conjugate morphine with sulfate; dogs glucuronidate morphine. Meperidine is metabolized slower in dogs than in humans; procaine is more rapidly metabolized in humans than it is in horses.

Biotransformations of Selected Common Drugs

As a guide to some of the metabolic reactions undergone by commonly used drugs, brief summaries of biotransformation reactions of selected drugs are presented in Table 4.4.

TABLE 4.4. Biotransformation reactions of selected common drugs.*

Acetaminophen (Datril, Tylenol). Most of the drug is metabolized by hepatic microsomal enzymes; relatively little is excreted unchanged. The urine contains conjugates of glucuronic acid (about 60%), sulfuric acid (about 35%), and cysteine (about 3%). The remainder is various hydroxylated and deacetylated products. *N*-Hydroxylation by cytochrome P_{450} mixed function oxidase yields *N*-acetyl-benzoquinoneimine, an arylating metabolite that covalently binds to hepatic macromolecules, causing cell damage and necrosis. Normally, this compound is rapidly further metabolized to less toxic cysteine, and mercapturic acid conjugates via a pathway requiring glutathione. In acetaminophen poisoning, glutathione levels are depleted and liver injury may occur.

Alcohol

Ethanol. The majority (90% to 98%) of ethanol is oxidized in a multistep process that occurs mostly in the liver and to a lesser extent in the kidney. Most other tissues cannot oxidize alcohols. Ethanol is first biotransformed to acetaldehyde by one of two pathways: alcohol dehydrogenation (major route) and mixed function oxidase (minor route). The acetaldehyde formed in the initial reaction is then rapidly further metabolized to acetate and acetyl-CoA, which is eventually incorporated into the citric acid cycle.

Ethanol elimination normally follows zero-order kinetics, i.e., the rate of decline in blood level is constant (see Chapter 3), and the rate of elimination appears to be insensitive to nearly all good intentions to increase it by chemical intervention. Ethanol metabolism can be interrupted and this is the mechanism of action of disulfiram (Antabuse). Disulfiram inhibits acetaldehyde dehydrogenase, the enzyme that catalyzes the biotransformation of acetaldehyde. Acetaldehyde levels are normally low, even in excessive ethanol consumption, owing to the rapid rate of the dehydrogenase catalyzed reaction. With disulfiram present, acetaldehyde rises to levels that cause the unpleasant effects associated with the disulfiram/ethanol combination.

Methanol. The same enzymes that convert ethanol to acetaldehyde convert methanol to formaldehyde. The formaldehyde is toxic and is probably responsible for the retinal damage observed in methanol poisoning. Recent concern has been expressed over the possible production of methanol from aspartame, the artificial sweetener, when the latter is subjected to high temperatures.

Barbiturates. Numerous metabolic pathways yield alcohols, ketones, phenols, and carboxylic acid. All of these products can undergo further biotransformation to glucuronides. Additional metabolites result from *N*-hydroxylation and opening of the ring structure. The *N*-allylbarbiturates are *N*-dealkylated to active compounds (e.g., mephobarbiturate to phenobarbiturate and methabarbiturate to barbital).

Benzodiazepines. Oxazepam (Serax) and lorazepam (Ativan) are mostly glucuronidated. Other benzodiazepines are biotransformed to active products via *N*-dealkylation or other oxidation pathways. Diazepam (Valium), chlordiazepoxide (Librium), and chlorazepate (Azene, Tranzene) share a common active metabolite—desmethyldiazepam (nordiazepam). Clorazepate (relatively inactive) is biotransformed to this active product nonenzymatically in gastric acid. Most of the benzodiazepines are excreted primarily through the kidney as oxidized or glucuronidated metabolites. Several of the intermediate metabolites of diazepam are active compounds.

Digitalis Glycosides

Digoxin (Lanoxin) is primarily excreted unchanged in the kidney. A few individuals metabolize a portion of the drug to dihydrodigoxin, an inactive product.

Digitoxin (Crystodigin, Purodigin) is extensively metabolized by hepatic microsomal enzymes to several products, including digoxin (see above). The rate of metabolism of digitoxin is accelerated by hepatic enzyme inducers, but is not greatly decreased by hepatic disease.

Enflurane (Ethrane). Most (about 95%) of the drug is eliminated unchanged in expired air or by some other route. The small amount that is metabolized appears as difluoromethoxydifluoroacetic acid and as the fluoride ion.

TABLE 4.4. *Continued.*

Estrogens. The rate and extent of biotransformation of the estrogens depend a great deal on whether the administered drug is an endogenous estrogen or a nonsteroidal synthetic agent. The naturally occurring estrogens and their esters are metabolized in the liver through the same pathways as the endogenous hormones. The nonsteroidal estrogens are degraded at a much slower rate. For the natural estrogens, glucuronides and sulfates of estradiol, estrone, and estriol are the major urinary excretion products, appearing with small amounts of a large number of other derivatives.

Fentanyl (Sublimaze). The major metabolic pathways of fentanyl involve oxidation (to norfentanyl) and hydrolysis (to desproprionolfentanyl). Sufentanyl undergoes these reactions plus *O*-demethylation.

Halothane (Fluorthane). The majority (about 85%) of the drug is expired unchanged. The remainder is metabolized by the cytochrome P_{450} mixed function oxidase system to several products, including trifluoroacetic acid, trifluoroacetylethanolamide, fluoride ion, and bromide ion.

High-Ceiling Diuretics. Drugs of this category are rapidly excreted in the urine. Ethacrynic acid (Edecrin) appears in the urine in approximately equal amounts of unchanged drug, a cysteine adduct, and an unidentified unstable metabolite. Furosemide (Lasix) is eliminated via the feces to a significant degree (about 30%) as well as the kidney (unchanged and as free or glucuronidated metabolites).

Ibuprofen (Motrin, Brufen). Nearly all of the drug is metabolized, little free drug is found in the urine. The major metabolites are a hydroxylated and a carboxylated product of the parent compound. The metabolites are excreted in the urine in the free or conjugated form.

Indomethacin (Indocin). 10% to 20% of the drug is excreted unchanged in the urine. The rest is *O*-demethylated (about 50%) and glucuronidated (about 10%) by hepatic microsomal enzymes and *N*-deacylated by a nonmicrosomal pathway. Free and conjugated metabolites appear in the urine, bile, and feces.

Insulin. A significant first-pass effect eliminates about 50% of an administered dose of this drug before it can reach the systemic circulation. The rest is destroyed mainly in the liver and kidney. A good deal of the drug is internalized by the cells of the liver and other organs (possibly by a "coated pit" process) and is destroyed by lysosomes. Additional amounts of the drug are apparently destroyed at the membrane surface and by two enzyme systems: a proteolytic enzyme that cleaves the molecule into peptides and amino acids and glutathione-insulin transhydrogenase, which reduces the disulfide bridges holding the subunits of the molecule together.

Ketamine (Ketalar, Ketaject). Ketamine is demethylated (via cytochrome P_{450}) to norketamine followed by hydroxylation, dehydration, and other reactions. The parent compound is also hydroxylated directly. All products also appear as the glucuronides.

Levodopa (Bendopa, Dopar, Larodopa, etc). More than two dozen metabolites of this drug have been reported, some of which are biologically active and contribute to the drug's actions and toxicity. Biotransformation in the periphery is counterproductive to its CNS actions. Without appreciable inhibition of metabolic degradation in the periphery, 1% or less is available to penetrate the blood-brain barrier. The rest is carboxylated by ubiquitous aromatic *L*-amino acid decarboxylase. High concentrations of this enzyme in the liver account for the significant first-pass effect. The principal metabolic pathway of levodopa is to dopamine (aromatic *L*-amino acid decarboxylase), which is subsequently biotransformed by monoamine oxidase and aldehyde dehydrogenase to 3,4- dihydroxyphenylacetic acid (DOPAC) and then by catechol-*O*-methyltransferase to homovanillic acid: 3-methoxy-4-hydroxyphenylacetic acid (HVA). DOPAC and HVA are the major urinary excretion products of levodopa, accounting for about half the administered dose. Other metabolites include 3-*O*-methyldopa, 3-methoxytyramine, norepinephrine, epinephrine, and melanin.

TABLE 4.4. *Continued.*

Meperidine (Demerol, Pethadol). A significant first-pass effect limits the amount of administered drug that reaches systemic circulation to about 50%. Only a small amount of the drug is excreted unchanged, the rest is metabolized principally by the liver. The metabolic products in humans are composed mainly of *N*-demethylated derivatives (including normeperidine), meperidinic acid (via hydrolysis), and their conjugated derivatives.

Methoxyflurane (Penthrane). The high lipid solubility of methoxyflurane promotes slow release from fatty stores and, hence, appreciable (50% to 75%) metabolism. Biotransformed products include methoxydifluoracetic acid, dichloracetic acid, oxalic acid, formaldehyde, and chloride and fluoride ions.

Methylxanthines

Caffeine is primarily metabolized in the liver; only about 1% is excreted unchanged in the urine. The major metabolites are 1-methyluric acid and 1-methylxanthine. 1,3-dimethyluric acid, 7-methylxanthine, and 1,7-dimethylxanthine are also present in the urine, but to a much less extent. Theophylline, like caffeine, is primarily metabolized in the liver; about 10% is excreted unchanged in the urine. The major metabolite is 1,3-dimethyluric acid, but appreciable quantities of 1-methyluric acid and 3-methylxanthine also appear in the urine.

Morphine. Numerous biochemical pathways are potentially available for opiate biotransformation and inactivation. Morphine participates in several metabolic reactions, including conjugation, *N*-methylation, and oxidation. Of these, the major metabolic pathway of morphine in humans appears to be conjugation with glucuronic acid to form morphine-3-glucuronide. *N*-Demethylation (to normorphine) and oxidation (to pseudomorphine) might occur, but to an appreciably less, even negligible, extent.

Nitrous Oxide. This gaseous anesthetic is excreted almost entirely unchanged in expired air, through the skin, etc. Minor metabolic reactions have been reported.

Phenacetin. Less than 1% is excreted unchanged in the urine. In the normal subject, 75% to 80% is rapidly biotransformed to acetaminophen. Extensive first-pass effect contributes to multiple metabolites, which include, in addition to acetaminophen, at least a dozen other products resulting from *N*-deacetylation to para-phenetidin and from hydroxylation. In genetically predisposed individuals, a decreased ability to metabolize phenacetin to acetaminophen gives rise to toxic metabolites that can result in methemoglobin formation and hemolysis.

Progesterone. Metabolism of this drug occurs mainly in the liver and excretion primarily in the urine (50% to 60%) and feces (about 10%). Pregnanediol is a major intermediate product in the biotransformation of progesterone and appears in the urine free or as the glucuronide. Levels of "pregnanediol" and derivatives vary with the stages of the menstrual cycle and during pregnancy.

Propranolol (Inderal). The first-pass effect biotransforms up to two thirds of propranolol, leaving only one third to enter the systemic circulation. Metabolic products include α-hydroxypropranolol (active, but has short half-life), naphthoxylactic acid, isopropylamine, and propranolol glycol. A large percentage of the metabolites appear in the urine as glucuronide conjugates.

Quinidine. The route and extent of the metabolism of this drug vary appreciably from individual to individual. Most of the drug is biotransformed in the liver, but a significant portion (about 20%) is eliminated by renal excretion. The major metabolites consist of mono-hydroxylated products (either on the quinoline or on the quinuclidine ring). Dihydroxylated products appear to a lesser extent. Some of these metabolites are thought to be cardioactive.

Sulfinpyrazone (Anturane). This drug is excreted in the urine in the unchanged form (about 90%) and as the *N'*-*p*-hydroxyphenyl metabolite.

TABLE 4.4. *Continued.*

Tricyclic Antidepressants. Generally, the tricyclic antidepressants are eliminated relatively slowly from the body. Biotransformation to active products (e.g., imipramine to desipramine; amitriptyline to nortriptyline) enhances or prolongs their actions. The final metabolic pathway of these compounds usually occurs in two steps: phase I, oxidation (microsomal enzymes); phase II, glucuronidation. The oxidation reactions yield 2-hydroxy (imipramine and desipramine) and 10-hydroxy (amitriptyline and nortriptyline) metabolites, which are subsequently glucuronidated.

*For each drug the material gathered from references 7, 14, 21, 24, 26, and 30, has been summarized.

REFERENCES

1. Adriani J: *The Pharmacology of Anesthetic Drugs.* Springfield, Ill, Charles C. Thomas, 1970, p 1–16.
2. Baden JM, Rice SA: Metabolism and toxicity of inhaled anesthetics, in Miller RD (ed): *Anesthesia*, New York, Churchill Livingstone, 1981, p 383–424.
3. Bentley JB: Deuterated volatile anesthetics, in Brown BR Jr (ed): *New Pharmacologic Vistas in Anesthesia*, Philadelphia, FA Davis Co, 1983, p 19–26.
4. Brenner RR: Metabolism of endogenous substrates by microsomes. *Drug Metab Rev* 1977; 6:155–212.
5. Brown BR: Hepatic microsomal enzyme induction. *Anesthesiology* 1973; 39:178–187.
6. Caldwell J: Conjugation reactions in foreign compound metabolism: definition, consequences, and species variations. *Drug Metab Rev* 1982; 13:745–777.
7. Cascorbi HF: Biotransformation of drugs used in anesthesia. *Anesthesiology* 1973; 39:115–125.
8. Ciaccio EI: Intimate study of drug action II: fate of drugs in the body, in Di Palma JR (ed): *Drill's Pharmacology in Medicine*, New York, McGraw-Hill, 1971, pp 36–66.
9. Conti A, Bickel MH: History of drug metabolism: discoveries of the major pathways in the 19th century. *Drug Metab Rev* 1977; 6:1–50.
10. Coon MJ: Drug metabolism by cytochrome P-450: progress and perspectives. *Metab Disposit* 1981; 9:1–4.
11. Csaky TZ: *Introduction to General Pharmacology.* New York, Appleton-Century-Crofts, 1969, pp 55–80.
12. Feinman L, Rubin E, Lieber CS: Adaptation of the liver to drugs, in Orlandi F, Jezequel AM (eds): *Liver and Drugs.* New York, Academic Press, 1972, pp 41–83.
13. Gibaldi M, Perrier D: Route of administration and drug disposition. *Drug Metab Rev* 1974; 3:185–199.
14. Goth A: *Medical Pharmacology.* St Louis, CV Mosby Co, 1984, pp 29–39.
15. Guenthner TM: Monoclonal antibodies to cytochrome P-450 isozymes. *Trends in Pharmacological Sciences* 1983; 4:5.
16. Hansch C: Quantitative relationships between lipophilic character and drug metabolism. *Drug Metab Rev* 1972; 1:1–14.
17. Hucker HB: Intermediates in drug metabolism reactions. *Drug Metab Rev* 1973; 2:33–56.
18. Jenner P, Testa B: The influence of stereochemical factors on drug disposition. *Drug Metab Rev* 1973; 2:117–184.
19. Kato R: Sex-related differences in drug metabolism. *Drug Metab Rev* 1974; 3:1–32.

20. LaDu BN: Genetic factors modifying drug metabolism and drug response, in LaDu BN, Mandel HG, Way EL (eds): *Fundamentals of Drug Metabolism and Drug Disposition.* Baltimore, Williams & Wilkins Co, 1971, pp 308–327.
21. Lawrence DR, Bennett PN: *Clinical Pharmacology,* ed 5, New York, Churchill Livingstone, 1980, pp 124–128.
22. Mandel HG: Pathways of drug biotransformation: biochemical conjugations, in LaDu BN, Mandel HG, Way EL (eds): *Fundamentals of Drug Metabolism and Drug Disposition.* Baltimore, Williams & Wilkins Co, 1971, pp 149–205.
23. Mannering GJ: Microsomal enzyme systems which catalyze drug metabolism, in LaDu BN, Mandel HG, Way EL (eds): *Fundamentals of Drug Metabolism and Drug Disposition.* Baltimore, Williams & Wilkins Co, 1971, pp 206–252.
24. Mayer SE, Melmon KL, Gilman AG: Introduction; the dynamics of drug absorption, distribution, and elimination, in Gilman AG, Goodman LS, Gilman A (eds): *The Pharmacological Basis of Therapeutics*, ed 6, New York, Macmillan Publishing, 1980, pp 12–20.
25. Preisig R, Bircher J (eds): *The Liver: Quantitative Aspects of Structure and Function.* Proc 3rd Intl Gstaad Symposium, September, 1978. Editio Cantor Aulendorf. pp 269–350.
26. Prescott LF, Critchley JAJH: The treatment of acetaminophen poisoning. *Ann Rev Pharmacol Toxicol* 1983; 23:87–101.
27. Short CR, Kinden DA, Stith R: Fetal and neonatal development of the microsomal monooxygenase system. *Drug Metab Rev* 1976; 5:1–42.
28. Stanski DR, Watkins WD: *Drug Disposition in Anesthesia.* New York, Grune & Stratton, 1982, pp 47–71.
29. Vesell ES: Individual variations in drug response, in Orlandi F, Jezequal AM (eds): *Liver and Drugs.* New York, Academic Press, 1972, pp 1–40.
30. Way EL, Adler TK: The pharmacologic implications of the fate of morphine and its surrogates. *Pharmacol Revs* 1960; 12:383–446.
31. White RE, Coon MJ: Oxygen activation by cytochrome P_{450}. *Ann Rev Biochem* 1980; 49:315–356.

5
Introduction to Specific Drug Action and Membrane Surface Phenomena

. . . we may, I think, without much rashness, assume that there is some substance or substances in the nerve endings or gland cells with which [drugs] are capable of forming compounds.

–J.N. Langley, 1878.

Drugs are believed to produce their effects on biological systems either by alteration of some physical property of the cell or by a specific chemical reaction between the drug and its receptor. Many drugs produce their effects by interacting with specific cellular receptors. A description of the mathematical analysis of the interaction of drugs with receptors can be found in Chapter 8. The present chapter presents only an outline of the general development of the drug-receptor concept and highlights those aspects of the development which are considered by many the "principles" underlying present conceptions of the drug-receptor interaction. A more recent development, the recognition of cell processes (e.g., membrane capping, coated pits, and coated vesicles) capable of modifying the number of cell-surface receptors, is described in more detail.

Nonspecific Drug Action

Although most drugs are specific, that is, act through specific receptors, some drugs seem not to behave this way. The most notable examples of these nonspecific drugs occur among the volatile anesthetics. They differ markedly in chemical structure, yet their effects are overtly similar. Evidence suggesting nonspecific activity of these agents comes from determinations of the anesthetic concentrations of the different compounds. Although these concentrations differ among the various compounds, they have strikingly similar values of relative anesthetic concentrations, that is, the ratio C/C_S, where C is the actual anesthetic concentration and C_S is the saturable, or maximum concentration (Table 5.1). Moreover, these compounds have different molecular structures and weights. The ratio C/C_S is a measure of the degree of saturation. This ratio is involved in the determination of the thermodynamic activity of a compound, and

The material on pp. 101–103, and portions of 104, 106, 107, 109–112 has been reprinted from TIPS, 6:133–136, 1985, with permission from Elsevier Biomedial Press.

TABLE 5.1. Anesthetic potencies*

Anesthetic	Anesthetic concentration (% by vol)	C/C_S at anesthetic concentration
Nitrous oxide	100	0.01
Diethyl ether	3.4	0.03
Chloroform	0.5	0.01

*Based on J. Ferguson.[21]

it may therefore be concluded that the biologic activity of these compounds depends on their thermodynamic activity. The foregoing is often referred to as Ferguson's principle.[21] Whenever the potency of a drug depends on a physiochemical property rather than on a specific chemical structure, it is suggestive of nonspecific (nonreceptor-mediated) action.

Specific Drug Action: The Development of the Concept of Receptors

LANGLEY

The concept of a highly specific drug-receptor interaction developed slowly. One of the earliest suggestions of the existence of receptors evolved from studies with antagonists. Langley[37] studied the blocking action of atropine on pilocarpine-induced effects and reasoned that the two drugs must react with the same substance. He further postulated conditions that should favor drug-receptor formation:

> To take the simplest case, if *a* and *b* are both able to form, with *y*, the compounds *ay*, *by* then *ay* and *by* are formed, quantity of *ay* and *by* depending on the relative chemical affinity to *y*.

HILL

The studies of A. V. Hill produced strong evidence favoring the receptor hypothesis. Studying nicotine-induced muscle contraction (frog rectus abdominis) and its antagonism by curare, Hill[31] showed that the dose-response curves and temperature dependencies he observed could be explained only by a chemical (involving chemical bonds), and not a physical, interaction of the drugs with the muscle tissue. In his early studies, Hill formulated many concepts about receptors that were ultimately adopted by subsequent theorists. The drug-receptor interaction was viewed as a reversible equilibrium reaction because the drug-induced muscle contraction could be terminated by removal of the stimulating drug. The observed effect (E_h) was assumed proportional to the quantity ($AR - M$), where AR is the drug-receptor complex and M the threshold amount of drug required for the first noticeable response. The steady-state effect E_h of a given drug concentration $[A]$ was given as

$$E_h = [k_1 r_t [A]/(k_2 + k_1[A])] - M,$$

where r_t represents the total amount of what was called "receptive substance."

Clark

Another important extension of the theory came from A. J. Clark,[9,10] who found that the shapes of the dose-response curves for acetylcholine were similar in two different preparations (frog rectus abdominis and isolated ventricle strip) and that these curves could be best described by equations of similar form, namely,

$$E_c = [A]^n/(K + [A]^m),$$

where $[A]$ is concentration of drug, E_c is the fractional effect, and K = constant. The experimental evidence supported a value of 1.0 for n and m.

Clark also noted the similarity between his equations describing drug action and those of Langmuir describing chemisorption of a gas on a solid surface.[38] Chemisorption is a special case of adsorption, characterized by high specificity and involving forces stronger than those normally encountered in simple physical adsorption. Physical adsorption consists of the binding of molecules to the surface of the adsorbent with relatively weak attraction, such as van der Waals' forces. In the adsorption process, molecules are altered only slightly, about to the extent that gas molecules are when condensed to the liquid state.

Chemisorption, on the other hand, is accompanied by major changes in the electronic distribution and bonding of the adsorbed molecules. The chemical changes of chemisorption are accompanied by a high heat of adsorption (5 to 100 kcal/g-mole) compared with physical adsorption (0.5 to 5 kcal/g-mole). These chemical changes brought about by chemisorption, and not physical adsorption, explain the catalytic effect of solid surfaces (or of the drug-receptor interaction), because the energy possessed by chemisorbed molecules can be substantially different from that of the molecules alone.[56]

The assumptions made in the derivation of the Langmuir isotherm have, for the most part, become incorporated into the present conceptualization of the drug-receptor interaction. Some of these assumptions are:

1. Adsorption occurs at discrete sites on the surface
2. Each site can accommodate only one molecule
3. All sites are identical
4. The energy of adsorbed species is everywhere the same on the surface
5. There is no interaction between adsorbed molecules
6. At most, a monolayer of adsorbed molecules can accumulate as opposed to physical adsorption in which several layers can build up

7. The rate of adsorption is given by $r_a = k_1[A](1 - f)$, where $[A]$ = concentration of adsorbed species in solution, f = fraction of total surface covered by absorbed molecules, and k_1 is a (rate) constant;
8. The rate of desorption is given by $r_d = k_2 f$.

With these assumptions surface coverage, or active site occupation (or receptor occupation), is given by $f = K[A]/(1 + K[A])$, where $K = k_1/k_2$. This equation is similar to that observed by Clark for acetylcholine action.

From an analysis of his own results, Clark[9] concluded that "... it is impossible that acetylcholine should act by forming a continuous layer over the surface of the heart cells, or by covering any larger area inside the cells." Thus, the theoretical concept of the existence of receptors was again supported by experimental findings.

Applicability of Mass Action

The assumption that the law of mass action (prominent in classic drug-receptor theory) sufficiently describes enzyme-substrate (or drug-receptor) interactions has been questioned.[12] The mass-action law is based on a model in which reactants, at low concentrations, are dissolved in a liquid and move freely. However, some enzymes (and presumably most receptors) are bound to membrane surfaces, and, therefore, their interactions should be considered as occurring at a liquid-solid interface.[11] Whereas some of these reactions may be accurately described by the mass-action law, others may not fit such a model. In this regard, a recent report[32] is informative. These authors surveyed the biochemical literature encompassing the period 1965 to 1976 and catalogued nearly 1,000 papers reporting enzyme reaction data that did not fit Michaelis-Menten kinetics. Since this number represented such a high percentage of the total, they concluded that not more than a handful of enzyme-substrate reactions have been shown to follow the Michaelis-Menten equation closely over a wide variety of experimental conditions.

Recent Ideas

Many modern receptor theories are actually special cases of the Langmuir treatment in which one or more of the original assumptions have been relaxed. Because of its relative simplicity, the Langmuir isotherm is usually the major one considered in pharmacological contexts, although there are many other isotherms available.[44] An appropriate isotherm for biological systems might be that of Fruendlich, who allowed for the possibility of heterogeneous active sites of different adsorption energies.[17] Indeed, studies have been reported on the adsorption of drugs to solids (e.g., reference 25) in which this isotherm has been applied.

Some recent views of the chemisorption process are particularly relevant to the drug-receptor interaction. Although the typical chemisorption binding is often covalent or ionic in nature, more complicated binding may be involved in situations in which the solid surface presents a complex electron distribution, such as conducting and semiconducting adsorbents. In this regard, the existence of collective electronic phenomena, called electromagnetic molecular electronic resonance, has already been demonstrated in at least one protein.[7] Along the same lines, effort has begun to plot the electrostatic field-lines around large molecules as a way of explaining drug-receptor recognition at these sites.[14,15] It is also becoming apparent that the heat of adsorption is seldom constant over the entire range of surface coverage, as assumed in the case of the Langmuir isotherm. A number of possibilities have been suggested to explain and incorporate this empirical information.[5] Some of these are:

1. Active sites might be heterogeneous, the most reactive being occupied first, the less reactive progressively later and with decreased strength of bonding.
2. Adsorbed molecules might be mutually attractive or repulsive, especially if they acquire or lose a net charge upon adsorption.
3. Adsorption might proceed with a net exchange of electrons between adsorbed molecule and the surface, so that the surface may become increasingly resistant to further reaction (because of exhaustion of an electron reservoir or sink).

A particularly interesting result is obtained if the first two conditions are true, because of the possible application of solid-state physics to the concept of drug action. The theoretically derived expression for the rate of adsorption in this case is[56]

$$r_a = \alpha P (1 - f)e^{(-E/RT)}/(2\pi m k_B T)^{1/2},$$

where E is the activation energy of adsorption, T is absolute temperature, R is the gas constant, m is the molecular mass, k_B is Boltzmann's constant, and P is pressure. This equation is a combination (actually the product) of three expressions: rate, availability, and energy:

$$\text{rate} = P/(2\, m k_B T)^{1/2},$$

$$\text{availability} = \alpha\,(1 - f),$$

$$\text{energy} = e^{(-E/RT)},$$

The experimental data, however, often do not fit the theoretical prediction, but instead yield adsorption rates more accurately described by the equation,

$$r_a = \alpha f P (1 - f)\, e^{(-E/RT)}/(2\pi\, m k_B\, T)^{1/2},$$

or, in many cases, by the simpler,

$$r_a = \beta\, P e^{(-zf)},$$

where β and z are constants determined experimentally.

This last expression, known as the Elovich equation, was first used in solid-state physics applications. It has recently been extended to several biological phenomena,[12] but it has not yet been specifically applied to the drug-receptor interaction.

Coated Pits and Coated Vesicles

It was convenient for early theorists to model the interaction between drugs and receptors in terms of relatively stationary and static receptors. The interaction between drug and receptor was considered to be initiated by motion of the drug molecule. This view was adopted principally because it simplified the mathematics and permitted useful assumptions to be made.[2,9,10,24] The view was reinforced by contemporary ideas about the "lock and key" fit of enzymes and substrates and by the similarity of shape between typical dose-response curves (hyperbolic) and Langmuir's isotherm, which described the interaction of gas molecules with a stationary, static metal surface.[38] Mainly for practical reasons, therefore, drug-receptor theory began with the drug molecule having the more dynamic role (see historical treatments in references 3, 4, and 16).

Modification of this view evolved slowly, aided by experimental and mathematical techniques that allowed for relaxation of some of the initially stringent assumptions about the drug-receptor interaction.[23,52,58,59] It has subsequently been proposed, for example, that the receptor can undergo a conformational change induced by the drug molecule,[6,26,36] can exist in allosteric forms,[34,40,60] and is mobile in a fluid-mosaic membrane.[13] Generally, though, the integrity of the receptor has been tacitly assumed to be conserved throughout the drug-receptor interaction. In this sense, the receptor serves a catalytic function and is not consumed in the reaction. Recent histological findings, however, may force a significant alteration in this concept with far-reaching consequences on current ideas about the drug-receptor interaction, receptor conservation, tachyphylaxis, and drug tolerance.

Electron microscopy (EM) has revealed specific subcellular structures that are believed to be associated with ligand-specific internalization of extracellular material (see recent reviews in references 1, 28, and 42). Some of these structures appear as invaginations or "pits" in the otherwise planar surface of the cell surface membrane. Other structures appear to be vesicles floating free in the cytoplasm. Some pits and vesicles possess characteristically electron-dense projections (emanating from the cytoplasmic face of their plasma membrane), which give rise to a "coated" appearance (Figure 5.1). Freeze-fracture techniques in which the membrane is split away from the cytoplasm clearly show that the "coat" is highly structured and consists of a basket-like array of interconnected polygonal structures (Figure 5.2).

Coated pits and vesicles are a relatively recent finding. They were first identified in toad spinal ganglion cells[48] and in mosquito oocytes.[49] Subsequently, they have been demonstrated in cells of higher animals.[19,22]

From the beginning it was recognized that coated structures appear to be closely associated with internalization of extracellular material. More than a dozen compounds are now known to enter cells by this specialized form of endocytosis, including insulin, epidermal growth factor, triiodothyronine (T_3), low-density lipoprotein, and some toxins.[42] Coated pits respond to the proper stimulus (the binding of a specific ligand or the incorporation of a ligand-receptor

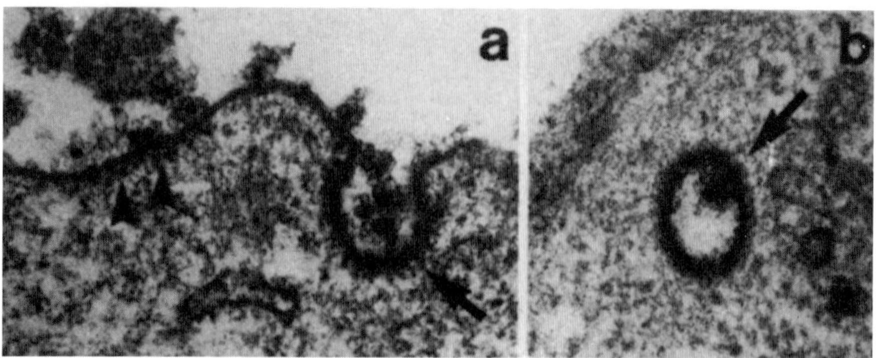

FIGURE 5.1. Illustrated here are the typical stages in the internalization of ligand into cells by receptor-mediated endocytosis. In the earliest phase, the segment of plasma membrane involved in endocytosis is often identified by a bristle-coating (a, double arrowheads), presumably clathrin, on the cytoplasmic leaflet. Subsequently, a coated pit (a, arrow) forms, which eventually detaches from the plasma membrane as a coated vesicle (b), arrow. At this point, the ligand and its receptor are contained within the coated vesicle and are within the cell. This specific example shows the endocytosis of human low density lipoprotein (LDL) by cultured granulosa cells from rat ovaries. The LDL particles are the pale, spherical structures surrounding a black dot, a 20 nm gold particle. Magnification 92 600 –. Courtesy of Dr. Laurie G. Paavola, Department of Anatomy, Temple University School of Medicine, Philadelphia, PA. (From Raffa RB: Coated pits and coated vesicles: histological findings and pharmacological implications. *Trends in Pharmacological Sciences* 1985, 6:133–136.)

complex) by budding off from the inner surface of the cell membrane and forming independent, free-floating vesicles. These vesicles remain "coated" for some variable time while they migrate through the cytoplasm to various destinations (or "targets"). Some targets identified to date include lysosomes, the Golgi apparatus, and, perhaps, the cell nucleus. The precise intracellular destinations of coated vesicles appear to be specific for specific ligands. Hence the contents of coated vesicles have varied fates. Some are enzymatically degraded; others are modified and subsequently secreted; still others are returned unchanged to the membrane surface or to the extracellular compartment.

Several functional roles have been suggested for the coated pit/vesicle system. These include:

1. Endocytosis, as mentioned above
2. Other transport (enzymes from Golgi apparatus to lysosomes, protein secretion by mammary epithelium, retrieval of excess cell surface membrane in presynaptic neurons)
3. Transportation of organelles that carry selected receptor-bound proteins into cells in a tightly controlled fashion
4. Limitation of the stimulus produced by one ligand-receptor interaction

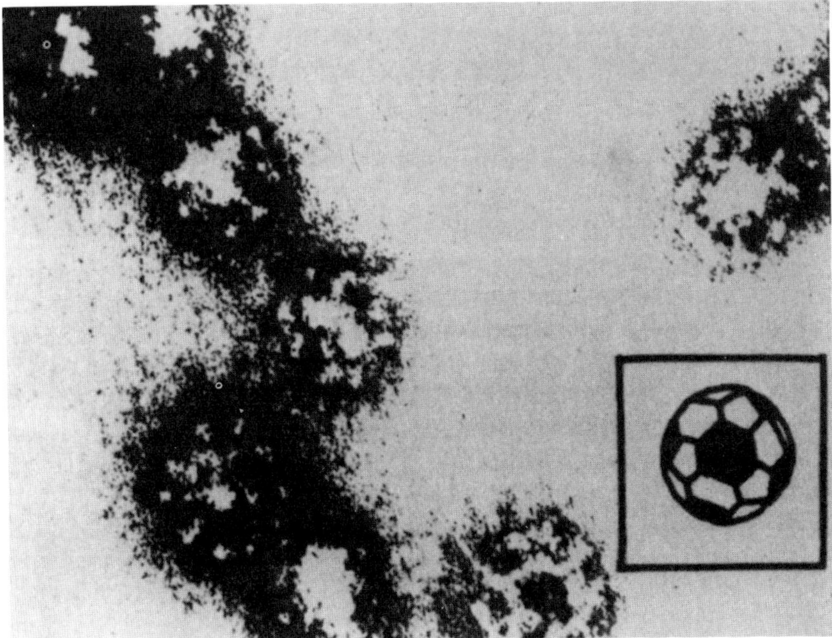

FIGURE 5.2. A magnified view of isolated coated structures. Note the organized and cage-like nature of the individual particles. An artist's rendering of the surface pattern formed by the coat components is depicted in the inset. The electron micrograph was generously supplied by Dr. James H. Keen, Fels Institute and Department of Biochemistry, Temple University School of Medicine. (From Raffa RB: Coated pits and coated vesicles: histological findings and pharmacological implications. *Trends in Pharmacological Sciences*, 1985, 6:133–136.)

5. Rapid clearance of hormones from the cell surface
6. Transportation of biologically active material to the nucleus
7. Exocytosis of secretory products from Golgi apparatus
8. Recycling of membrane components.

While at first coated pits and vesicles may seem to have little relevance for pharmacology, there appear to be many aspects of this phenomenon that could contribute to the current concept of pharmacological receptors. In this regard, it is interesting to note that in many instances a prerequisite for internalization of extracellular material via this mechanism is the recognition and binding of the extracellular material to highly selective receptors on the cell surface. Interaction between the extracellular ligand and the cell surface receptor initiates the series of physiological events comprising the process of endocytosis. Hence, the relevance of coated pits and coated vesicles to pharmacology is the existence of histological evidence for specific cell surface structures that are capable of internalizing drugs, receptors, or both. The ramifications of such a process include a mechanism by which drugs possessing intracellular sites of action can be internalized; a mechanism by which drugs possessing cell surface sites of action are limited to finite impact; and a mechanism by which receptor number or density can be modified during exposure to drug molecules (such as in tachyphylaxis or tolerance).

Coated Structures and Endocytosis

Many, if not all, cells internalize variable amounts of their extracellular environment during endocytosis. The internalization of extracellular material by cells functions both as a defense mechanism and as a means of obtaining nutrients present in the extracellular fluid. Harmful organisms can be internalized and destroyed (e.g., by lysosomal enzymes) and useful nutrients can be ingested and utilized. Endocytosis is conventionally divided into phagocytosis (in which large particulate material is internalized) and pinocytosis (in which liquid is ingested). The process of pinocytosis can be further divided on the basis of specificity. In *nonspecific* pinocytosis, molecules are internalized in proportion to their extracellular concentration and not necessarily to their physiological importance. A large amount of fluid (macropinocytosis) or a small amount of fluid (micropinocytosis) can be involved. An example of macropinocytosis occurs when a membrane ruffle falls back upon the cell surface and, in so doing, traps extracellular fluid. The resultant fluid inclusions are termed macropinososomes and typically range from 0.5 to 3 μm. These inclusions are usually rapidly attacked by phase-dense lysosomes and torn into small pieces by a process colorfully termed "piranhalysis." Micropinocytosis, on the other hand, occurs predominantly through small indentations in the cell surface (caveolae). Micropinososomes are typically on the order of about 800 Å.

Specific endocytosis occurs when there is a coupling of membrane receptor activity to internalization of macromolecules. In this case the term receptor-mediated endocytosis is applied, and the internalized packets of fluid are called "receptosomes." Endocytosis by this route can be substantial.[1] For example, it has been estimated that at least 1,500 to 3,000 coated vesicles can form per minute per cell (accounting for about 2% of the cell surface). Indeed, cells may internalize the equivalent of 150% of their surface per hour. Macrophages in culture have been shown to internalize 0.0001 ml of culture per hour per 10^6 cells.

Rosenbluth and Wissig[47] were among the earliest to identify coated pits and vesicles. Interested in examining the transport of molecules through satellite cell sheaths into ganglion cells, they intraperitoneally injected toads with aqueous ferritin as a tracer (water soluble, electron opaque, a known molecular size of 95 Å, and low toxicity). In addition to their other findings, the authors observed clusters of ferritin particles aggregated in localized invaginations of the plasmalemma. These invaginations were coated on their cytoplasmic surface with a radially striated, felt-like material. They termed the EM appearance of this material a "coat" and distinguished coated structures attached to the surface membrane (pits) from coated structures floating free in the cytoplasm (vesicles).

Roth and Porter[49] observed the same phenomenon in mosquito oocytes. The mosquito oocyte is a good model to study endocytosis because there is selective removal of protein from the insect's blood to support rapid yolk development and because there is a relative lack of subcellular structures to interfere with EM observation. These authors described the presence of "pits" or "wells" (140 µm diameter) dispersed irregularly on the oocyte surface or free in the cortex of the ovary. There were also "bristle-coated vesicles" (140 µm) present. A mechanical function for the bristle coat on these vesicles was suggested, namely, that a natural repulsion between the outer ends of each bristle would stabilize the spherical shape of these structures. Significantly, coated structures appeared to have a functional role because there were many more pits on the oocyte surface during active yolk deposition (approximately 300,000) as compared with "rest" (approximately 20,000).

Rosenbluth and Wissig[48] tracked ferritin disposition in vivo and in vitro as it traveled from the connective tissue spaces in toad spinal ganglia into the neurons. In the course of this study, they observed indentations (0.1 to 0.2 µm) along the neuronal surface and a "felt-like coating" approximately 120 Å thick. The coat was lost in permanganate-fixed tissue.

Fawcett[19] reviewed the surface specializations of absorbing cells and highlighted the known differences in the time course of events between vesicles that possessed a coat and those that did not possess such a coat. In general, noncoated micropinocytomes had more often been observed near the cell surface. Only a relatively few were found floating free or in some intermediate location. The conclusion was that the dissociation of this type of vesicle from the surface must be slow, but that the subsequent steps are rapid. In comparison, few coated vesicles had been observed near the surface, but many more were observed in intermediate locations. Thus, coated vesicles appear to form and depart at rather constant rates.

Friend and Farquhar[22] explored the modes of transport between Golgi, lysosomes, and the cell surface using a combined morphological and cytochemical approach with peroxidase as a tracer for protein absorption and acid phosphatase and thiamine pyrophosphatase as markers for lysosomes and Golgi, respectively. Two types of coated vesicles were described, distinguishable by size. Large vesicles ($>1{,}000$ Å) were located near the membrane surface and possessed 18 to 25 bristles (150 to 200 Å). Smaller vesicles (750 Å) were located nearer the Golgi apparatus, were more granular, and contained dense material. The small vesicles had only 8 to 13 bristles (150 to 200 Å).

Composition of Coated Structures

The harvesting of coated structures was first attempted from nervous tissue[33] and later improved by Pearse,[43] who named the major constituent of the coat "clathrin." Clathrin is now known to be a 180,000 molecular weight (mol wt) polypeptide that is capable of spontaneously forming cage-like structures, even in the absence of a membrane template. Assembly polypeptides probably mediate

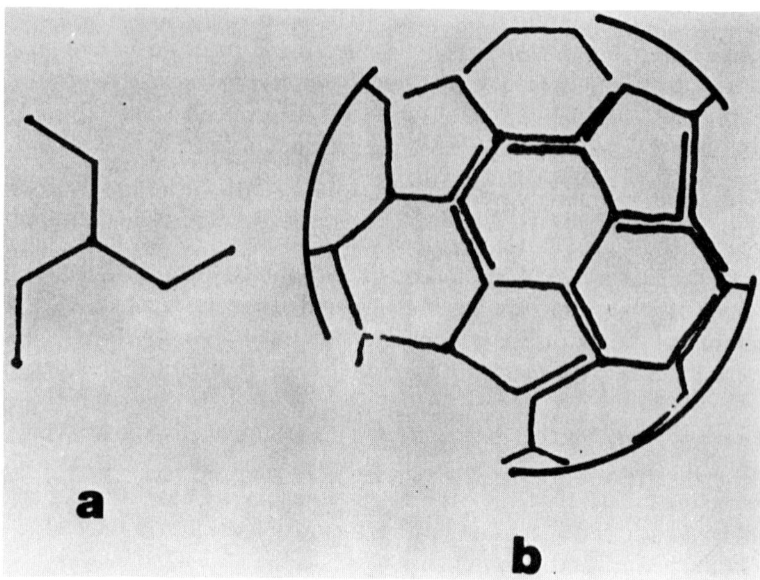

FIGURE 5.3. Schematic representation of a single "triskelion" (a) and a collection of triskelions (b) arranged to simulate the surface pattern observed in electron micrographs of coated structures. (From Raffa, RB: Coated pits and coated vesicles: histological findings and pharmacological implications. *Trends in Pharmacological Sciences*, 1985, 6:133–136.)

this reassembly.[62] Coat material isolated from a variety of animals has been found to be composed predominantly of clathrin, but it is now recognized that other polypeptides are also associated with coated vesicles. Molecules of 110,000, 55,000, and 33,000 to 36,000 mol wt have been identified. Recent studies have suggested that tubulin[35] and an acid glycoprotein[41] are also molecular components of coated vesicles. These components combine to form characteristic three-legged structures having the contours of triskelions (see Fig. 5.3a). Each leg of the triskelion projects from its vertex a distance of about 44 nm. About 16 nm from the vertex, there is a kink in each leg, bending it at an angle of 60 to 75 degrees, but maintaining it approximately in the plane of the proximal portion. In any one triskelion, all three legs are bent in the same direction. A typical triskelion is about 630,000 mol wt and consists of three heavy chains (180,000 each) and three light chains (32,000 to 36,000). Although the term clathrin was originally used to designate the 180,000 mol wt component of triskelions, it has recently been proposed[61] that the term clathrin be used to refer to the entire triskelion-shaped protein molecule.

Triskelions can be aligned in such a way as to form polygons (Figure 5.3b). Coated pits and vesicles are constructed from these polygons, which are arranged in cage-like lattice structures with a distance from vertex to vertex being about

18.6 μm. A particular coat can be composed of several different types of polygons (from pentagons to heptagons), but hexagons appear to predominate in planar portions of the membrane and pentagons appear to predominate in indented membrane areas. Thus, the complicated arrangement of a coated pit may develop in vivo in a stepwise manner. Initially, there exists a planar hexagonal arrangement of clathrin below the membrane surface. This sheet then folds over a developing pit and the rest of the structure becomes filled in with pentagons transformed from hexagons.[33]

Kaneseki and Kadota[33] referred to coated vesicles by perhaps the most colorful name, "vesicles in a basket," and likened the hexagonal and pentagonal arrangement of coated vesicles to a soccer ball (see Figure 5.3b). They also used the picturesque word "coronet" to describe the vesicle coat. Other terms that have been used to describe these structures are bristle-coated structures, rhopheosomes, rhopheocytic vesicles, complex vesicles, alveolate vesicles, acanthosomes, amorphous-coated structures, and wells.

A vesicle's coat and its contents are apparently independent,[33] such that the coat acts only as a temporary housing for the encased material. The clathrin coat is probably noncovalently bound to the coated-vesicle membrane since it can be removed by treatment with urea or protonated amines. A polypeptide of 100,000 mol wt has been implicated as the site of this binding.

The lipid composition of some coated pits is mainly phosphatidylcholine (40%); and phosphatidylethanolamine (30%). Overall, the cholesterol/phospholipid ratio in coated pits is 0.1 to 0.3, which is generally less than most membranes. This may have implications for the fluidity of the membrane in the immediate vicinity of these structures.

Components of the membrane surface have been observed to move at the rate of 3 to 9 $\times$ 10^{-10} cm^2 sec^{-1}.[53] Presumably, unoccupied receptors move at this speed but do not accumulate in coated pits. It seems likely that the proper ligand changes the receptor in some manner that causes the complex to get trapped in the coated pits. Several factors may be involved in regulating this binding. For examples, calmodulin has been implicated in the control of recruitment of clathrin underneath patches of cross-linked receptor-IgM in the plasma membrane of human lymphoblastoid cells.[50]

Membrane Capping

During the course of immunological research in the early 1970s, it was discovered that radiolabeled anti-immunoglobulin antibody binds to the cell surface membrane of B-lymphocytes and initiates a chain of events that ultimately results in the concentration of label at one pole of the cell. This process has come to be called "membrane capping" (see review in reference 54).

In addition to its potential value for diagnostic differentiation of clinically similar disorders,[45] the capping process is of general theoretical interest because the attachment of antibody to the B-lymphocyte in membrane capping is not simply a general physical binding, but is a highly specific bonding that results in a highly specific biological response. It is analogous to the drug-receptor interaction.

Background

Lymphocytes have their origin from stem cells located in the bone marrow. The newly formed, and still inactive, cells pass (either prenatally or a few months postnatally) to two major sites of activation: the thymus gland, giving rise to T-lymphocytes; and an as yet unidentified location in mammals, giving rise to B-lymphocytes. Following activation, both types of lymphocytes are transported to the lymph nodes, where they are trapped by a reticular cell mesh. It is here that they produce antibody or sensitized lymphocyte clones highly specific for antigen. Following initial exposure to an antigen, subsequent encounter results in a series of transformations of dormant lymphocytes to lymphoblasts, plasmoblasts, immature plasma cells, and finally mature plasma cells (which release γ-globulin antibodies, i.e., Ig immunoglobulins).

Antigen binding is decreased or eliminated by exposure of B-lymphocytes to anti-Ig antibodies or by covering or removing surface Ig. It has been concluded from this type of information that antigen binding occurs at the sites of surface Ig. At the surface, a portion of Ig is imbedded in the membrane and another (larger) portion is exposed to the outside. Several types of Ig have been isolated, but the types principally involved in capping are IgM and IgD. Whichever type occurs on a given cell, however, it is highly homogeneous and highly specific for a particular antigen. It has been estimated that there are about 100,000 Ig molecules (or receptors) per B-lymphocyte. Surface Ig is diffusely distributed on the cell surface and is, for the most part, randomly arranged. Surface Ig is synthesized by the B-lymphocyte and is actively transported to the cell surface membrane. New Ig can be inserted in the membrane within a few hours.

Immediately following the formation of Ig-antigen complexes, and preceding cap formation, the complexes aggregate in diffuse clusters in a process known as "patching." Microclusters rapidly migrate in a coordinated manner toward one pole of the cell. There is little interaction between the microclusters until they are joined at the cap. The capping process takes three to four minutes at 37°C, which is too rapid to be explained by simple diffusion. Eventually, all complexes move to the cap. A thermodynamic explanation of patching has been proposed, based on the difference in free energy between "free" complex and that in a patch.[27] The surface tension involved in a patch would keep surface Ig separated until cross-linking by antigen increased the radius of the complex to a critical size.

Capping is an energy-dependent process, whereas patching is not. Patching can occur at 4°C; capping cannot occur below 20°C. Patching is independent of the respiratory chain or glycolysis; capping is totally dependent on both. Differences in susceptibility to drugs have also been noted.

Shortly after completion of cap formation, pieces of the cap are broken off and internalized in vesicles and are usually transported to the Golgi region where they fuse with lysosomes and are destroyed. This process is rapid, requires energy, and is favored by cross-linking. The capping process removes essentially all the Ig receptors from the cell surface. Following this endocytosis, new receptors are produced (except in young animals) and transported to the cell surface. This process is usually complete within 24 hours.

Capping and Coated Structures

Salisbury et al.[50] demonstrated that, for at least some ligands, the processes of membrane capping and endocytosis by a coated-vesicle pathway are united. These authors used a human B-lymphoblastoid cell line to study mobility and endocytosis of the surface-bound IgM-ligand complex. Fluorescein (used for light microscopy) or ferritin (for EM)-labeled antibody was observed to be initially uniformly dispersed on the cell surface, and then cap over the Golgi region (50% in 15 minutes, 80% to 90% in 30 minutes). The following sequence of events was established:

1. Binding of multivalent ligand diffusely over the cell surface
2. Clustering (patching) of ligand-receptor complex (not affected by calmodulin-directed trifluoperazine or actin-directed dihydrocytochalasin B)
3. Recruitment of clathrin coats to cytoplasmic surface opposite ligand-receptor clusters to form coated pits (sensitive to trifluoperazine, but not dihydrocytochalasin B)
4. Assembly
5. Internalization of coated pits to make vesicles (dihydrocytochalasin B sensitive, not affected by trifluoperazine)
6. Delivery to large vesicular compartment (partly lysosomal) in the Golgi-lysosome region.

Dihydrocytochalasin B was chosen for this study because of its actin-directed action. Contractile proteins have been seen to redistribute during capping.[8,55] In the presence of this agent, conversion of pits to vesicles is decreased. Trifluoperazine (Stelazine) was chosen because of its calmodulin-directed action. Although the role of Ca^{2+} in membrane capping is not fully understood, several pieces of information suggest that surface Ig and cytoplasm contractile elements are linked. Evidence for the role of Ca^{2+} in capping has also been presented from studies using tertiary amine anesthetics, which, along with increasing membrane volume and fluidity, also displace membrane-bound Ca^{2+} via a reversible competition for Ca^{2+} binding sites. These anesthetics inhibit cap formation (partially overcome by increasing extracellular Ca^{2+} concentration) and disperse already formed caps. Additionally, calmodulin has been detected in purified coated vesicles from pig brain.[39] In the presence of 25 μm trifluoperazine, capping proceeds normally, but endocytosis is dramatically decreased greater than 50%. Ligand-receptor clusters remain on the surface, suggesting that trifluoperazine produces a decrease in recruitment of coat material to the membrane, but does not have an effect on subsequent steps of the process of endocytosis.

The results of these investigations were that capping can be inhibited without inhibition of coated pit formation and the internalization of pits and capping are both inhibited by dihydrocytochalasin B. Therefore, both events, though independent, require actin-microfilament interaction with the ligand-receptor complex.

Receptor Recycling

Evidence has been found for the endocytosis of a transferrin receptor into K562, a human erythroid cell line.[18] The internalization of transferrin, an iron-binding serum protein, along with its specific cell surface receptor, is thought to be the major mechanism by which iron is transported into many types of cells. Also reported was endocytosis of transferrin and its receptor into rat reticulocytes.[29] In addition, their data suggest the recycling of ligand and receptor back to the cell surface. An average receptor recycle time of about 30 minutes was estimated.

There is strong evidence for the receptor-mediated endocytosis of insulin into rat hepatic cells[46] and for recycling of the receptor to the cell surface.[20]

Heuser and Reese[30] presented evidence for recycling of synaptic vesicle membrane during transmitter release. They stimulated the nerve of isolated frog sartorius muscle at 10 Hz and observed that synaptic vesicles became transiently depleted (redistribution rather than disappearance, since the total amount of membrane remained constant). The vesicles reappeared after a 15-minute rest period. These authors concluded ". . . that synaptic vesicle membrane added to the surface during exocytosis is retrieved by coated vesicles and recycled into new synaptic vesicles by way of intermediate cisternae." Whether or not acetylcholine is recycled via a coated-vesicle pathway is still open to question.[51]

For a detailed review of the evidence for recycling of receptors and other surface membrane components, see reference 57.

Speculation

If receptors are indeed internalized by a process of endocytosis triggered by binding of selective extracellular ligands and are either destroyed intracellularly or recycled to the cell surface, then the number of receptors on a cell's surface would reflect the net contribution of receptor generation and receptor degradation (Figure 5.4). It can be presumed that cellular control mechanisms maintain receptor number at some equilibrium level in the absence of ligand. In the presence of ligand, however, receptor number could be modulated:

1. No change
   a. Receptors are internalized and recycled at a rapid rate, with no net change in receptor number on the cell surface.
   b. Receptors are internalized and destroyed, but the cell generates new receptors at a rapid rate.

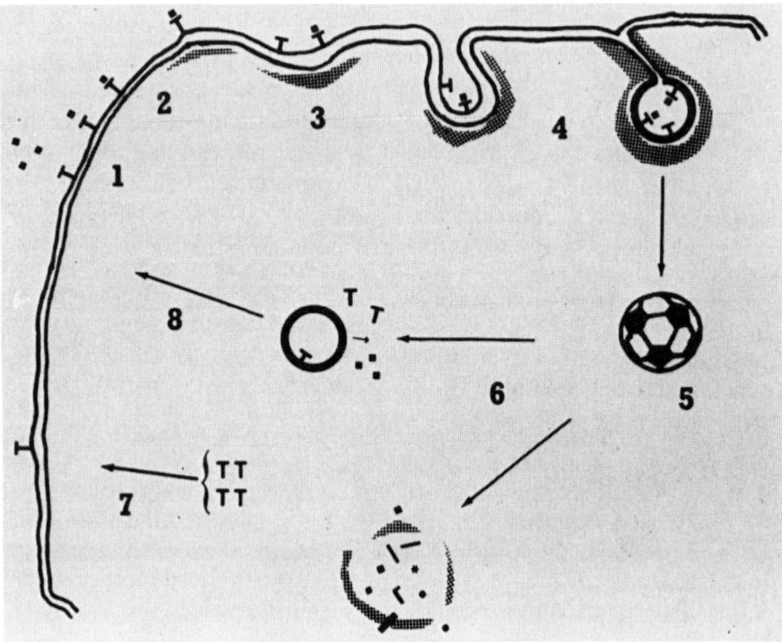

FIGURE 5.4. Hypothetical pathways involved in receptor generation, degradation, and recycling.

2. Increase
   a. Internalized receptors stimulate an enhanced generation of de novo receptor synthesis that exceeds receptor destruction or potentiates receptor recycling.
   b. The ligand-receptor complex is less susceptible to the normal degradation process.
3. Decrease
   a. Receptors are internalized and destroyed permanently (e.g., disease states).
   b. Receptor recycling or generation lags receptor internalization for a relatively short (tachyphylaxis) or long (tolerance) period of time.

It seems quite likely that the individual steps depicted in Figure 5.4 could be selectively modified by drugs, hormones, toxins, antigen-antibody interactions, and other factors.

Conclusion

It is now well established that there exists a highly selective (i.e., ligand specific) receptor-mediated process of endocytosis on many (if not all) cells. It is also established that certain ligands bind to and cap on cell membranes prior to being internalized via "coated" structures. There is also strong evidence for the recycling of cell surface membrane components including, perhaps, receptors.

A provocative hypothesis is that small drug molecules might also participate in cell surface reactions such as capping and coated vesicle formation. The implications of such a process, if true, would possibly shed light on some puzzling drug-receptor phenomena. Specifically, receptor "down regulation," receptor sensitivity, fade, and the development of tachyphylaxis and/or tolerance would be easily explained by internalization and destruction or recycling of drugs, receptors, or both.

References

1. Anderson RGW, Kaplan J: Receptor-mediated endocytosis, in: *Modern Cell Biology.* New York, Alan R Liss Inc, 1983, pp 1–52.
2. Ariëns EJ: Affinity and intrinsic activity in the theory of competitive inhibition. *Arch Int Pharmacodyn Ther* 1954; 99:32–50.
3. Ariëns EJ, Beld AJ: The receptor concept in evolution. *Biochem Pharmacol* 1977; 26:913–918.
4. Ariëns EJ: Receptors: from fiction to fact. *Trends In Pharmacological Sciences* 1979; 1:11–15.
5. Barrow GM: *Physical Chemistry.* New York, McGraw-Hill, 1966, pp 753–768.
6. Belleau B: Conformational perturbation in relation to the regulation of enzymes and receptor behavior. *Adv Drug Res* 1965; 2:89–127.
7. Biscar JP: Photon enzyme activation. *Bull Math Biol* 1976; 38:29–38.
8. Bourguignon LYW, Singer SJ: Transmembrane interactions and the mechanism of capping of surface receptors by their specific ligands. *Proc Natl Acad Sci USA* 1977; 74:5031–5035.
9. Clark AJ: The reaction between acetyl choline and muscle cells. *J Physiol (Lond)* 1926; 61:530–546.
10. Clark AJ: The antagonism of acetylcholine by atropine. *J Physiol (Lond)* 1926; 61:547–556.
11. Cope FW: A theory of enzyme kinetics based on electron conduction through the enzymatic particles, with applications to cytochrome oxidases and to free radical decay in melanin. *Arch Biochem Biophys* 1963; 103:352–365.
12. Cope FW: A review of the applications of solid state physics concepts to biological systems. *J Biol Phys* 1975; 3:1–41.
13. Cuatrecasas P: Membrane receptors. *Ann Rev Biochem* 1974; 43:169–214.
14. Dean PM: Drug-receptor recognition: electrostatic field lines at the receptor and dielectric effects. *Br J Pharmacol* 1981; 74:39–46.
15. Dean PM: Drug-receptor recognition: molecular orientation and dielectric effects. *Br J Pharmacol* 1981; 74:47–60.
16. DeMeyts P, Rousseau GG: Receptor concepts – a century of evolution. *Circ Res* 1980; (suppl I) 46:I3–I9.
17. Eggers DF Jr, Gregory NW, Halsey GD Jr, et al: *Physical Chemistry.* New York, John Wiley & Sons, 1964, pp 739–741.
18. Enns CA, Larrick JN, Suomalainen H, et al: Co-migration and internalization of transferrin and its receptor on K562 cells. *J Cell Biol* 1983; 97:579–585.

19. Fawcett DW: Surface specializations of absorbing cells. *J Histochem Cytochem* 1965; 13:75–91.
20. Fehlman M, Carpenter J-L, LeCam A, et al: Biochemical and morphological evidence that the insulin receptor is internalized with insulin in hepatocytes. *J Cell Biol* 1982; 93:82–87.
21. Ferguson J: The use of chemical potentials as indices of toxicity. *Proc Soc (Lond)* 1939; 127B:387–404.
22. Friend DS, Farquhar MG: Functions of coated vesicles during protein absorption in the rat vas deferens. *J Cell Biol* 1967; 35:357–375.
23. Furchgott RF: The use of β-haloalkylamines in the differentiation of receptors and in the determination of dissociation constants. *Adv Drug Res* 1966; 3:21–25.
24. Gaddum JH: The action of adrenaline and ergotamine on the uterus of the rabbit. *J Physiol (Lond)* 1926; 61:141–150.
25. Ganjian F, Cutie AJ, Jochsberger T: In vitro adsorption studies of cimetidine. *J Pharmaceut Sci* 1980; 69:352–353.
26. Gero A: Interactions of narcotics and their antagonists with human serum esterase—IV. drug-receptor interaction at the acceleratory site. *Arch Int Pharmacodyn Ther* 1973; 206:41–46.
27. Gershon ND: Model for capping of membrane receptors based on boundary surface effects. *Proc Natl Acad Sci USA* 1978; 75:1357–1360.
28. Goldstein JL, Anderson GW, Brown MS: Coated pits, coated vesicles, and receptor-mediated endocytosis. Nature 1979; 279:679–685. .
29. Harding C, Heuser J, Stahl P: Receptor-mediated endocytosis of transferrin and recycling of the transferrin receptor in rat reticulocytes. *J Cell Biol* 1983; 97:329–339.
30. Heuser JE, Reese TS: Evidence for recycling of synaptic vesicle membrane during transmitter release at the frog neuromuscular junction. *J Cell Biol* 1973; 57:315–344.
31. Hill AV: The mode of action of nicotine and curari determined by the form of the contraction curve and the method of temperature coefficients. *J Physiol (Lond)* 1909; 39:361–373.
32. Hill CM, Waight RD, Bardsley WG. Does any enzyme follow the Michaelis-Menten equation? *Mol Cell Biol* 1977; 15:173–178.
33. Kaneseki T, Kadota K: The "vesicle in a basket". *J Cell Biol* 1969; 42:202–220.
34. Karlin AJ: On the application of a "plausible model" of allosteric proteins to the receptor for acetylcholine. *J Theor Biol* 1967; 16:306.
35. Kelly WG, Passaniti A, Woods JW, et al: Tubulin as a molecular component of coated vesicles. *J Cell Biol* 1983; 97:1191–1199.
36. Koshland DE: *The Enzymes*, vol 1; Boyer PD, Myrback K, Lardy H (eds) New York, Academic Press, 1958, p 305.
37. Langley JN: On the physiology of the salivary secretion, pt II. *J Physiol* 1878; 1:339–369.
38. Langmuir I: The adsorption of gases on plane surfaces of glass, mica and platinum. *J Am Chem Soc* 1918; 40:1361–1403.
39. Linden CD, Roth TF, Dedman JR: The association of calmodulin with coated vesicles. *J Cell Biol* 1979; 83:289a.
40. Monod J, Wyman J, Changeux JP: On the nature of allosteric transitions: a plausible model. *J Mol Biol* 1965; 12:88–118.
41. Murphy TL, Decker G, August JT: Glycoproteins of coated pits, cell junctions, and the entire cell surface revealed by monoclonal antibodies and immuno-microscopy. *J Cell Biol* 1983; 97:533–541.

42. Pastan IH, Willingham MC: Receptor-mediated endocytosis of hormones in cultured cells. *Ann Rev Physiol* 1981; 43:239–250.
43. Pearse BMF: Coated vesicles from pig brain: purification and biochemical characterization. J Mol Biol 1975; 97:93–98.
44. Perry RH, Chilton CH, Kirkpatrick SD: *Chemical Engineer's Handbook.* New York, McGraw-Hill, 1963, p **16**–8.
45. Pickard NA, Gruemer H-D, Verrill HL, et al: Systemic membrane defect in the proximal muscular dystrophies. *N Engl J Med* 1978; 299:841–846.
46. Pilch PF, Shia MA, Benson RJJ, et al: Coated vesicles participate in the receptor-mediated endocytosis of insulin. *J Cell Biol* 1983; 93:133–138.
47. Rosenbluth J, Wissig SL: The uptake of ferritin by toad spinal ganglion cells. *J Cell Biol* 1963; 19:91A.
48. Rosenbluth J, Wissig SL: The distribution of exogenous ferritin in toad spinal ganglia and the mechanism of its uptake by neurons. *J Cell Biol* 1964; 23:307–325.
49. Roth TF, Porter KR: Yolk protein uptake in the oocyte of the mosquito aedes aegypti L. *J Cell Biol* 1964; 20:313–332.
50. Salisbury JL, Condeelis JS, Satir P: Role of coated vesicles, microfilaments, and calmodulin in receptor-mediated endocytosis by cultured B lymphoblastoid cells. *J Cell Biol* 1980; 87:132–141.
51. Salpeter MM, Harris R: Distribution and turnover rate of acetylcholine receptors throughout the junctional folds at a vertebrate neuromuscular junction. *J Cell Biol* 1983; 96:1781–1785.
52. Schild HO: pA, a new scale for the measurement of drug antagonism. *Br J Pharmacol* 1947; 2:189–206.
53. Schlessinger J, Shechter Y, Cuatrecasas P, et al; Quantitative determination of the lateral diffusion coefficients of the hormone-receptor complexes of insulin and epidermal growth factor on the plasma membrane of cultured fibroblasts. *Proc Natl Acad Sci USA* 1978; 75:5353–5357.
54. Schreiner GF, Unanue ER: Membrane and cytoplasmic changes in B lymphocytes induced by ligand-surface immunoglobulin interaction. *Adv Immunol* 1976; 24:37–165.
55. Schreiner GF, Fujiwara K, Pollard TD, et al; Redistribution of myosin accompanying capping of surface Ig. *J Exp Med* 1977; 145:1393–1398.
56. Smith JM: *Chemical Engineering Kinetics.* New York, McGraw-Hill, 1970, pp 329–335.
57. Steinman RM, Mellman IS, Muller WA, et al: Endocytosis and the recycling of plasma membrane. *J Cell Biol* 1983; 96:1–27.
58. Stephenson RP: A modification of receptor theory. *Br J Pharmacol* 1956; 11:379–393.
59. Tallarida RJ, Harakal C, Rusy BF, et al: Theoretical basis for the determination of the molecularity of drug-receptor reactions and affinity of agonists. *Curr Mod Biol* 1968; 2:249–253.
60. Thron CD. On the analysis of pharmacological experiments in terms of an allosteric receptor model. *Mol Pharmacol* 1973; 9:1–9.
61. Ungewickell E, Branton D: Triskelions: the building blocks of clathrin coats. *Trends In Biochemical Sciences* 1982; 7:358–361.
62. Zaremba S, Keen JH: Assembly polypeptides from coated vesicles mediate reassembly of unique clathrin coats. *J Cell Biol* 1983; 97:1339–1347.

6
Drugs and Receptors: Chemical Bonding

Corpora non agunt nisi fixata. (Drugs do not act unless they bind).

—Paul Erlich, 1913.

General Principles*

The interaction of drug molecules with biological material—whether with protein, lipid, cell membrane, or receptor—is highly complex and is understood in only the most rudimentary way. A fully detailed, yet practical, understanding of the nature of drug molecules, biological material, and the interaction between them does not exist. Although sophisticated theories that describe the electronic nature of molecules do exist (e.g., quantum mechanical approaches), they are difficult to apply to large drug molecules. Further, whereas the biological material can be well characterized anatomically, the interaction of this material with drug molecules is still speculative (proton tunneling, analogies to solid-state physics, etc.). Although the details of the advanced analysis of these phenomena are beyond the scope of this book, some basic ideas of long standing are still useful in visualizing the drug–tissue interaction and are summarized in this chapter.

A drug's biological activity and toxicity are determined by the number and type of chemical bonds that the drug forms with its surroundings. Drugs that bind to receptors produce (or block) the effects mediated by the receptor. Drugs that bind to critical macromolecular components can interfere with normal cell function, producing toxic effects. Most clinically useful drugs combine reversibly with receptors and produce transitory effects. In these cases the reversible binding between drugs and receptors typically involves weak intermolecular associations such as those produced by van der Waals' or London forces, dipoles, hydrophobic interaction, and hydrogen bonding.

In contrast to these easily reversed bonds, *covalent* bonding between a drug and a receptor, or some other cell component, results in a coupling that is difficult to

*For each section of this chapter the material gathered from references 1, 2, 4–6, 9, 12–14, and 16–18 has been summarized.

reverse. Such bonding is generally not a favorable property of therapeutic agents, but can be of great value experimentally in identifying receptors. Drugs that bind irreversibly (or only very slowing reversibly) with their receptors have found application in radioligand and autoradiographic studies.[3,19] For example, quinuclidinylbenzilate (QNB) has high affinity ($K = 10^{-11}$ *M*) for the muscarinic acetylcholine receptor and has been used for receptor localization and characterization. Other high-affinity ligands include alprenolol ($K = 10^{-8}$ *M*) and iodohydroxybenzylpindolol ($K = 10^{-10}$ *M*) for β-adrenoceptors, strychnine ($K = 10^{-9}$ *M*) for glycine receptors, spiroperidol ($K = 10^{-10}$ *M*) for dopamine receptors, and dihydroergocryptine ($K = 10^{-9}$ *M*) and the antagonist WB-4101 ($K = 10^{-10}$ *M*) for α-adrenoceptors.

Covalent binding of drugs to nonreceptor sites can have toxic consequences as exemplified by parathion and other thiono-sulfur (C=S and P=S) containing compounds used as insecticides.[15] Biotransformation of these compounds generates reactive intermediates and metabolites that form covalent bonds with cell macromolecules. This binding is thought to be responsible for several of the toxic actions of these compounds, including tissue necrosis.*

In all situations of drug action (therapeutic or toxic), the extent and duration of the action are governed by the number, types, and strengths of the chemical bonds that can form between the drug and the components of biological material.

The well-known skeletal muscle blockers, neostigmine and physostigmine, both carbamic esters, irreversibly inhibit acetylcholinesterase by forming a covalent bond with the enzyme. Organomercurial diuretics also form covalent bonds with receptors, probably involving one or more sulfhydryl groups, and the chemotherapeutic action of penicillin is believed to be due to its ability to form covalent bonds with a transpeptidase involved in cell-wall synthesis. Also, many anticancerous agents are believed to form covalent bonds with certain proteins or nucleic acids. These examples are actually the exception, rather than the rule, since most drug–receptor bonds are relatively weak and their effects readily reversible. Generally, the bonds formed between a drug and a receptor are the weaker kinds: ionic bonds, hydrogen bonds, hydrophobic bonds, and van der Waals' interactions. Some discussion of these seems in order, but first we consider the essential thermodynamics of bond energies.

Thermodynamics: The Free Energy

In understanding chemical bonding it is helpful to draw on the thermodynamic concept of free energy. For example, the formation of a covalent bond is often characterized by a decrease in free energy of 40 to 110 kcal/mol. In contrast, the much weaker van der Waals' interactions between drug and receptor occur with a free energy release of 0.5 to 1 kcal/mol.

*For an excellent review of the mechanisms involved in cell necrosis, see reference 10.

Under any set of conditions of temperature and pressure, a compound has a particular free energy, denoted G. A chemical reaction is, accordingly, characterized by a change, ΔG, between products and reactants. If a compound is unstable, it is high on the free-energy scale. A compound is stable when its free energy is low. If a chemical reaction proceeds spontaneously at constant temperature and pressure, and no energy is put in, then $\Delta G < 0$. If ΔG of a reaction is more than 0, then energy must be provided from another source.

The value of ΔG depends on the chemical structures and the concentrations of the compounds involved. Under standard conditions ΔG is denoted $\Delta G°$. But at other conditions of temperature and pressure the value ΔG, not $\Delta G°$, must be used. The importance of the free energy (at constant temperature and pressure) is that it is the maximum energy free to do work from the reaction.

The free-energy change should be distinguished from the other thermodynamic parameter ΔH of the reaction, which is the maximum heat released. These are related according to the equation

$$\Delta H = \Delta G + T \cdot \Delta S,$$

where ΔS is the change in entropy.

The free-energy change of a reaction is related to the equilibrium constant K_e. For the reaction

$$\mathrm{A + B \rightleftharpoons C + D}$$

$$\Delta G = \Delta G° + RT \ln \frac{\mathrm{(C)\,(D)}}{\mathrm{(A)\,(B)}}$$

At equilibrium $\Delta G = 0$; thus

$$\Delta G° = -RT \ln \frac{\mathrm{(C)\,(D)}}{\mathrm{(A)\,(B)}} = -RT \ln K_e.$$

Electronic Nature of Molecules

It is generally agreed that the principal factor governing the interaction of matter is the electronic structure of the atoms or molecules of which the matter is composed. The electronic structure, in turn, is dictated by the distribution of the electrons and protons comprising the atoms or molecules. In all cases the distribution of these subatomic particles is nonuniform. That is, the negative charges (electrons) are separated from the positive charges (protons) by a relatively large distance (on an atomic scale). Hence, even neutral atoms or molecules (i.e., those for which the number of protons equals the number of electrons) contain electric charges separated in space and can interact electrostatically with other particles.

Electrons encircle the nucleus at various distances (orbits) from the center and form a "cloud" of negative charge that partially shields the nucleus from interaction with other particles. The nucleus is not without importance in chemical interactions, however. As atoms or molecules approach, at least three sets of electrostatic interaction occur: (1) positively charged nuclei repel one another,

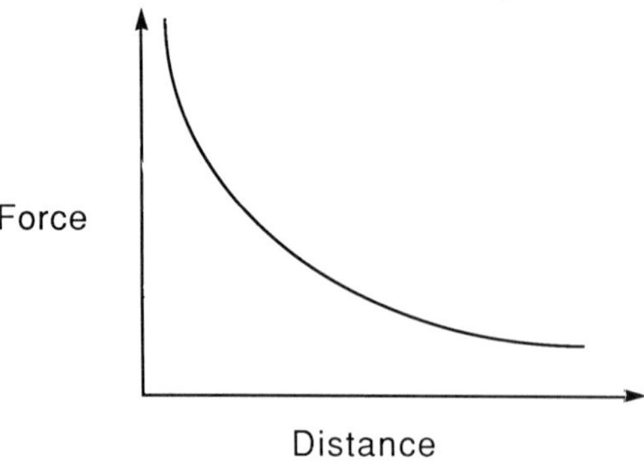

FIGURE 6.1. Graph of Coulomb's law.

(2) negatively charged electrons repel one another, and (3) oppositely charged nuclei and electrons attract one another.

If the net result of these interactions is favorable to bond formation, the distance between the nuclei of the bound atoms or molecules (i.e., the length of the chemical bond) will be the balance between these attractive and repulsive forces.

The electrostatic interaction between atoms or molecules can be analyzed in an elementary way by application of Coulomb's law. According to this law, developed by Priestly, Cavendish, and Coulomb, the force (F) of attraction or repulsion between two point charges (q and q') is directly proportional to the product of the magnitude of the charges and inversely proportional to the square of the distance (L) between them. This relationship is expressed mathematically as,

$$F = k(q)(q')/L^2, \qquad \textit{Coulomb's law}$$

where the units of distance are meters and $k = 9 \times 10^9$ when the units of charge are expressed in coulombs. The electrostatic force between two charged particles drops off rapidly as the distance between the particles is increased, as shown in Figure 6.1.

Atomic diameters are of the order 1×10^{-8} cm to 5×10^{-8} cm (i.e., 1 to 5 Å). Nuclear diameters, on the other hand, are of the order of 10^{-13} cm. If two atoms of the same element are considered point charges, each having a charge q and nuclear diameter 10^{-13} cm, and are separated by a distance of 2×10^{-8} cm, then the electrostatic force between them can be estimated by Coulomb's law. In the absence of electrons, the nuclei could approach one another until separated by a distance of about 1×10^{-13} cm. The electrostatic force (F_1) between these nuclei would then be,

$$F_1 = k(q)(q')/1 \times 10^{-13})^2.$$

On the other hand, with an electron cloud present, the nuclei could approach to within only about 2×10^{-8} cm of each other and the electrostatic force (F_2) between them would be

$$F_2 = k(q)(q')/(2 \times 10^{-8})^2.$$

The relative magnitude of the electrostatic forces in these two situations can be compared by examining the ratio F_2/F_1,

$$\frac{F_2}{F_1} = \frac{k(q)(q')/(2 \times 10^{-8})^2}{k(q)(q')/(1 \times 10^{-13})^2} = \frac{1 \times 10^{-26}}{4 \times 10^{-16}} = 5.0 \times 10^{-11}$$

Thus, with the electron cloud present, the nuclei experience only a small fraction of the electrostatic repulsion that they would experience in the absence of the electron cloud.

If we accept the model of an atom as a nucleus surrounded by electrons that behave as discrete solid particles, then chemical bond formation between atoms can be viewed as the exchange or sharing of electrons. Experimental measurements indicate that chemical bonds are most stable when electrons are shared or exchanged in such a way that each atom acquires the electron structure of the noble gas nearest to it in the periodic table. Since each noble gas, except for helium, has eight electrons in the highest principal energy level, chemical bonds are said to satisfy the "octet" rule. Bonds of this type are the strongest of the chemical bonds.

Types of Bonds

Ionic Bonds

Ionic bonds are formed between two atoms when one atom yields electrons and the other atom gains electrons in such a way that each atom of the bound pair obeys the octet rule (Figure 6.2). This transfer of electrons occurs between atoms that are initially neutral (equal number of protons and electrons). Hence, the atom that gains electrons becomes negatively charged and the atom that loses electrons becomes positively charged. The resulting charged atoms (ions) exert an electrostatic attraction for each other. It is this electrostatic attraction that comprises the ionic bond.

The strength of such a bond can be estimated using Coulomb's law for two separated point charges of opposite sign, namely,

$$\text{strength} \propto 1/L^2.$$

The strength of ionic bonds is of the order of 5 to 10 kcal/mol and is of intermediate strength in relation to other types of chemical bonds (see Table 6.1). Bond strengths of this magnitude are generally reversible under physiological conditions. Thus, ionic bond formation between drug and receptor yields a complex that is generally transient in nature.

The tendency for the atoms of drug and receptor molecules to exchange electrons and, hence, participate in ionic bond formation is characterized by a number called "electronegativity."

The more electronegative an atom, the greater is the likelihood that it will gain electrons. Examples of atoms with high electronegativity are fluorine (4.0), oxygen (3.5), chlorine (3.0), and nitrogen (3.0). Carbon has an electronegativity

TABLE 6.1. Approximate strengths of various types of bonds.

Bond	Strength (kcal/mol)
Covalent	50–150
Ionic	5–10
Ion-dipole	2–5
Dipole-dipole	2–5
Hydrogen	2–5
Hydrophobic interaction	1–2
van der Waals	0.5–1.0

of 2.5. Hydrogen has an electronegativity of 2.1. The electronegativities of other atoms commonly found in biological material have been determined. Chemical groups that attract electrons more strongly than hydrogen (i.e., electron acceptors) include:

$-NH_3+$ $-CHO$ $-Br$ $-CH{=}CH_2$

$-NO_2$ $-C{=}O$ $-OH$ $-CR{=}CR_2$

$-C{\equiv}N$ R $-OR$ $-C{\equiv}CH$

$-COOH$ $-F$ $-SH$

$-COOR$ $-Cl$ $-SR$

Chemical groups that attract electrons less strongly than hydrogen (i.e., are electron donors) include:

$-CH_3$ $-CHR_2$

$-CH_2R$ $-CR_3$

It is pointed out later in this chapter that the greater the difference in electronegativity between atoms, the greater is the likelihood that the bond between them is "ionic" in character.

Covalent Bond

Pure Covalent Bonds

In covalent bonding, two atoms unite in such a way as to satisfy the octet rule by sharing (rather than exchanging, as in ionic bonding) electrons. A covalent bond, then, consists of a pair of electrons shared between two atoms, occupying two stable orbitals, one of each atom. One, two, or even three, pairs of electrons can be shared between atoms, giving rise to single, double, and triple bonds, respectively (see Figure 6.3). The number of covalent bonds that an atom is capable of forming is often termed the "covalency" of the atom.

Covalent bonds are the strongest of all chemical bonds (in the range 50 to 150 kcal/mol). Because of the high strength of covalent bonds, formation of a covalent

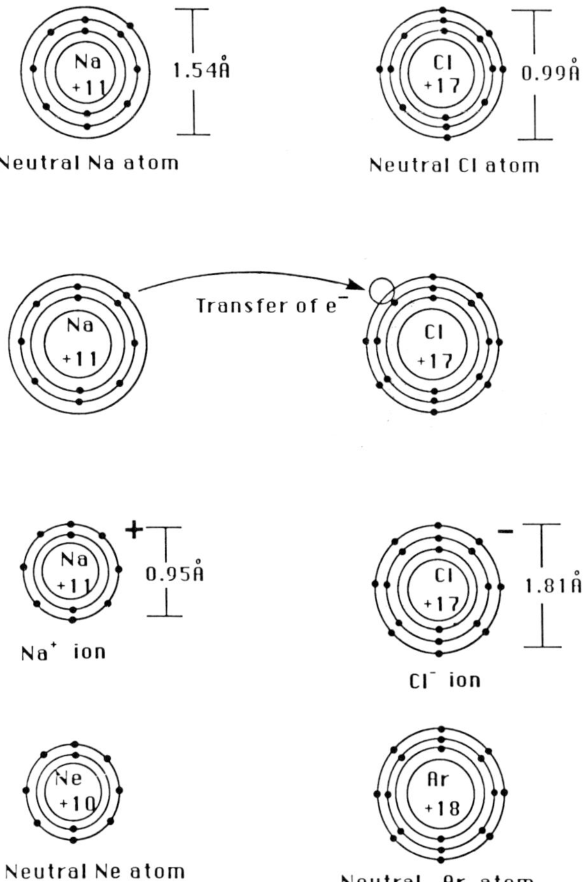

FIGURE 6.2. Formation of sodium and chlorine ions from their natural atoms during ionic bond formation. The ions obey the octet rule (eight electrons in outermost orbital) and have the same electronic configuration as the nearest noble gas (neon and argon) in the Periodic Table. Note the difference in diameter between a neutral atom and its ion.

bond between a drug and receptors may be nearly irreversible at the temperatures of physiological processes and in the absence of the catalytic action of enzymes.

Examples of drugs that are believed to form covalent bonds with receptors are phenoxybenzamine (an irreversible α-adrenoceptor antagonist) and echothiophate (an irreversible acetylcholinesterase inhibitor). Such drugs are difficult to dislodge from the receptor and tend to have long durations of action.

Percentage Ionic Character

The electrons that constitute a covalent bond need not be necessarily shared equally between the two covalently bound atoms. Because chemical elements differ with respect to both electron distribution and number of protons, the

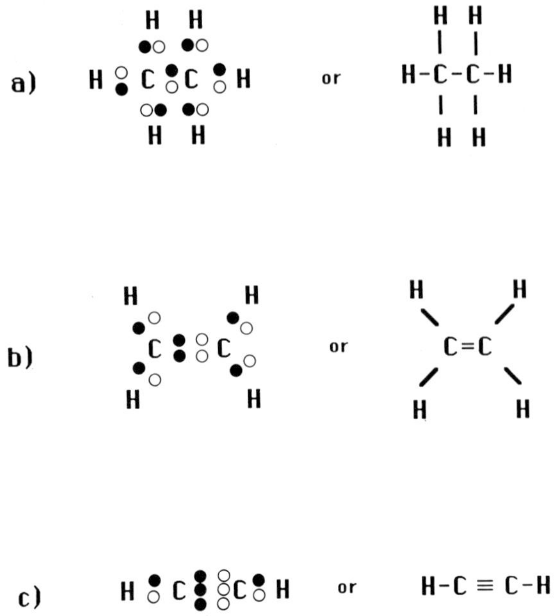

FIGURE 6.3. Covalent bonding between hydrogen and carbon (a). A covalent bond consists of a pair of shared electrons. More than one pair of electrons can be shared, leading to multiple covalent bonds as shown in (b) and (c).

electrons are not always equally shared when atoms of different elements are united in a covalent bond. One atom may attract the electrons with a slightly stronger pull. This atom will develop, as a consequence of this greater electron pull, a fractional negative charge. The other atom of the bound pair will develop a net positive charge. When this happens, the covalent bond that forms is termed "polar," that is, the center of positive charge does not coincide with the center of negative charge.

The strength with which an atom attracts electrons is related to its electronegativity. In a covalent bond, the degree to which an electron is attracted to one atom more than the other atom depends on the difference in electronegativities between the two atoms.

The pure ionic bond and the nonpolar covalent bond are actually two extremes of a spectrum of chemical bonds that can result from the distribution of a pair of electrons between two bound atoms. Chemical bonds with properties intermediate between ionic and covalent bonds are common. Hence, the transition from an ionic bond to a covalent bond does not have a sharp boundary. Most bonds are not exclusively covalent or exclusively ionic. Rather, they are said to have some "percent ionic character."

It is possible to estimate the percent ionic character of chemical bonds by comparing the electronegativities of the bound atoms. The greater the magnitude

TABLE 6.2. Electronegativity percent ionic character

A. Values of electronegativity (Linus Pauling units) for selected atoms.

Atom	H	Li	C	N	O	F	Na	Mg	P	S	Cl	K	Ca
Electronegativity	2.1	1.0	2.5	3.0	3.5	4.0	0.9	1.2	2.1	2.5	3.0	0.8	1.0

B. Conversion of the difference in electronegativity between two atoms to the % ionic character of the chemical bond formed between them.

Difference in electronegativity	Percent ionic character	Difference in electronegativity	Percent ionic character
0.1	0.5	1.7	51
0.2	1	1.8	55
0.3	2	1.9	59
0.4	4	2.0	63
0.5	6	2.1	67
0.6	9	2.2	70
0.7	12	2.3	74
0.8	15	2.4	76
0.9	19	2.5	79
1.0	22	2.6	82
1.1	26	2.7	84
1.2	30	2.8	86
1.3	34	2.9	88
1.4	39	3.0	89
1.5	43	3.1	91
1.6	47	3.2	92

of the differences in electronegativities, the greater is the percent ionic character. Thus one can, as a first approximation, determine the type of bond that will form between two atoms, based on the difference in their electronegativities. Of course, multi-atom drug molecules are a composite of bonds and bond types and might not be analyzed so simply. Values of electronegativities, along with the conversion of electronegativity differences into percent ionic character, are commonly available in various periodic tables. The figures from one such tabulation are presented in Table 6.2. As an example of the use of such information, if two atoms differ in electronegativity by only 0.1 (Linus Pauling units), they have approximately equal pull on electrons, and the bond between them would be only 0.5% ionic in character—essentially a nonpolar covalent bond. At the other extreme, a difference in electronegativity of 3.2, indicating quite unequal pull on electrons, is equivalent to a bond that is 92% ionic in character, an almost pure ionic bond.

Molecular Orbital Approach

The covalent bond has been described, to this point, based on the early view of electrons as hard spheres that encircle the nucleus in orbits of fixed energy levels at fixed distances from the nucleus. Although in some respects this concept is still appealing and useful, recent research on the nature of electrons (such as quantum mechanical analysis) has produced some new ideas. It seems more realistic (unfortunately, not always more practical) to view the electron as having properties of both particles and waves. In some ways an electron behaves as if it is a small spinning particle with some mass and a unit negative charge. In other ways, an electron behaves as if it had a wave character. The wave nature of electrons suggests that the negative charge surrounding the nucleus of an atom is smeared into a diffuse "cloud." Alternatively, the concept of electrons as solid spheres can be maintained if the electron "cloud" is considered to represent the distribution of the probabilities for finding the electron in a particular location around the nucleus. In this case, the electron location must be expressed in terms of a probability function because of the inability to know precisely both the location and the velocity of an electron (Heisenberg uncertainty principle).

According to some of the newer theories, covalent bonds form when there is overlap of the electron clouds (or probability functions) of two atoms. The overlap is the equivalent of a shared pair of electrons and thus constitutes the covalent bond. The bond length is still the balance between attractive forces (electron–nucleus) and repulsive forces (electron–electron and nucleus–nucleus). In this model electrons are viewed as distributed around the bound atoms in patterns quite different from the patterns around the individual atoms, that is, electrons travel in paths that form around the entire molecule rather than around the individual atoms. The actual distribution of the electrons around the molecule is the one that results in the most stable molecule. Such orbitals are known as molecular orbitals, and this approach to chemical bonds is known as molecular orbital theory. The strength of covalent bonds comes from the mutual sharing of electrons by several nuclei of the molecule. In an atom there is an electrostatic attraction between the electron and a single nucleus. In a molecule there is electrostatic attraction between an electron and many nuclei. Such an arrangement results in a lower energy state of the molecule compared with the separated atoms and, hence, a more stable state.

There are many variations of molecular orbital theory, and several methods of calculating molecular orbitals. For all but the simplest molecules, however, the precise solution of the relevant equations is not always possible. Approximate solutions are therefore necessary. One of these approximations is also useful for conceptualizing the covalent bond. It is the "linear combination of atomic orbitals," or LCAO method, and it asserts that a molecular orbital (U_{MO}) of bound atoms is simply the linear combination of the atomic orbitals (U_A and U_B) of the individual atoms, i.e.,

$$U_{MO} = U_A + U_B,$$

where the square of each U term is related to the electron charge density (or the probability of finding an electron at a given location) around the individual and bound atoms. The full expression for U_{MO} is then

$$U_{MO}^2 = U_A^2 + 2\,U_A\,U_B + U_B^2.$$

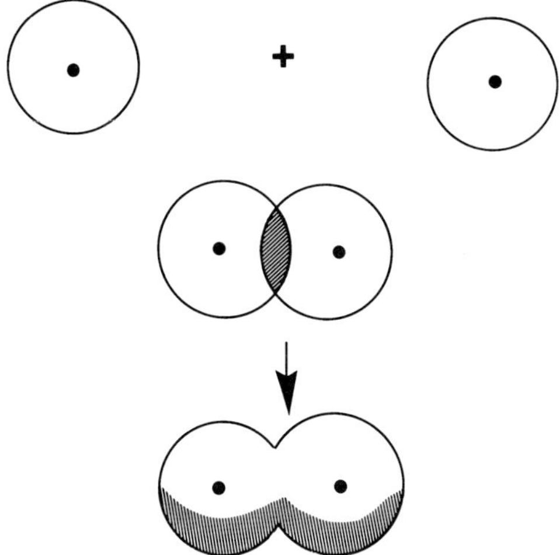

FIGURE 6.4. Overlap of atomic orbitals of two atoms. The portion of overlap (high-charge density) comprises the covalent bond. The strength of the covalent bond is related to the extent of the overlap of atomic orbitals.

The "overlap" term, 2 $U_A U_B$, represents the covalent bond (see Figure 6.4). The larger this term, the greater is the overlap of atomic orbitals (and the large density between nuclei) and the stronger (more stable) is the bond.

A covalent bond is formed when three conditions are met:

1. The two atoms must be positioned such that the electron orbitals of one atom overlap the electron orbitals of the other above.
2. Each orbital must contain one, and only one, electron.
3. The two electrons can only be "paired" if they have opposite spins (Pauli exclusion principle).

The number and type of covalent bonds that form between atoms can affect the shape of a molecule. For example, the shape of molecules such as methane (CH_4) and carbon tetrachloride (CCl_4), is known to be tetrahedral, i.e., the four atoms attached to the central carbon atom occupy each of the four corners of a regular tetrahedron. Molecular orbital theory attempts to account for the shape of molecules by postulating the existence of bond orbitals that are hybrids of atomic orbitals.

DIPOLES (POLAR MOLECULES)

Whether an electron is equally or unequally shared by the two atoms participating in a covalent bond may seem an esoteric matter, important only on a subatomic scale. However, this is not the case. If the electrons are predominantly with one atom (or the electron density is highest near one atom), the molecule will have a small negative charge localized near that atom. Since the molecule as a whole is neutral, there must be an equal and opposite charge near the atom with a weaker pull on the electrons. Thus, the overall neutral molecule has, on a submolecular level, two opposite charges separated by a set distance—in other words, the molecule is a miniature electric dipole.

Molecules that possess electric dipoles are termed "polar" molecules. Polar molecules tend to be soluble in water (hydrophilic) and other polar environments of biological tissues. "Nonpolar" molecules, on the other hand, tend to be soluble in lipid (hydrophobic) environments, such as biological membranes. For a molecule to be nonpolar, two criteria must be met. First, it must be electrically neutral; second, the center of negative charge (of the electrons) must exactly coincide with the center of positive charges (of the nuclei).

Molecular dipoles are often represented by the symbol

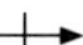

where the head of the arrow points toward the negative charge, and the length of the arrow suggests the relative magnitude of the dipole. In diatomic molecules, the direction of the dipole is toward the more electronegative of the two atoms. For example, in the case of hydrochloric acid,

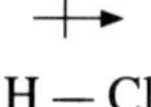

there is a greater density of electrons at the chloride end of the molecule than at the hydrogen end. In this case the center of the negative charge of the electrons does not coincide with the center of the positive charge of the protons. Therefore, the HCl molecule is polar.

The electric dipole of a bond can be quantitated in terms of two characteristics, both of which are incorporated in the "dipole moment." The dipole moment (μ) is defined as the product of charge (q) and charge separation (δ).

$$\mu = q\,\delta.$$

Note that different molecules may have the same dipole moment, that is, the dipole moment is not necessarily unique for each molecule. For example, the dipole moment resulting from twice the charge, but separated by one-half the distance, would be the same,

$$\mu = (2q)(\delta/2) = q\,\delta.$$

The existence of electric dipoles on certain molecules allows them to form chemical bonds that are somewhat similar to ionic bonds, only generally weaker. In addition, two atoms need to be close together for these bonds to exert any significant force. The strength of such a bond drops off rapidly with increasing separation between the dipoles:

$$\text{strength} \propto 1/(\text{distance})^7.$$

Dipoles can interact with positively or negatively charged ions. Dipole-ion bonds may also form. Such bonds are involved in solution processes, especially the dissolution of ionic compounds in water or other polar solvent.

Hydrogen Bonds and Water

In pharmacology the importance of molecular dipoles is apparent in the physical and chemical properties of water. The water molecule is electrically neutral, but the centers of positive and negative charge do not overlap. Thus, there is an electronic dipole associated with each water molecule,

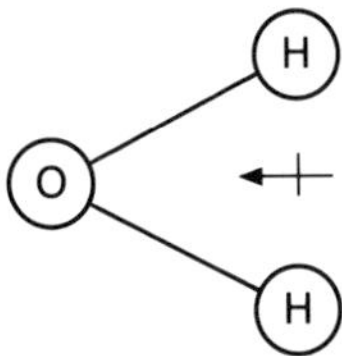

The dipole nature of the water molecule has several consequences in pharmacology: (1) water makes an excellent solvent for ionic drugs, and (2) the separation of charges on the water molecule allows for attraction between water molecules.

The positive end of one water molecule is attracted to the negative end of another water molecule. Since a small hydrogen atom forms the bridge between the two large electronegative oxygen atoms, water molecules can approach each other close enough to produce an attraction sufficiently strong (approximately 3 to 10 kcal/mol) to be considered a chemical bond. This specialized dipole–dipole bond is called a hydrogen bond and can be intra- as well as intermolecular. In pharmacology such bonds are most often associated with -OH, -NH, and -SH groups, although hydrogen bonds can form with other chemical groups as well.

In liquid water, both of the two hydrogen atoms on a water molecule may participate in hydrogen bonding with other water molecules. Thus, several hydrogen bonds can develop. Extensive hydrogen bonding between water molecules in liquid water results in an arrangement of the water molecules into a nonrandom, structured network. This network extends diffusely throughout the fluid. Hence, water molecules in the liquid state are not totally independent in their movement or in their interaction with biological materials, ions, or drugs.

The exact nature of the structure of water has not been determined. Nevertheless, the fact that water has a structured arrangement has important implications in understanding drug action. A drug molecule dissolved in water may be exposed to a microenvironment quite different from our macroscopic perception of water (as, for example, neutral and of low viscosity). This is especially true as the drug molecule approaches receptors on biological surfaces. Many biological membranes contain hydrophilic molecules such as proteins, which interact with water molecules through various attractive forces to form rather stable attachments such as hydrogen bonds.

Water molecules tend to line up near hydrophilic surfaces of biological material, with the molecules nearest the surface being most strongly bound and molecules far from the surface only loosely bound. It has been estimated that the influence of the surface extends into the bulk medium sufficiently far to maintain a relatively stable layer of closely bound water molecules approximately four layers thick. The existence of such a structured layer around a receptor located on a membrane surface would certainly influence the mechanism and rate of access of a drug molecule with the receptor. Diffusion of the drug through this layer might even be the rate-limiting step in the overall drug-receptor interaction. The thickness of the structured water layer has been estimated to be about 10 or 11 Å. This implies that water molecules located between hydrophilic surface layers less than 22 Å apart are completely structured. It is interesting, in this regard, that the typical cell membrane is only 75 to 100 Å wide, the typical synapse is only 200 to 300 Å wide, and membrane pores are thought to be on the order of 8 Å in diameter.

Hydrophobic Interaction

Another important type of interaction between water molecules and biological material is hydrophobic bonding—or, perhaps more precisely, hydrophobic attraction—that tends to aggregate nonpolar material. Common hydrophobic surfaces are lipid membranes, intracellular organelles, and portions of proteins and nucleic acids that contain aliphatic chains (e.g.,-$[CH_2]_n$-). Such interactions stabilize proteins and other macromolecules.

The attractive interaction between organic nonpolar molecules, such as hydrocarbons, in water is unusually strong. This "hydrophilic interaction" is responsible for the low solubility of hydrophobic molecules in water and has a central role in micelle formation, biological membrane structure, and in determining the conformation of proteins. It was once believed that because the interaction is so strong there is a hydrophilic "bond" associated with it, but it is now believed that the interaction involves the configurational rearrangement of water molecules as two hydrophobic species come together and is, therefore, of longer range than a typical covalent bond.

In the biophase the drug and receptor molecules are each linked to water molecules by hydrogen bonding. These bonds must be broken before any drug (D)-receptor (R) interaction can occur. The sequence of events could be

$$D\text{-}H_2O \rightarrow D + H_20$$

$$R\text{-}H_2O \rightarrow R + H_2O$$

$$D + R \rightarrow DR$$

$$DR + H_2O \rightarrow DR\text{-}H_2O.$$

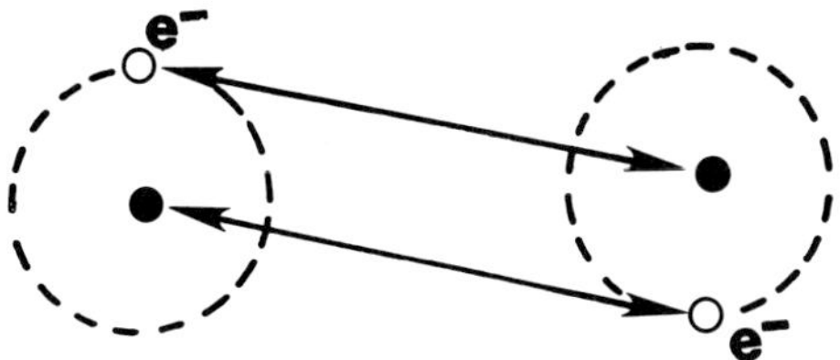

FIGURE 6.5. Development of attractive forces between two neutral atoms. Electron motion transiently imbalances charge distribution and creates a temporary electric dipole.

VAN DER WAALS' OR LONDON FORCES

It might be expected that bonds could not form between two nonpolar molecules. However, it is known that all gases can be liquefied, including the noble gases. Therefore, some kind of attractive forces must exist between these molecules.

There are several types of forces that have been postulated to explain the attraction between two nonpolar atoms. Such forces result in "bonds" of low strength (0.5 to 1.0 kcal/mol) that drop off rapidly with distance [$1/(\text{distance})^7$].

One mechanism by which such forces are postulated to develop is as follows. The electron distribution around nonpolar molecules is such that the molecule is neutral, and the centers of positive and negative charges overlap (no dipole). However, the electrons are constantly in motion. Hence at any given instant, electron motion may result in a temporary imbalance of charge distribution around the molecule. Such an imbalance is extremely short lived, but allows a nonpolar molecule to be momentarily "self-polarized." During the short periods of intermittent polarization, the molecule can induce a dipole in a neighboring molecule, and the two can exert a mutual attractive force owing to dipole–dipole interaction (Figure 6.5).

Bond Formation in the Drug–Receptor Interaction

It is difficult to determine precisely the types of bonds that occur in the interaction between drugs and receptors. Limitations in technical ability and limitations in the ability to analyze the complex array of forces involved preclude simple description. However, many aspects of the drug-receptor interaction can be inferred from what is known about the intensity and duration of drug action and from our knowledge of enzymes and substrates.

Some drugs appear to form strong, nearly irreversible bonds with their receptors. These drugs, as discussed previously, probably form covalent bonds with their receptors. The bonds are very stable at physiological conditions and will persist in the absence of enzymes capable of breaking the bonds. The covalent bonds can have some "ionic" character, depending on the difference in electronegativity between the drug and receptor molecules. Further, various hydrogen

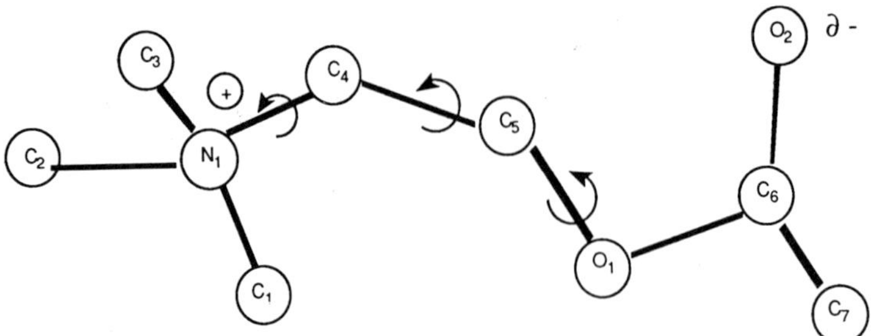

FIGURE 6.6. Stick-and-ball representation of the acetylcholine molecule emphasizing the multiple weak bonds that can form between a drug and its receptor.

and van der Waals' bonds may form between drug and receptor, and hydrophobic attraction may further add to the strength of these bonds. Thus, if the drug molecule is large and has a heterogeneous surface, a combination of all the bonds discussed above may form. The sum total of the number and strength of bonds that a drug can form with a receptor accounts for the affinity of a drug for that receptor. The geometrical disposition of bond-forming surface on the receptor accounts for the stereoselectivity of drug binding.

The majority of therapeutically useful drugs bind reversibly to their receptors. In these cases the bonds that are formed are weaker than covalent bonds and consist of some combination of ionic, hydrogen, van der Waals', or other bonds. Although a single bond of this type is generally too weak to maintain sufficient contact, the cumulative effect of several of these bonds along the drug molecule permits sufficient bonding. The drug is held in place at the receptor, even with these relatively weak bonds, because the drug and receptor possess complementary chemical groups that allow bond formation.

An example of a drug that binds to its receptor by forming multiple weak bonds is acetylcholine (Figure 6.6). This type of arrangement explains the high degree of specificity shown by receptors for drug molecules. Only drug molecules with the proper steric potential will bind with a sufficient number of complementary sites on the receptor to be effective.

Some of the implications of reversible drug-receptor interaction (transient occupancy) include the following (see Figure 6.7):

1. The drug effect is transient, i.e., drug molecules that leave the receptor are free to return to the general circulation and are subject to metabolic breakdown and elimination.
2. The drug effect is reversible, i.e., other compounds, agonists, or antagonists with affinity for the receptor, can successfully compete for receptor sites.
3. Agonists that bind weakly to receptors could still be strong agonists, particularly if the rate of drug-receptor interaction (rate theory) were the principal determinant of drug action. (See "rate theory," Chapter 8.)

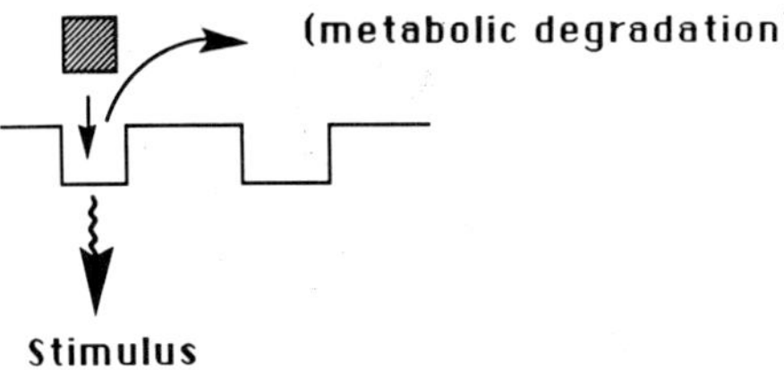

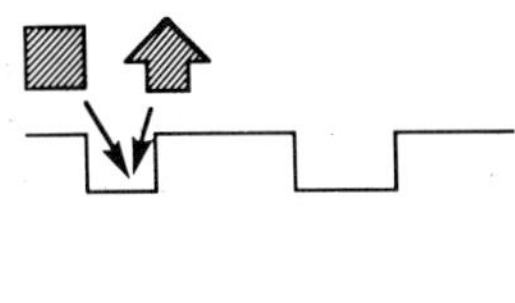

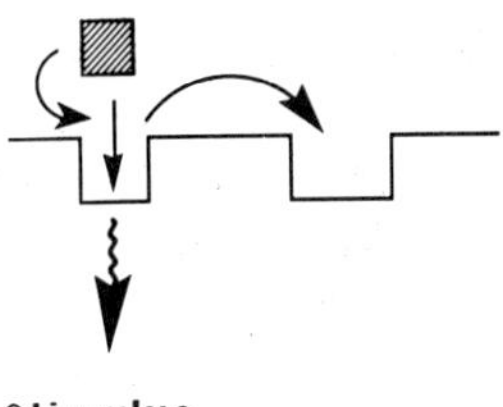

FIGURE 6.7. Some implications of the reversibility of many drug-receptor interactions: (a) transient drug effect–the drug molecule does not remain on the receptor, (b) competition–multiple ligands (agonists or antagonists) can interact with the same receptor, and (c) recombination–the potential for multiple drug-receptor interactions (e.g., rate theory).

Computerized analysis of the interaction of drugs with receptors has been undertaken in recent years. In one analysis,[7,8] the surface of the drug molecule presenting to the biological tissue on which the receptor is located is represented as a three-dimensional electrostatic field. If the electrostatic field near the receptor is known, the drug-receptor interaction can be modeled. Because electrostatic fields are vector quantities, the computerized computational procedures yield information on the direction as well as the magnitude of the forces between drugs and receptors (Figure 6.8). The direction of force is an integral part of the recognition process that occurs between a drug molecule and its receptor.

As a way of summarizing some of the chemical forces involved in the interaction of drugs with receptors presented in this chapter and by other authors (particularly Goldstein et al.[11]), Figure 6.9 is presented. This figure emphasizes the fact that the actual binding step in the drug-receptor interaction is only the final step in a sequence of events leading to drug-receptor coupling. Other factors

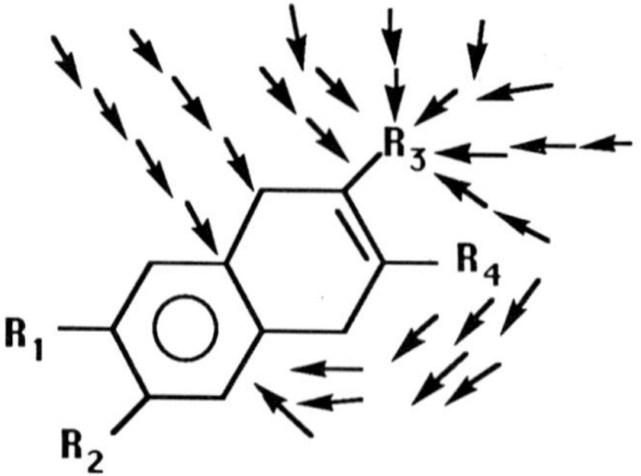

FIGURE 6.8. Hypothetical results of a computerized computational analysis of the force fields surrounding a drug molecule as it combines with its receptor. The magnitude and direction of electrostatic attraction and repulsion can be determined by this type of analysis. This figure is intended only to indicate the type of information that is attainable by this technique. For actual application of this method, see references 7 and 8.

that are important in this process include the transport of the drug to the receptor site, diffusion to the biophase, and approach to the receptor. Any one of these steps can be the rate-determining step of the drug-receptor interaction (discussed in detail in Chapter 7). Additionally, the drug molecule is assumed to have a water molecule cage surrounding it and is attached by weak bonds. Similarly, the receptor surface must be assumed to be covered by one or more layers of orderly arranged water molecules. The drug must pass through this layer, pushing the water molecules aside, to interact with the receptor.

Once near the receptor, the following sequence of events presumably takes place[11]:

1. Coulombic interaction (attraction or repulsion) occurs between drug and receptor. These forces are the first ones experienced by the approaching drug molecule because they extend the furthest from the receptor surface (strength $1/L^2$)
2. If the coulombic forces are attractive, the drug molecule approaches the receptor through the layer of ordered water molecules. Disruption of the ordered arrangement of the water molecules presumably increases the entropy sufficiently to account for drug binding in the presence of an unfavorable change in enthalpy.
3. Ionic bond(s) may begin to form between drug and receptor. A single ionic bond may not be sufficiently strong to maintain drug-receptor contact because physiological temperature (37°C) is high enough to disrupt a single ionic bond that is not reinforced by some other means.
4. The drug comes under the influence of shorter-range forces (such as van der Waals). These "accessory" or "secondary" bonds reinforce the primary ionic bonds already formed and help position the molecules for covalent bonding.

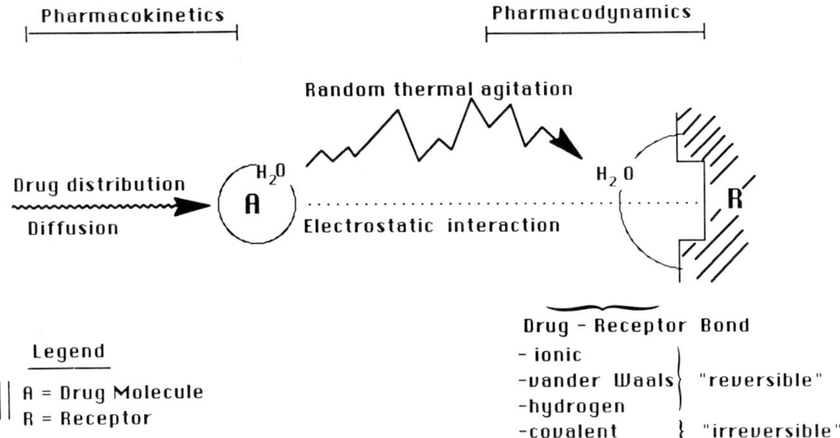

FIGURE 6.9. Total drug-receptor interaction. The drug molecule (surrounded by a water lattice) reaches the biophase at a time and concentration determined by the route of administration and other pharmacokinetic parameters. The drug molecule interacts with the receptor via a complex interplay of attractive and repulsive electrostatic forces. Formation of weak bonds can be disrupted by processes such as thermal agitation and, hence, are reversible. The formation of covalent bonds is a more stable arrangement.

5. The resultant effort of the multiple forces involved in the drug-receptor interaction position the drug at the receptor site in such a way as to allow either a good or a poor fit of the drug to the receptor. The receptor may undergo a conformational change at this point in response to drug binding.

A good fit between drug and receptor will occur if the concerted effort of bonds aligns the drug with the receptor in such a way that complementary groups of the drug and receptor are brought into close approximation. Such a fit will lead to receptor activation (intrinsic activity) and is characteristic of strong agonists. Partial fit may be characteristic of partial agonists or antagonists.

The sum effect of multiple "weak" bonds (ionic, hydrogen, dipole–dipole, van der Waals, etc.) can be sufficient to maintain contact between drug and receptor long enough for the production of the biological stimulus that through a chain of intermediate steps, produces the observed drug effect.

REFERENCES

1. Ariëns EJ: A general introduction to the field of drug design, in Ariëns EJ (ed): *Drug Design*. New York, Academic Press, 1971, pp 1–270.
2. Barlow RB: *Quantitative Aspects of Chemical Pharmacology*. Baltimore, University Park Press, 1980, pp 181–185.

3. Barnard EA: Visualization and counting of receptors at the light and electron microscope levels, in O'Brien RD (ed): *The Receptors.* New York, Plenum Press, 1979, pp 247–310.
4. Barrow GM: *Physical Chemistry.* New York, McGraw Hill, 1966, pp 263–331.
5. Brescia F, Arents, J, Meislich H, et al: *Fundamentals of Chemistry.* New York, Academic Press, 1966, pp 206–235.
6. Companion AL: *Chemical Bonding.* New York, McGraw-Hill, 1964, pp 1–113.
7. Dean PM: Drug-receptor recognition: electrostatic field lines at the receptor and dielectric effects. *Br J Pharmacol* 1981; 74:39–46.
8. Dean PM: Drug-receptor recognition: Molecular orientation and dielectric effects. *Br J Pharmacol* 1981; 74:47–60.
9. Dickerson RE, Gray HB, Haight GP Jr: *Chemical Principles.* Menlo Park, CA, Benjamin/Cummings Publishing, 1979, pp 331–352.
10. Farber J: Biology of Disease: Membrane injury and calcium homeostasis in the pathogenesis of coagulative necrosis. *Lab Invest* 1982; 47:114–123.
11. Goldstein A, Aronow L, Kalman SM: *Principles of Drug Action: The Basis of Pharmacology.* New York, John Wiley & Sons, 1974, pp 3–25.
12. Israelachniki J, Pashley R: The hydrophobic interaction is long range, decaying exponentially with distance. *Nature* 1982; 300:341–342.
13. Korolkovas A: *Essentials of Molecular Pharmacology.* New York, John Wiley & Sons, 1970, pp 1–320.
14. Morrison RT, Boyd RN: *Organic Chemistry.* Boston, Allyn & Bacon, 1966, pp 5–26.
15. Neal RA, Halpert J: Toxicology of Thiono-sulfur compounds. *Ann Rev Pharmacol Toxicol* 1982; 22:321–339.
16. Pauling L: *General Chemistry.* San Francisco, WH Greeman & Co, 1970, pp 148–204.
17. Schueler FW: *Chemobiodynamics and Drug Design.* New York, McGraw-Hill, 1960, pp 199–212.
18. Tollenaere JP: Muscarinic pharmacophore identification. *Trends Pharmacol. Sci.* 1984; 5:85–86.
19. Yamamura HI, Enna SJ, Kuhar MJ: *Neurotransmitter Receptor Binding.* New York, Raven Press, 1978, pp 113–126.

Appendix A. Physical Constants

	Symbol	Value
Avogadro's number	N	6.023×10^{23} (particles) mol^{-1}
Curie	Ci	3.70×10^{10} disintegrations s^{-1}
Dalton	–	1.661×10^{-24}g
Faraday's constant	F	96,487 coul mol^{-1}
		23,062 cal $volt^{-1}$ mol^{-1}
Gas constant	R	8.314 J mol^{-1} K^{-1}
		1.987 cal mol^{-1} K^{-1}
Planck's constant	h	6.626×10^{-34} J s
		1.584×10^{-34} cal s
Velocity of light	c	2.998×10^{10} cm s^{-1}

$\pi = 3.1416$

$e = 2.718$

$\ln(x) = \log_e(x) = 2.303 \log(x)$

$1.0 \text{ J} = 0.239 \text{ cal} = 10^7 \text{ ergs} = 1 \text{ W-s}$

Units

10^{12}	tera	(T)	10^{-3}	milli	(m)
10^{9}	giga	(G)	10^{-6}	micro	(μ)
10^{6}	mega	(M)	10^{-9}	nano	(n)
10^{3}	kilo	(K)	10^{-12}	pico	(p)
10^{2}	hecto	(h)	10^{-15}	femto	(f)
10^{-1}	deci	(d)	10^{-18}	atto	(a)
10^{-2}	centi	(c)			

Appendix B. Comparison of Atomic, Ionic, and Hydrated Radii of Some Chemical Elements

Element	Atomic radius (Å)	Crystal ionic radius (Å)	Effective hydrated radius (Å)
Barium	2.22 (Ba)	1.35 (Ba^{+2})	3.7
Calcium	1.97 (Ca)	0.99 (Ca^{+2})	4.5
Carbon	0.77 (C)	–	–
Chlorine	0.99 (Cl)	1.81 (Cl-)	–
Copper	1.28 (Cu)	0.96 (Cu)	4.5
Fluorine	0.64 (F)	1.36 (F-)	–
Hydrogen	0.37 (H)	–	–
Lithium	1.35 (Li)	0.60 (Li^{+})	4.5
Magnesium	1.30 (Mg)	0.65 (Mg^{+2})	5.9
Nitrogen	0.70 (N)	1.71 (N^{+3})	–
Oxygen	0.66 (O)	1.40 (O^{-2})	–
Phosphorus	1.10 (P)	2.12 (P^{-3})	–
Potassium	1.96 (K)	1.33 (K^{+})	2.2
Sodium	1.54 (Na)	0.95 (Na^{+})	3.4
Sulfur	1.04 (S)	1.84 (S^{-2})	–
Zinc	1.38 (Zn)	0.74 (Zn^{+2})	4.5

Note that cations are smaller than the corresponding neutral atom and that anions are larger than the corresponding atom. Hydration greatly increases the size of ions.

Appendix C. Structures of Drug Groups.

CH_3CO – acetyl
H_2N – amino
$CH_3(CH_2)_4$ – amyl
$C_6H_5CH_2$ – benzyl
$CH_3(CH_2)_3$ – butyl
H_2NCO – carbamyl
$OC =$ carbonyl
HOOC – carboxyl
$CH_3(CH_2)_{10}CH_2$ – dodecyl
R–C(–O–)C–R′ epoxy
$CH_3\ CH_2$ – ethyl
HO-hydroxyl
NH – imino (imido)
$(CH_3)_2\ CH$ – isopropyl
HS – mercapto or sulfhydryl
CH_3 – methyl
O_2N – nitro
ON – nitroso

Ether	$R-O-R$
Amine	$R-NH_2$
Aldehyde	$R-\underset{\underset{H}{\vert}}{C}=O$
Ketone	$R-\underset{\underset{R}{\vert}}{C}=O$
Carboxyl	$-\underset{\underset{O}{\Vert}}{C}-OH$
Carboxylic a.	$R-\underset{\underset{OH}{\vert}}{C}=O$
Ester	$R-\underset{\underset{O}{\Vert}}{C}-OR$
Amide	$R-\underset{\underset{O}{\Vert}}{C}-NH_2$

$CH_3(CH_2)_7$ – octyl
$CH_3(CH_2)_{14}CO$ – palmitoyl
C_6H_5O – phenoxy
C_6H_5 – phenyl
$CH_3CH_2CH_2$ – propyl
$-OCCH_2CH_2CO$ – Succinyl
–S – thio
C_2H_5O – ethoxy

7
The Rate of Drug–Receptor Interactions

Introduction

The rate of a drug–receptor reaction, like that of most chemical reactions, is generally not predictable, even if all the reactants and their concentrations are known. In almost all cases the reaction rate must be measured experimentally. This is particularly true in biological systems, where the rate of a chemical reaction can be strongly influenced by the local environment in which the reaction occurs. Adding to the difficulty of uncovering the true rate of the drug–receptor interaction is the limitation imposed by measurement techniques. Unlike most chemical reactions, the changes in concentration of two of the components of the drug–receptor interaction (i.e., the receptors and the drug–receptor complex) are generally not easily monitored. Furthermore, the rate-limiting step of the overall process may actually be the response time of the measurement equipment.

The overall rate of a drug's action is influenced by many factors, in addition to interaction with its receptor. These include diffusion barriers, steric hindrance at membrane surfaces, pH, temperature, and catalytic action by enzymes, to name a few. In certain situations, for example, in the presence of a large diffusion barrier, the role played by these factors may actually predominate in the control of the overall reaction rate. That is, the overall reaction would occur more rapidly in the absence of such influences and, therefore, the observed rate is limited by this step termed the "rate-limiting step" of the overall reaction. In drug–receptor interactions, the combination of drug with receptor may or may not be the rate-determining step of the overall reaction.

Measuring the Rate of Chemical Reactions

The rate of a chemical reaction can be quantitatively expressed in many ways. One of the most convenient is the rate at which the number of molecules of one component of the reaction changes with time. As an example, for a general chemical reaction involving reactants A and B and products C and D, related according to the formula,

$$A + B \rightarrow C + D,$$

the reaction can be expressed as the rate of change of the number of moles (1 mole = Avogadro's number of molecules = 6.023×10^{23}) of any component of the reaction. Hence, in terms of component C the change in the number of moles of C (m_C) per unit volume (V) of solution is given by

$$\text{rate} = (1/V)(dm_C/dt). \tag{7.1}$$

The rate may also be expressed, equally correctly, as the rate of change in the number of moles of any other component of the same reaction. Therefore,

$$\text{rate} = (1/V)(dm_D/dt) = (1/V)(dm_A/dt) = (1/V)(dm_B/dt).$$

Note that by this definition the rate of reaction is positive for products of the reaction (i.e., the number of product molecules increases with time) and negative for the reactants (the number of reactant molecules decreases with time).

It is often more convenient to express the reaction rate in terms of concentration rather than number of moles or molecules. Because the number of moles is equal to the product of concentration and the volume of the reaction mixture [moles = (moles/vol) × (vol)], the reaction rate shown in equation (7.1) can be rewritten in terms of the concentration [C] of component C as,

$$\text{rate} = (1/V)\,(d[\text{C}]V/dt). \tag{7.2}$$

For reactions that occur in a constant volume, such as is the case with many biological processes, equation (7.2) can be further simplified to,

$$\text{rate} = d[\text{C}]/dt.$$

Thus, reaction rates can be expressed as the time rate of change in concentration of any one of the components of the reaction.

For the more general reaction of form,

$$a\text{A} + b\text{B} \rightarrow c\text{C} + d\text{D},$$

the relative rates at which the mass of each reactant and product change with time is related to the stoichiometry of the reaction. The reaction rate for this reaction can be expressed in terms of one of the reactants or products, so that,

$$\text{rate} = -d[\text{A}]/dt = -(a/b)d[\text{B}]/dt = +\,(a/c)d[\text{C}]/dt = (a/d)d[\text{D}]/dt,$$

where, by convention, the minus sign denotes reactants (concentration decreases with time).

The Law of Mass Action

Quantitative measurements of the rates of irreversible homogeneous reactions (those occurring in a single phase) by Guldberg and Waage in 1879 led to the generalization that chemical reactions often proceed at rates that are proportional to the concentrations of the reactants raised to some power. This generalization has become known as the "mass-action law" or the "law of mass action." Although this "law" is often invoked in situations where it does not apply (discussed below), it remains a useful foundation for the study of reaction rates.

Using the same example of an irreversible chemical reaction as above, that is,

$$aA + bB \rightarrow cC + dD,$$

the law of mass action states that the reaction rate has the form,

$$\text{rate} = [A]^x [B]^y,$$

where x and y are the powers to which the concentration of reactants A and B must be raised in order to match the reaction rate observed experimentally. This reaction is said to be of *order* x with respect to reactant A and of *order* y with respect to reactant B. The overall reaction order is defined as the sum of the individual orders. In the case of the example above, the overall reaction order n is simply

$$n = x + y.$$

The numerical value of the exponents of the rate equation, x and y, must be obtained by observation of the rate of the reaction. These values cannot be deduced from the written chemical reaction.

It must be stressed that the exponents of the rate equation, x and y, need not be the same as the stoichiometric coefficients, a and b, of the overall reaction. In fact, the exponents in rate equations need not even be positive integers. They can be fractions, can be positive or negative, or can even be zero. Additionally, the rate equation may include terms of chemical species not explicitly stated in the chemical equation (such as catalysts). Consider the reaction,

$$H_2 + Br_2 \rightarrow 2\ HBr.$$

The observed rate of this reaction, expressed as the rate of formation of HBr, is given by

$$\frac{d[HBr]}{dt} = \frac{[H_2][Br_2]^{\frac{1}{2}}}{\text{Constant} + [HBr]/[Br_2]}.$$

Certainly there is no obvious relationship between order and stoichiometry for this reaction.

In situations where the order of the reaction does not correspond to the stoichiometry of the chemical equation, it is prudent to suspect that the reaction, as written, does not describe an elementary reaction. An *elementary reaction* is one in which the molecular events of a chemical reaction proceed exactly as represented by the chemical equation. For example, the reaction,

$$H_2 + O \rightarrow H_2O,$$

if truly an elementary reaction, would imply that a water molecule is formed by the collision and uniting of a hydrogen molecule with an oxygen atom. This is very unlikely, the actual process probably proceeds through a series of more fundamental steps.

The rate law for nonelementary reactions, unlike for elementary reactions, cannot often be deduced from its stoichiometry. Hence, reaction *order* is defined differently from molecularity. The *molecularity* of a reaction is defined as the number of species (e.g., atoms, ions, drug molecules) that participate in an elementary reaction to form the products. On this basis, reactions can be classified as unimolecular, bimolecular, or trimolecular. Molecularities greater than three are possible, but the probability of the simultaneous collision of more than three particles is so low that these events generally occur at negligibly slow rates.

The formation of final products during a nonelementary reaction occurs through a series of elementary reactions. The sequence of steps that leads from initial reactants to final products is termed the reaction *mechanism*. Because the individual steps usually occur at different rates, the experimentally observed (overall) reaction rate is determined principally by the rate of the slowest step in the sequence (the rate-determining or rate-limiting step).

The constant of proportionality in rate equations is termed the "rate constant." For the elementary step,

$$\mathrm{A} + \mathrm{B} \rightarrow \mathrm{C},$$

the rate equation is given by,

$$\text{rate} = k\,[\mathrm{A}][\mathrm{B}],$$

and k is the reaction rate constant. Note that the kinetic rate constant would be equal to the overall reaction rate if [A] = [B] = 1.0. The rate constant has units appropriate for the units of concentration of the reaction components (see Table 7.1).

Rates of Equilibrium Reactions

Most drug-receptor interactions are assumed to occur in an elementary, bimolecular, reversible reaction represented by the equation

$$\mathrm{A} + \mathrm{R} \underset{k_r}{\overset{k_f}{\rightleftharpoons}} \mathrm{AR},$$

where k_f is the rate constant of the forward reaction, and k_r is the rate constant of the reverse reaction.

The rate of the forward reaction (expressed as rate of formation of *AR*) is

$$d\,[\mathrm{AR}]/dt = k_f[\mathrm{A}][\mathrm{R}].$$

TABLE 7.1. Units of rate constants for reactions of various order.

Order of reaction	Units of k
1	s^{-1}
2	M^{-1} s^{-1}
3	M^{-2} s^{-1}
.	.
.	.
.	.
n	M^{1-n} s^{-1}

Similarly, the rate of the reverse reaction (expressed as the rate of disappearance of AR) is given by,

$$d\,[\mathrm{AR}]/dt = -k_r\,[\mathrm{AR}].$$

The net change in AR concentration is the difference between the rates of formation and disappearance of AR, that is,

$$d\,[\mathrm{AR}]/dt = k_f[\mathrm{A}][\mathrm{R}] - k_r[\mathrm{AR}]. \tag{7.3}$$

This equation can be solved for [AR] as a function of time.

At equilibrium, the forward and reverse rates are equal, so there is no net change in [AR]. Thus, at equilibrium,

$$d\,[\mathrm{AR}]/dt = 0 = k_f[\mathrm{A}]_e\,[\mathrm{R}]_e - k_r[\mathrm{AR}]_e.$$

(The subscript e here means equilibrium concentrations.)
Then

$$k_r/k_f = [\mathrm{A}]_\mathrm{e}\,[\mathrm{R}]_\mathrm{e}/[\mathrm{AR}]_\mathrm{e}.$$

Note that the ratio $[\mathrm{A}]_\mathrm{e}\,[\mathrm{R}]_\mathrm{e}/[\mathrm{AR}]_\mathrm{e}$ is also the dissociation constant (reciprocal of the equilibrium constant) of this reaction:

$$K_\mathrm{d} = \frac{1}{K_e} = \frac{k_r}{k_f} = \frac{[\mathrm{A}]_e\,[\mathrm{R}]_e}{[\mathrm{AR}]_e}.$$

Factors That Affect the Rate Constant

1. Rate constants can be a function of several conditions of the biological environment such as temperature and pH. Most rate constants are a function of at least temperature. In fact, rate constants usually vary exponentially with temperature. The direction of this change, that is, whether a particular reaction proceeds faster with increasing or decreasing temperature, depends on whether the reaction is endothermic ($\Delta H > 0$, i.e., requires heat input) or exothermic ($\Delta H < 0$, i.e., gives off heat).

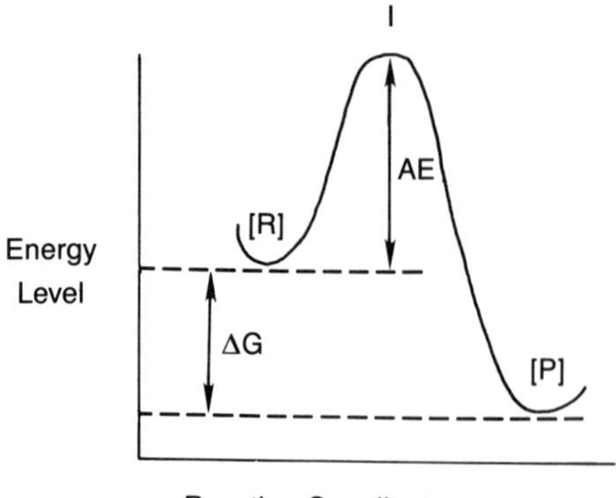

FIGURE 7.1. Schematic representation of a chemical reaction having a negative ΔG, but also having an energy barrier, AE, that reactants (R) must overcome in order to proceed to products (P). AE = activation energy; I = transient intermediate, or activated complex.

2. Particularly relevant to the drug–receptor interaction is that the rate constant may be a function of local conditions near a membrane surface (wall effects). In these situations, the rate constant can be expected to vary with both the nature and size of the membrane surface.
3. A negative ΔG (Gibbs free energy) is a necessary, but not sufficient, requirement for a chemical reaction to proceed at a reasonable rate. Many well-known reactions have negative ΔG values, but proceed at imperceptibly slow rates. One such reaction is the formation of water from hydrogen and oxygen. In the absence of a catalyst, only negligible quantities of water are produced, despite a relatively large ΔG (113 kcal/mol at 25°C).

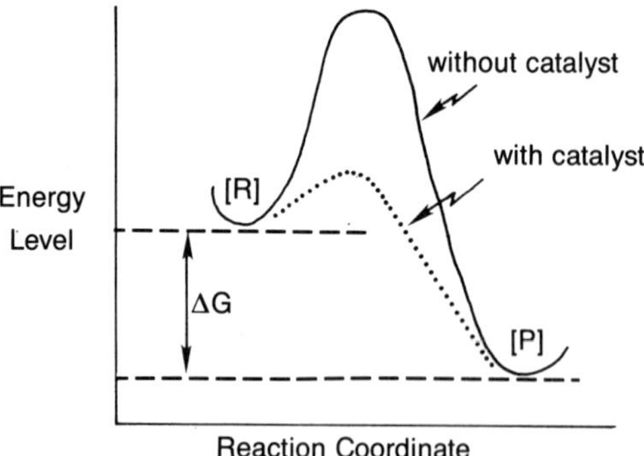

FIGURE 7.2. The effect of a catalyst on the energy barrier for the reaction $P = R$. Note that the energy barrier of the reverse reaction, as well as the forward reaction, is reduced.

The reason that some reactions proceed slowly, despite large ΔG values, is that ΔG is merely a measure of the distance that a reaction is from equilibrium and does not indicate the magnitude of the energy barriers the reactants must overcome to reach equilibrium. Large energy barriers can exist even for "spontaneous" reactions (those with negative ΔG). This concept is illustrated in Figure 7.1. In this figure the ordinate represents the energy level of the relevant molecules, either the reactants (R) or the products (P). The overall reaction is said to be "spontaneous" because the energy level of the products is less than the energy level of the reactants (i.e., negative ΔG). However, for the reaction to actually proceed, a transient energy input is required to move the reactants through the activation-complex stage (intermediate state between reactants and products) represented by I in the figure. The energy input necessary to take the reactants through the activation-complex stage is termed the "activation energy" (AE). This energy is imparted to the bonds of the reactant molecules and distorts them sufficiently to permit conversion to product molecules. In the case of reactions with negative ΔG, the activation energy (and more) is recovered when products are formed so that the net energy change is negative.

For a reaction at specific conditions (such as temperature or pH), it is the height of the activation-energy barrier that determines the rate at which the reaction occurs. Reactant molecules that do not possess the required energy cannot overcome the barrier and are not converted to product molecules, despite the fact that such a conversion is thermodynamically favorable.

To be complete, we should add that quantum-mechanical calculations predict that there is a finite probability that molecules possessing less energy than the activation energy can still traverse the barrier. The probability of this occurring is very low, particularly for particles other than a hydrogen nucleus (proton). In those situations in which this phenomenon has been postulated to occur, it is termed "quantum-mechanical tunneling." There has been some speculation that quantum-mechanical tunneling may be involved during some drug–receptor interactions.

There are several ways by which the transition from reactant to product can be accelerated. Energy can be added to the reactant molecules by, for example, increasing the temperature. By this mechanism, the average energy content of the reactant molecules is increased and consequently more molecules possess the required activation energy. For many reactions, the rate doubles for every 10°C change in temperature. Alternatively, the reaction rate can be accelerated by lowering the activation energy barrier. This is accomplished by the use of catalysts. Catalysts provide an alternative reaction mechanism, one that has a lower activation energy (Figure 7.2). The exact mechanism by which catalysts lower the activation energy is different for different catalysts, but may be as simple as providing a large surface area conducive to the reaction. The catalyst participates only in the transition state of the reaction and is thus not consumed in the reaction. In the case of a reversible reaction, the catalyst does not affect the equilibrium (dissociation) constant, only the rate at which the reaction approaches equilibrium. This is because the catalyst lowers the activation energy of the reverse reaction to the same extent as the forward reaction. Thus, in the conversion of reactants (R) to products (P) according to

$$R \underset{k_r}{\overset{k_f}{\rightleftharpoons}} P,$$

catalysts enhance the k_f to the same degree as k_r. Hence, since $K_{eq} = k_f/k_r$, the value of K_{eq} remains unchanged when k_f and k_r are altered.

Reaction Rate Equations

Most chemical reactions (and drug–receptor interactions) occur at rates that can be described by zero-, first-, or second-order kinetics.

Zero Order

In zero-order kinetics the reaction proceeds at a constant rate, that is, it is independent of concentration such that:

$$d\,[P]/dt = k \text{ for products and } -d\,[R]/dt = k \text{ for reactants.}$$

Integration of this form of differential equation yields:

$$[R] = [R]_o - kt \text{ for reactants and} \tag{7.5}$$

$$[P] = [P]_o + kt \text{ for products,} \tag{7.6}$$

where the subscript indicates initial concentration (usually $[P]_o = 0$). Graphical representation of these equations are shown in Figure 7.3.

Reactants	Products
$[R] = [R]_o - kt$	$[P] = [P]_o + kt$

First Order

In first-order kinetics the reaction proceeds at a rate that is proportional to concentration. That is:

$$-\frac{d\,[R]}{dt} = k\,[R]$$

Integration of this equation yields:

$$[R] = [R]_o e^{-kt} \tag{7.7}$$

which describes an exponential decline in reactant concentration with time.

The equation for the products of this reaction can be determined by substituting $[R] = [R]_o - [P]$ into the above equation, yielding:

$$[P] = [R]_o\,(1 - e^{-kt}). \tag{7.8}$$

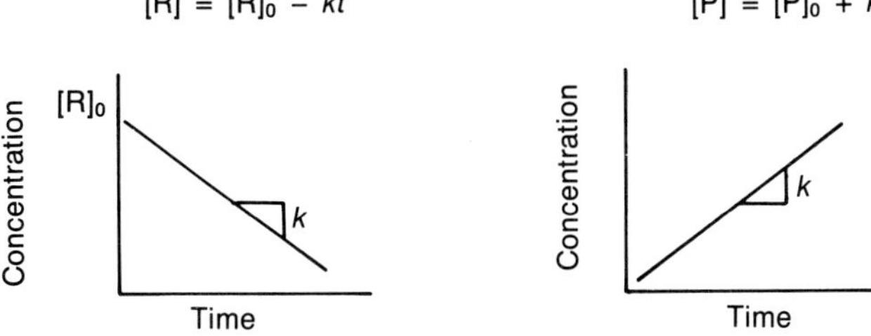

FIGURE 7.3. Kinetics of a zero-order reaction. (a) Linear decline of reactant concentration [*C*] with time. (b) Linear increase in product concentration with time.

The graphical representations of equations (7.7) and (7.8) are shown in Figure 7.4.

Second Order

In second-order kinetics the reaction proceeds at a rate described by the equation:

$$-\frac{d\,[\mathrm{R}]}{dt} = k\,[\mathrm{R}]^2 \tag{7.9}$$

or, for reactions of the type A + B → P,

$$\frac{\mathrm{d}\,[\mathrm{P}]}{dt} = k\,[\mathrm{A}][\mathrm{B}]\,. \tag{7.10}$$

In the first case [equation (7.9)], integration yields,

$$[\mathrm{R}] = \frac{[\mathrm{R}]_o}{1 + [\mathrm{R}]_o\,kt} \tag{7.11}$$

and in the second case,

$$\frac{dP}{dt} = k\,(A_o - P)\,(B_o - P)$$

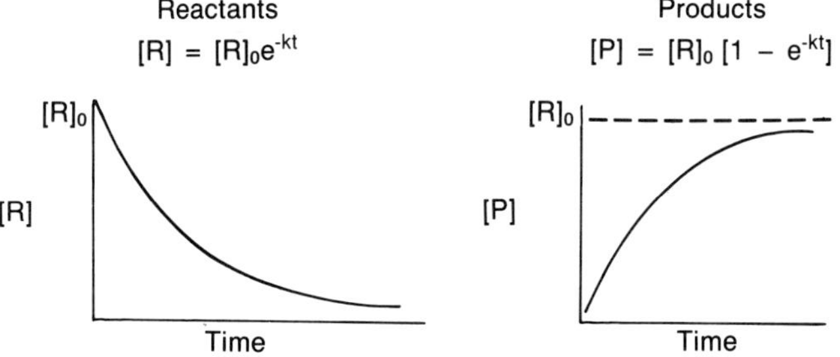

FIGURE 7.4. Kinetics of a first-order reaction.

and therefore

$$[P] = \frac{[A]_o [B]_o\{1 - \exp[-k([B]_o - [A]_o)t]\}}{[B]_o - [A]_o \exp[-k([B]_o - [A]_o)t]} \tag{7.12}$$

Pseudo-Order

Analysis of a reaction that has a complex rate equation can sometimes be made more manageable by judicious experimental manipulation. For example, if a reaction proceeds according to the equation

$$\text{rate} = k\,[A]^{\alpha}\,[B]^{\beta}\,[C]^{\gamma}, \tag{7.13}$$

the analysis could be made more simple if two of the components of the reaction were present in excess. If this were the case, the concentration of the components in excess would not vary much with time and, hence, could be incorporated into the rate constant, forming a new "lumped" rate constant (k'). Equation (7.13) would become,

$$\text{rate} = k'\,[C]^{\gamma} \tag{7.14}$$

which could be easily analyzed. It would appear, however, that the reaction was of order γ instead of the more complicated order of equation (7.13). Hence, γ is the "pseudo"-order of the reaction, because it only applies to the special case of [A] and [B] in excess.

Determination of Initial Rate

Experimental measurement of reaction rate often yields data that appear to be exponential—i.e., the initial rate is rapid and the rate then decreases to very low levels.

The true exponential nature of the data can be determined by graphing on semi-log paper. If the original data are, indeed, exponential, then the equation describing the data is of the form,

$$A = A_o e^{-kt} \tag{7.15}$$

where A_o is initial concentration and k is termed the "rate constant" (= 1/time constant) of the exponential decay. Taking logarithms of each side of equation (15), yields

$$\ln(A) = \ln(A_o) - kt \tag{7.16}$$

Plotting $\ln(A)$ against t yields a straight line (if the original data are truly exponential) with slope $-k$, x-intercept $\ln A_o/k$) and y-intercept $\ln(A_o)$.

A graph of this type is useful in determining the initial rate of reactions. If the rate is exponential, then the rate ($-dA/dt$) is given as a function of time as,

$$\frac{-dA}{dt} = kA_o e^{-kt} \tag{7.17}$$

Equation (7.17) can be used to determine the reaction rate for any given time. In the specific case of initial rate (i.e., $t \rightarrow 0$),

$$\frac{-dA}{dt} = k\,A_o.$$

where k and A_o may be found from a graph of equation (7.16).

Rate of the Drug–Receptor Interaction

The interaction of a drug (A) with its receptor (R) is often assumed to occur in a bimolecular, reversible reaction represented by the model,

$$\mathrm{A} + \mathrm{R} \underset{k_2}{\overset{k_1}{\rightleftharpoons}} \mathrm{AR} \rightarrow \text{effect.}$$

It is further assumed that this equilibrium reaction occurs as an elementary step, so that the rate of the reaction can be written,

$$d[\mathrm{AR}]/dt = k_1[\mathrm{A}][\mathrm{R}] - k_2[\mathrm{AR}].$$

Letting $x = [\mathrm{AR}]$, the concentration of drug–receptor complex, this equation becomes (see Chapter 8)

$$dx/dt = k_1\mathrm{A_o}\,(r_t - x) - k_2 x,$$

where $\mathrm{A_o}$ is initial drug concentration and r_t is total concentration of receptors. Rearrangement of this equation yields,

$$dx/dt = k_1\mathrm{A_o}\,r_t - (k_1\mathrm{A_o} + k_2)x. \tag{7.18}$$

If the chemical reaction between drug and receptor is the rate-limiting step of the overall drug–receptor interaction, then equation (7.18) accurately describes the rate of formation of the drug–receptor complex. Furthermore, equation (7.18) can be integrated to yield an equation for the concentration of drug–receptor complex as a function of time. Integrating equation (18) yields,

$$-(k_1\,\mathrm{A_o} + k_2)^{-1} \ln\,[k_1\mathrm{A_o}r_t - (k_1\mathrm{A_o} + k_2)x] = t + c \tag{7.19}$$

where c is the constant of integration. To evaluate c, we take the case of $t = 0$, where we know $x = 0$, from which

$$x = \frac{k_1\mathrm{A_o}r_t}{\mathrm{k_1A_o} + k_2}\,\{1 - \exp\,[-\,(k_1\mathrm{A_6} + k_2)t]\} \tag{7.20}$$

Equation (20) is the integrated form of equation (18) and describes the formation of drug–receptor complex as a function of time (when the drug–receptor reaction is the rate-limiting step). Note that at equilibrium this equation reduces to

$$x = \frac{A_o\, r_t}{A_o + K_A}$$

which is presented in Chapter 8 (where $K_A = k_2/k_1$).

Unfortunately, equation (7.20) cannot be uncritically assumed to describe the rate of reaction observed in pharmacologic experiments. Equation (7.20) is a true description of the overall rate of drug–receptor interaction only if formation of the drug–receptor complex occurs as an elementary reaction and is the rate-limiting step. In biological processes, this may not always be the case.

Influence of Diffusion on Reaction Rate

In situations such as drug–receptor interaction, where the drug molecule must diffuse to the receptor site on the surface or within the cell, equation (7.20) might require modification to account for diffusion of drug into the biophase. In the case of whole-body administration, the diffusion barriers may be obvious (e.g., gastrointestinal tract or blood–brain barrier). In this case, the concentration of drug at the receptor site might be simply some fraction of the administered dose. Hence, the concentration term of equation (7.20), A_0, could be replaced by some fraction of this value, say aA_0, where $0 < a < 1.0$. Then equation (7.20) would be

$$x = \frac{ak_1 A_0 r_t}{k_1 A_0 + k_2}\,[1 - e^{-(k_1 a A_0 + k_2)t}].$$

Note that analysis of the constants k_1 and k_2, using this equation, could yield significantly different values than would be obtained by using equation (20).

As drug molecules get near the membrane surface in their approach to receptor sites, diffusion barriers may be less obvious, but, nevertheless, equally important. Even if the receptor is located on the outer membrane surface of a cell, diffusion of the drug molecule to the receptor site is still necessary. This is because a concentration gradient develops from the bulk fluid (high concentration of drug molecules) to the membrane surface (low concentration of drug molecules). If it were not for this gradient, drug molecules could not move from the bulk fluid to the surface. Stirring the bulk fluid will decrease the width of the diffusion layer adjacent to the surface, but some diffusion will always be required. To illustrate the potentially significant role that diffusion may play in the overall rate of a chemical reaction, consider the simple case of an irreversible reaction of order n. The rate of the chemical reaction at the membrane surface (r_R) is given by

$$r_R = k_R\,([A]_S)^n, \tag{7.21}$$

where k_R is the reaction rate constant. The rate of diffusion (r_D) of the drug molecule toward the membrane surface is proportional to the concentration difference of drug from the bulk fluid ($[A]_B$) to the surface ($[A]_S$),

$$r_D = k_D([A]_B - [A]_S), \tag{7.22}$$

where k_D is a proportionality constant, also known as a mass transfer coefficient.

In situations such as the drug–receptor interaction, where both diffusion (to the receptor) and surface reaction (at the receptor) are involved in the overall reaction, the rate of one of these processes may predominate. Two extreme causes can be considered: case 1, the surface reaction is the rate-limiting step and case 2, the diffusion step is rate limiting.

Case 1: Surface reaction is rate limiting. The assumption that the surface reaction is rate limiting is commonly used in drug-receptor theory. Under these circumstances, k_D is much greater than k_R and, thus, drug molecules diffuse to the membrane surface faster than they are consumed in the surface reaction. As a consequence, the concentration gradient from bulk fluid to membrane surface diminishes, and the concentration of drug at the surfaces, $[A]_S$, approaches that in the bulk fluid, $[A]_B$. In this situation, r_D becomes negligible in comparison to r_R, and the overall reaction rate is approximated by equation (7.21), namely,

$$r = k_R\,([A]_S)^n$$

Case 2: Diffusion is rate limiting. Under these circumstances, k_R is much greater than k_D and, thus, drug molecules participate in the surface reaction at a rate that is faster than the rate that they can be replenished by diffusion from the bulk fluid. Consequently, the concentration of drug at the surface, $[A]_S$, decreases to near zero. In this situation, the rate of diffusion to the surface

$$r = k_D\,([A]_B - [A]_S),$$

dominates the overall reaction rate.

When Case 2 describes the observed overall rate of drug–receptor interaction, errors are incurred by using equation (7.20) to describe the concentration of drug–receptor complex as a function of time.

In conclusion, it is not possible to predict the rate of drug–receptor interactions unless the details of the elementary steps of the surface effects are known and can be quantified. Usually, the necessary information is not available, and the reaction rate must be measured experimentally. For the experimental procedure to be valid, the drug–receptor reaction must be the rate-determining step of the overall process. In particular, the measurement apparatus must be able to respond at a rate at least as fast as the drug–receptor reaction, and care must be taken to ensure that reaction rate, and not *diffusion* rate, is being measured.

Suggested Reading

Barlow RB: *Quantitative Aspects of Chemical Pharmacology.* Baltimore, University Park Press, 1980.

Campbell JA: *Why do Chemical Reactions Occur?* Englewood Cliffs NJ, Prentice-Hall, Inc, 1965.

Engel PC: *Enzyme Kinetics: The Steady State Approach.* London, Chapman and Hall, 1977.

Guldberg CM, Waage P: *J Prakt Chem*[2], 1879; 19:69.

Jordan PC: *Chemical Kinetics and Transport.* New York, Plenum Press, 1979.

Smith JM: *Chemical Engineering Kinetics.* New York, McGraw-Hill, 1970.

Wilkinson F: *Chemical Kinetics and Reaction Mechanisms.* New York, Van Nostrand Reinhold, 1980.

8
Pharmacodynamics: The Interaction of Drugs with Receptors

Pharmacologic Receptors

The distinction between affinity and intrinsic activity therefore seems of general importance.

—*E.J. Ariëns, 1954.*

The mathematical methods used in bioassays have become so complicated that few pharmacologists can keep track of them.

—*J.H. Gaddum, 1953*

Drugs with diverse biological actions yield dose–response curves that are rather similar in shape. Whether a drug's effect is on vascular smooth muscle, the central nervous system, the heart, or some other tissue, the relationship between the observed drug effect and the drug concentration is relatively uniform. The question of why the dose–response curves of diverse agonists appear similar led early theorists to seek a common mechanism by which drugs produce their effects. From this search the existence of specific receptors and the interaction between drug and receptor as a chemical reaction evolved.

The concept of a pharmacologic receptor was introduced by Langley[35] in 1878. Noting that some compounds lack biological actions of their own, but can block the actions of biologically active compounds, he reasoned that the two compounds react with the same "receptive substance" on the biological tissue. He even stated the conditions that would determine the relative influence of the active compound (agonist) and the blocking compound (antagonist). The relative degree of binding of either compound to the receptor would be a function of the amount of each compound (i.e., mass or concentration) and the relative affinity of each compound for the receptor. In later experiments, Langley[36] observed that skeletal muscle twitched in response to the application of nicotine to localized areas of the muscle surface. The receptive substance therefore must be localized to these areas. Independently, Ehrlich[15] developed similar ideas about receptor regions on biological tissue in order to explain observations that some cells are stained more deeply or differently than other cells. From these ideas theoretical schemes that would account for the selective action of drugs emerged.

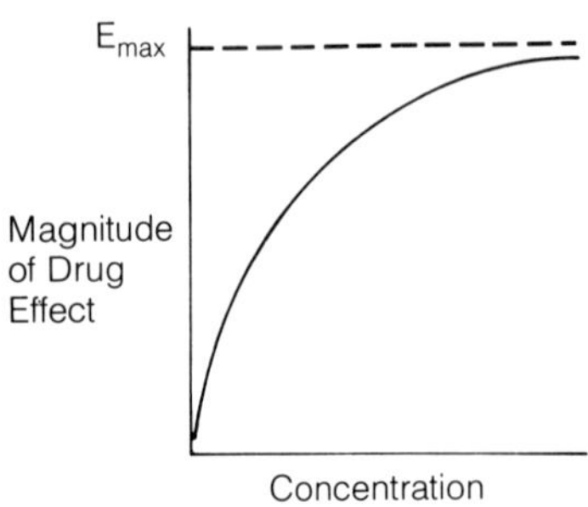

FIGURE 8.1. Drug effect plotted against concentration of drug.

The most general definition of a receptor is that *it is the component of a cell with which a drug molecule combines to produce an effect.* Although relatively little is known about the chemical or physiochemical makeup of the receptor, many indirect studies have given general acceptance to the receptor concept, and several classes and subclasses of receptors have been identified. Furthermore, valuable therapeutic agents have been successfully designed and developed based on their presumed action at postulated receptors.

It has been observed in many experimental protocols that a drug's effect is a hyperbolic function of drug concentration. That is, drug effect (E) is related to drug concentration (A) by the equation,

$$E = \frac{E_{\text{max}}\,[A]}{[A] + \mathrm{C}}, \tag{8.1}$$

where C is a constant (see Figure 8.1). When the drug effect is plotted against the logarithm of drug concentration, a common procedure in expressing dose–response curves, the sigmoidal-shaped curve of Figure 8.2 is obtained.

As mentioned, the question of why the dose–response curves of diverse agonists are qualitatively similar led to the concept of the receptor. The question remained of how dose–response curves can differentiate between one agonist and another. The answer lies in those terms in equation (8.1) that are free to vary with

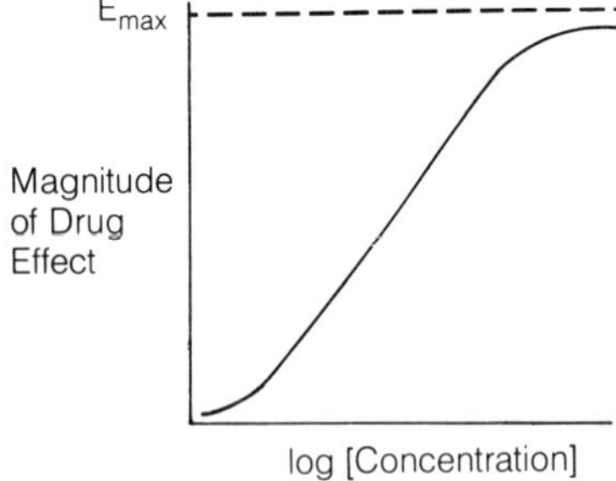

FIGURE 8.2. Drug effect plotted against logarithm of drug concentration.

different drugs. That is, although the general shape of the dose–response curve is given by equation (8.1) and is similar for all agonists, the details of the curve will be governed by the quantities E_{max} (efficacy), $[A]$ (related to potency), and C (a constant). Hence, agonists can differ in their potency, their efficacy, and in their value of C (discussed in more detail later in this chapter).

Formation of the Drug–Receptor Complex

The binding of drugs to their receptors is a stereoselective process. The analogy has often been made to the "lock and key" fit of enzyme and substrate. Indeed, the similarity of drugs and receptors to substrates and enzymes has produced a valuable interchange of ideas and mathematical models.

In the simplest case, the interaction between drug (A) and receptor (R) is viewed as occurring in a bimolecular, reversible reaction

$$\mathrm{A} + \mathrm{R} \underset{k_2}{\overset{k_1}{\rightleftharpoons}} \mathrm{AR} \rightarrow \mathrm{S} \rightarrow \rightarrow \cdots \rightarrow \mathrm{E},$$

where k_1 and k_2 are the forward and reverse rate constants, respectively, AR is the drug–receptor complex that gives rise to a biological stimulus S (Stephenson)[45] that leads, through a series of intermediate steps, to the observed effect (E).

If x denotes the number of drug receptor complexes at any time t, r_t the total number of receptors, and A the total number of drug molecules, then the rate of the forward reaction (V_f) follows from the mass action law*:

$$V_f = k_1\,(A - x)(r_t - x).$$

Similarly, the rate of the reverse reaction V_r (dissociation of complex) is proportional to the amount of complex;

$$V_r = k_2 x.$$

The net rate of complex formation per unit time (dx/dt) is given by the difference between V_f and V_r:

$$\frac{dx}{dt} = V_f - V_r = k_1(A - x)(r_t - x) - k_2 x. \qquad (8.2)$$

At equilibrium (steady state), the rates of the forward and reverse rate constants are, by definition, equal. Hence, $dx/dt = 0$, and from equation (8.2):

$$k_1(A - x_e)(r_t - x_e) = k_2 x_e. \qquad (8.3)$$

*The law of mass action, Guldberg and Waage (1864), states that for an elementary bimolecular reaction, the rate of the reaction is proportional to the concentrations of unreacted reactants.[27] For a more detailed discussion, see Chapter 7.

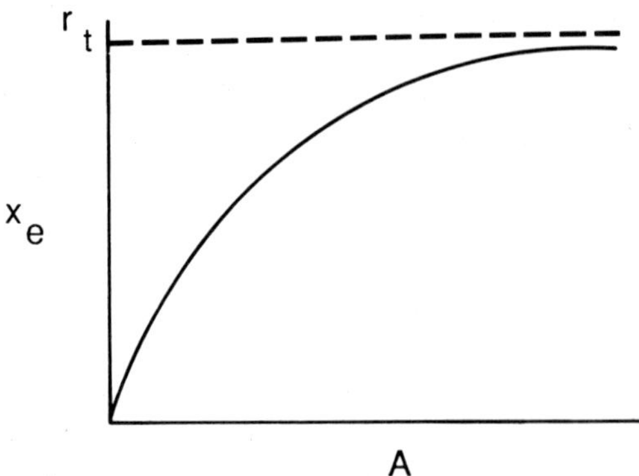

FIGURE 8.3. Hyperbolic curve of equation (8.4).

where the subscript e denotes equilibrium conditions for x. Since x is small compared with A, the amount of free drug $(A - x_e)$ is approximately the same as A. Thus equation (8.3) becomes

$$k_1 A(r_t - x_e) = k_2 x_e$$

or

$$x_e = \frac{A r_t}{A + k_2/k_1} \tag{8.4}$$

The hyperbolic shape of many dose–response curves and the similarity of these curves for different agonists to the graph of equation (8.4) is readily apparent (see Figure 8.3). It should be noted, however, that equation (8.4) relates X_e to A, whereas the hyperbolic curves [described by equation (8.1)] relate effect E to A. One *cannot* conclude, therefore, that the constant C of equation (8.1) is the ratio k_2/k_1.

Since at equilibrium, $k_1/k_2 = \frac{[AR]}{[A][R]}$, by rearrangement of equation (8.3), and this is also the definition of the equilibrium constant (K_e), the ratio k_2/k_1 is the reciprocal of the equilibrium constant, known as the dissociation constant $K = k_2/k_1$).

Prior to attaining equilibrium, the concentration of the drug–receptor complex depends on time and may be obtained by solving equation (8.2) for X. Since $A \gg X$, $A - X \doteq A$, and equation (3.2) becomes

$$\frac{dx}{dt} = k_1 A(r_t - x) - k_2 x.$$

Solving for x yields

$$x = \frac{Ar_t}{A + K}\left\{1 - \exp[-(k_1A + k_2)t]\right\},$$

which is the expression for the concentration of drug–receptor complex (x) as a function of time (t). Note that the dependent variable here is the concentration of drug–receptor complex (generally not directly measurable) and not the observed effect. This equation cannot be used to relate the rate of onset of observed drug effect in time unless specific conditions about the dose–response interaction are known, e.g., that the formation of drug–receptor complex is the rate-determining step in the overall drug–receptor interaction (see Chapter 7).

Note that x rises exponentially to a plateau value, $Ar_t/(A + K)$, which is the equilibrium value described by equation (8.4).

The rate of association, V_{assoc}, is $k_1A(r_t - x)$ or, expressing x in terms of t,

$$V_{\text{assoc}} = k_1A\left(r_t - \frac{Ar_t}{A + K}\left\{1 - \exp[-(k_1A + k_2)t]\right\}\right)$$

$$= \frac{Ar_t}{A + K}\left\{k_2 + k_1A\exp[-(k_1A + k_2)t]\right\}.$$

As seen, V_{assoc} is largest at $t = 0$ and decreases to the steady-state value $Ar_tk_2/(A + K)$. A further discussion of this result will accompany the "Rate Theory", (p).

In practice, the units of A, r_t, and x_e are those of *concentration*. Numbers of molecules may be converted to concentrations by dividing by the volume. The units of the rate constants and the dissociation constant are a function of the molecularity of the reaction. For a biomolecular reaction, the units of the forward rate constant (k_1) are those of time^{-1} × concentration^{-1} and of the reverse rate constant (k_2) are those of time^{-1}. Hence K_A ($= k_2/k_1$) has the units of concentration for a biomolecular reaction. The units of K_A for reactions with different molecularity would differ.

The graph of the theoretically derived equation (8.4), shown in Figure 8.3, closely resembles the graphs of experimentally obtained dose–response curves shown in Figure 8.1. This similarity suggests a simple relationship between the concentration of drug–receptor complex and the magnitude of drug-induced effect. As already pointed out, however, the effect may be several steps removed from the drug–receptor complex, and even if the effect is intimate, the mathematical relationship between x_e and effect is generally unknown because of an inability to measure x_e or r_t. Furthermore, administered drug dose need not be the same as the drug concentration in the vicinity of the receptor (the "biophase"). Hence, some assumptions need to be made about the interaction between drug and receptor and the functional relationship between AR complex and drug effect.

Classical Theory

One of the oldest theories of drug action that explicitly related the relationship between biological effect and the concentration of drug–receptor complex was proposed by A.J. Clark.[9] The theory as formulated by Clark was extended and refined by E.J. Ariëns[1,2] and co-workers. These early formulations are now often referred to as "classical theory." Although there have been modifications to classical theory, as we will see subsequently, the Clark-Ariëns view is a useful beginning in our discussion of theories of drug action.[24]

Recognizing the limitations inherent in postulating a priori the relationship between drug effect (measurable) and receptor occupancy (unmeasurable), Clark nevertheless realized the practical advantages of specifying this relationship as a first approximation.

Two major assumptions constitute the foundation of classical theory. First, it is assumed that the magnitude of a drug's effect (E) is directly proportional to the concentration (x) of drug–receptor complex, i.e.,

$$E = \alpha x, \tag{8.5}$$

where α designates the "intrinsic activity" of an agonist, i.e., its ability to produce a biological stimulation after binding to a receptor.

Second, as a natural extension of the first assumption, the maximal drug effect is said to occur when *all* the receptors are occupied. At full receptor occupation the concentration of drug–receptor complex is equal to the total receptor concentration r_t. Hence,

$$E_{\max} = \alpha r_t. \tag{8.6}$$

Several additional assumptions of the classical theory were borrowed from the work of Langmuir[37] on the adsorption of gas molecules to metal surfaces. Some of these assumptions were: each binding site can accommodate only one molecule, all binding sites are identical, and there is no interaction between bound molecules.

When equations (8.5) and (8.6) are combined with equation (8.4), the following relation between effect and drug concentration results:

$$E = \frac{\alpha r_t A}{A + K} = \frac{E_{\max} A}{A + K}, \tag{8.7}$$

which is identical to equation (8.1).

From equation (8.7) it follows that K is numerically equal to the concentration that produces a half maximal effect (the A_{50} value). The limitations accompanying the application of this simple theory apply as well to using A_{50} values as measures of apparent dissociation constants for agonist compounds.

In equation (8.7) E is the magnitude of the (equilibrium) effect produced by concentration A, and $E_{\max}$ is the maximum effect. The constant K is the dissociation constant of the drug–receptor complex (more properly, K is the *apparent* dissociation constant, since the true concentration at the receptor is unknown). The reciprocal of K is a measure of the *affinity* of the drug for the receptor.

With the introduction of the concept of intrinsic activity [the constant of proportionality, α, in equations (8.5), (8.6), and (8.7)], Ariëns added another parameter for quantitating drug action. The first parameter was K, the dissociation constant. With the addition of intrinsic activity, agonists could now be characterized by two constants instead of one, expanding the applicability of the theory and increasing the number of phenomena that could be mathematically modeled. In this scheme, for a drug to exert an effect on a tissue, it must not only combine with a receptor, but it must have the ability to interact in an "effective" way. Agonists, then, must possess both affinity for the receptor and intrinsic activity, whereas pure antagonists have affinity for the receptor, but do not possess intrinsic activity.

Arguments against the assumptions that lead to equation (8.7) have resulted in several modifications of classical theory. Among the major objections to this theory (recognized from its inception) is its assumption of linearity between receptor occupancy and drug effect [equation (8.5)]. This assumption is especially suspect for drug effects that are composites of multiple cellular processes.

The view often attributed to classical theorists such as Clark and Ariëns – that a simple proportionality exists between drug effect and the number of drug–receptor complexes – was implied, but probably not intended to be a general rule. There is reason to believe from Clark's own writing, for example, that he doubted its universal applicability. Clark said, "it seems fair to assume as a general principle that if a pharmacological reaction appears simpler than an analogous reaction in non-living systems, the simplicity must be apparent rather than real."[9] Ariëns[2] is more explicit in qualifying the use of the direct proportion, saying it is "the simplest although not the most probable case." Also, experimental evidence suggests that for many drugs, maximum effects can be achieved with something less than full receptor occupancy.[41,45] These findings have led to the idea of *spare receptors*, i.e., to the realization that a maximal effect may be reached without receptor saturation.

In general, advances in drug receptor theory have corresponded to sequential relaxation of the stringent assumptions of classical theory. In most cases, the stringent assumptions were not relaxed unless equally useful applications could be demonstrated. For example, allowance for a nonlinear relation between effect and drug–receptor complex was accepted more readily when a means for determining K (a major benefit of classical assumptions) was demonstrated. Several modifications of classical theory are presented later in this chapter.

Interestingly, in spite of the objections, a great deal of experimental results are still interpreted within the framework of the classic theory of Clark and Ariëns. There are probably several reasons for this. Among them is the observation that the theory holds reasonably well for *some* drug-effect combinations. Further, in radioligand studies, where the effect is measured in terms of binding rather than pharmacologic response, classical theory is more likely to apply. Another reason that the classical theory is important is that its kinetics are virtually identical with those that govern enzyme–substrate interactions. Thus, receptor theory has benefited from advances in enzyme technology and research. In any event, the formulation of the theory by Clark (and its promotion and application by Ariëns) represented the first important attempt to develop the receptor concept quantitatively and provided a background against which to interpret drug–receptor data. It also provided a basis for subsequent theorists, such as Gaddum,[22,23] who later formulated a theory of competitive drug antagonists.

Alterations in Classical Drug–Receptor Theory and Alternative Approaches

This section briefly presents several receptor theories, hypotheses, and special cases that differ in some important way from those of classical theory. Like classical theory, none of them totally accounts for all observed drug phenomena and, thus, may not have met with universal acceptance. However, since even the most widely accepted theories are not fully satisfactory, the inclusion of these alternative ideas is useful. Also, it is possible that drug–receptor interactions may not be amenable to the description of any single simple theory, requiring instead a variety of approaches.

An early modification of classical drug–receptor theory appeared in 1956 in an important paper by R.P. Stephenson[45] of the University of Edinburgh. The modification basically consisted of the following three postulates regarding drug action:

1. An agonist effect can produce a maximum effect by occupying only a fraction of the total receptor population.
2. The magnitude of the effect produced by an agonist is some unknown function of the number of receptors occupied. This function need not be assumed to be the simple direct proportion, $E = \alpha AR$, of the classical theory.
3. Each drug–receptor complex provides a biological stimulus (S) to the tissue that is directly proportional to the fraction of receptors occupied: i.e., $S = \varepsilon Y$, where Y is the fraction of receptors occupied, and ε is termed efficacy. The effect, then, is an unknown function f of the stimulus: $E = f(S)$.

Note that Stephenson retained the concept that the effect depends on the amount of drug–receptor complex, thus preserving the occupation model.

In addition to relaxing the requirement of linearity between effect and occupancy, there are several conceptual points that represent significant departures from classical theory. For example, postulate 1 above states that a maximal response can occur even with low receptor occupancy. This suggests the existence of "spare" receptors, a concept of great theoretical and practical importance. Drugs that can produce a maximal tissue response with appreciable spare receptor capacity have come to be known as strong agonists or full agonists. For these agents, fractional receptor occupancy, Y in the relation $S = \varepsilon Y$, is small and

ε, the efficacy, is very large. The opposite is true of weak agonists. Notice that the concept of efficacy is similar to the concept of intrinsic activity of Ariëns. Indeed, it is not unusual to see the terms "efficacy" and "intrinsic activity" used synonymously in the literature. There is an important distinction, however, that should not be lost. Intrinsic activity relates drug effect to receptor occupancy, whereas efficacy relates drug-induced stimulus to receptor occupancy. Thus, drugs of different efficacy produce different stimuli, but the relation between stimulus and effect is a property of the tissue and not the drug. In other words, stimulus is a drug-independent property.

Partial agonists are drugs of low efficacy that produce a response that is less than the maximum even when they are occupying all, or nearly all, of the receptors. In such cases, the spare receptor capacity is low or zero.

Partial agonists compete for, and occupy, the same receptors as full agonists. Hence, they diminish the effect of a full agonist when both are present simultaneously. Partial agonists are, therefore, agents that possess properties intermediate between full agonists and pure antagonists.

From Stephenson's postulates 2 and 3 we have, $E = f(S)$ and $S = \varepsilon Y$, where Y is determined from the mass action law [equation (8.4)],

$$Y = \frac{X_e}{r_t} = \frac{A}{A + K}.$$

Thus, in contrast to classical theory, the function relating E to A divides the total process of drug-induced effect into two portions. There is a linear, drug-dependent portion describing the stimulus produced by drug interaction with receptors and represented by $S = \varepsilon Y$ and there is another portion, drug-independent and probably nonlinear, that describes the events distal to the receptor. This latter portion is represented by $E = f(S)$. A theory such as this has numerous advantages. It allows for the separate description of events that involve only the drug and the receptor (characterized by the dissociation constant) and those events that are a property of the system and independent of the drug (characterized by the stimulus–effect relation). Thus, quantitative characterization can be made of compounds that act on the same type of receptor in different tissues. The dissociation constant is a useful parameter for answering certain questions such as:

1. When two or more compounds produce similar effects, are these compounds acting on the same receptor?
2. When a single compound produces more than one effect, are the separate effects mediated by the same or by separate receptors?

Likewise, compounds with overtly similar pharmacological actions can be distinguished on the basis of their ability to produce stimuli. The efficacy of an agonist is a measure of the intrinsic power of the compound to produce the effect.

A drug effect represents a change in the state of the biological system. The effect can be far removed from the site of the drug–receptor interaction and grossly observable, such as a change in respiration after a barbiturate or opiate drug is administered, or a more intimate event, such as muscle membrane depolarization following the administration of a muscle relaxant. Because of the variety of effects that can result from drug administration and the number of intermediate events that separate the observed effect from the original stimulus, it is generally not possible to formulate a theory of drug action that relates the magnitude of the effect to the concentration of the drug–receptor complex for all drugs. Hence, the magnitude of a drug effect can only be expressed as some (unknown) function of the drug–receptor complex: i.e., $E = f(DR)$. A consequence of this restriction is that one cannot assume that the dissociation constant K is numerically equal to the A_{50} value obtained directly from the dose-response curve (as in classical theory). It is particularly relevant to point out this inequality since in many binding studies employing radiolabeled ligands, the K values obtained have been compared with the A_{50} or D_{50} values from pharmacologic experiments, presumably to validate the contention that binding sites are truly the receptors that mediate drug action. A comparison of that kind does not, unfortunately, constitute such proof.[18] Further aspects of Stephenson's theory and methods for determining K that do not use the assumptions of classical theory will be described subsequently.

For partial agonists it is necessary to distinguish between the E_{max} produced by a drug and the inherent E_{max} of the tissue. The term A_{50} will be used here to denote the concentration of drug A that produces a response equal to one half the tissue maximum.

The relation $E = f(S)$ between effect and stimulus is a property of the system, regardless of the source of the stimulus. The only necessary condition of the function f is that $E = 0$ when $S = 0$. The unit for the stimulus was taken (arbitrarily) by Stephenson to be that corresponding to A_{50}; that is, $S = 1$ at $A = A_{50}$ and $E = E_{max}/2$ when $S = 1$. Since $S = \varepsilon Y$, it follows that for drug A with efficacy ε_A and dissociation constant K_A that

$$S = \frac{\varepsilon_A A}{A + K_A}. \tag{8.8}$$

From the definition of the unit for stimulus, equation (8.8) gives $1 = \varepsilon_A A_{50}/(A_{50} + K_A)$. Thus,

$$\varepsilon_A = \frac{A_{50} + K_A}{A_{50}} = 1 + \frac{K_A}{A_{50}}. \tag{8.9}$$

The value of A_{50} can be determined directly from the dose–response curve of each agonist. K_A can be calculated using methods to be described in the following sections of this chapter. Thus, knowing these values, the efficacy ε_A can be determined from equation (8.9). Knowing ε_A and K_A, the stimulus versus concentration curve can be constructed using equation (8.8). In the case of a strong agonist (for which $A_{50} \ll K_A$), equation (8.9) yields

$$\varepsilon_A \doteqdot \frac{K_A}{A_{50}} . \tag{8.10}$$

Stephenson did not specify the molecular mechanism by which an agonist produces its stimulus. Part of the value of his theory is that knowledge of this mechanism is not required. Subsequent workers have speculated on what this mechanism might be, including the interesting idea that the drug molecule induces a conformational change in the receptor. If the receptor is an enzyme, the drug-induced change could transform a latent catalytic form of the enzyme to an active form, which, in turn, catalyzes some reaction that leads to the observed effect. Antagonist binding, on the other hand, would convert the enzyme to the less active form.

Allosteric Theory

It will be recalled that a plot of the fractional receptor occupancy, y, versus drug concentration, A, using a linear scale of concentration, yields a hyperbolic curve, $y = A/(A + K)$, where K is the dissociation constant. This relation follows from the mass action law, so that it is no surprise that this kind of relation applies to many biological reactions in addition to those between drugs and receptors. A common physiological example is the binding of oxygen to myoglobin, the oxygen-carrying protein of "red" muscle.

In certain situations, deviation from this simple rule is observed. For example, the binding of oxygen to hemoglobin in blood results in a relation whose graph is sigmoidal or S-shaped when plotted with linear scales. The interpretation of such data is that the binding of each oxygen to each of the four hemes is not independent of each other. The binding of one oxygen to heme is affected by the state of the other three hemes, such that the first oxygen binds relatively slowly, the second and third more rapidly, and the fourth binds very rapidly. This phenomenon is called *cooperativity* and nicely accounts for the S-shaped curve relating oxygen binding to hemoglobin. The example given is one of positive cooperativity, but examples of negative cooperativity are also known. When applied to reactions between enzymes and substrates, the term cooperativity means that the interaction of one substrate molecule to the enzyme affects the next substrate–enzyme interaction. Enhancement of subsequent interaction may result from induced configuration changes in the enzyme, a so-called allosteric effect.[39,40]

Allosteric theory was extended to drug–receptor interactions by the work of Changeux and co-workers,[8] of Karlin,[32] and of others. In certain of their preparations, such as the electroplax cells of the eel, these investigators found that a sigmoidal curve best represented the relationship and drug concentration. Such findings suggest a cooperativity similar to that exhibited by oxygen binding to a hemoglobin molecule. Katz and Thesleff[33] and Jenkinson[31] found sigmoidal dose–response curves relating membrane conductance changes of the frog motor endplate to acetylcholine concentration. Findings such as these have lent support for the allosteric theory in drug–receptor interactions.

A feature of allosteric theory is that receptors exist in two conformational states that, in Karlin's terminology, are called R and T. In the drug-free biological system the active form R and the inactive state T are in equilibrium,

$$\mathrm{T} \rightleftharpoons \mathrm{R}$$

and the equilibrium ratio of the two forms is given by L (known as the allosteric constant), where L = T/R. The R and T forms can interchange, such as

$$\mathrm{A} + \mathrm{R} \overset{K_{\mathrm{AR}}}{\rightleftharpoons} \mathrm{AR}$$

$$\mathrm{A} + \mathrm{T} \overset{K_{\mathrm{AT}}}{\rightleftharpoons} \mathrm{AT}$$

where K_{AR} and K_{AT} are the dissociation constants of the active and inactive forms, respectively. Drugs are agonists or antagonists, depending on their selective affinity for the R or T conformation.

Such a model of drug action is attractive because it provides a detailed view of molecular events at the receptor site.

Rate Theory

Probably the best-known alternative to classical receptor theory is the "rate" theory advanced in 1961 by Professor W.D.M. Paton of Oxford. According to the rate theory, the magnitude of a drug effect is proportional to the rate of association of drug and receptor.[42] The reaction

$$\mathrm{D} + \mathrm{R} \underset{k_2}{\overset{k_1}{\rightleftharpoons}} \mathrm{DR}$$

is characterized by specific rate constants k_1 for the forward reaction and k_2 for the reverse reaction. The affinity of a drug thus depends on the relative magnitude of k_1, the association rate constant; and k_2, the dissociation rate constant. The ratio k_2/k_1 is equal to K_{A}, the dissociation constant of the drug-receptor interaction. In contrast to classical theory, where k_1 and k_2 only influence the time course of agonist action, these values also influence the magnitude of drug action in the rate theory. According to rate theory, the measured effect (E) is directly proportional to the rate of association (V_{assoc}), such that,

$$E = \varphi\, V_{\mathrm{assoc}},$$

where φ is a proportionality constant. The rate of association for the drug in concentration A is $k_1\, A(r_t - x)$, where r_t is total receptor number and x is the receptor occupancy as discussed before. At equilibrium, the association rate, $k_1 A\ (r_t - x)$, equals the dissociation rate, $k_2 x$. Since $x = r_t\, A(A + k_2/k_1)$, the rate of association is (at equilibrium)

$$V_{\text{assoc}} = \frac{k_2 r_t A}{A + k_2/k_1}.$$

Thus, in rate theory, the equilibrium effect is

$$E_{\text{e}} = \frac{\varphi k_2 r_t A}{A + k_2/k_1}. \tag{8.11}$$

Note that equation (8.11) is formally similar to equation (8.7) of classical occupation theory. This similarity has made it difficult to design the critical experiment that would validate one of the two theories.

An attractive feature of rate theory is its simplicity. For example, differences in efficacies of drugs are simply related to the differences in their values of k_1 and k_2. Hence, there is no need for a third drug-dependent constant such as in equation (8.7). In the latter equation, from classical theory, different drugs have different values of α (intrinsic activity). In equation (8.11), rate theory, different drugs have different values of the rate constant k_2, but the value of φ is the same for all drugs acting on the same receptor.

Rate theory also permits a simple explanation for the differences between agonists and antagonists. Strong agonists are those compounds for which k_2 is large, meaning that the drug readily leaves the receptor, making further association possible. The faster this process occurs, the greater the drug effect. Partial agonists are drugs with moderate values of k_2 and antagonists are compounds with low values of k_2. According to rate theory, therefore, an antagonist is a compound that leaves the receptor slowly. This theory also accounts for the persistence of effect of an antagonist on a tissue. Further, it accounts nicely for the phenomenon of "fade," i.e., decline in tissue response from maximum, even in the presence of a constant drug concentration.

For conditions short of equilibrium, the rate of association is given by

$$V_{\text{assoc}} - \frac{A r_t}{A + K}\left\{k_2 + k_1 A \exp[-(k_1 A + k_2)t]\right\}.$$

Examination of this equation shows that the rate of association is largest at time $t = 0$ and decreases to its equilibrium value at a rate dependent on the exponent of e.

Another feature of rate theory is the ability to determine separate values of k_2 and k_1 (rather than just their ratio, K) for competitive antagonists from measurements of their reaction rates. It should be noted that k_2/k_1 ($= K$, the dissociation constant) in rate theory is numerically equal to the A_{50} concentration just as it is in classical theory.

Rate theory quite successfully accounts for several actions of agonists and antagonists on the isolated guinea-pig ileum and other preparations. Yet in other systems the support for the theory is less solid. In addition, several of the experimental results that are successfully explained by rate theory are equally well explained in other mechanisms. The details of the evidence for and against rate theory are summarized in the review by Waud.[57]

Flux-Carrier Model

Some drugs that act at the neuromuscular junction and on ganglia first produce a membrane depolarization, but then continue to act in the presence of membrane repolarization. This type of dual drug action is not easily explained by classical receptor theory. MacKay[38] attempted to interpret dual drug actions by advancing a hypothesis based on three postulates:

1. Influx of a drug across a cell membrane causes depolarization
2. This flux may be facilitated by carriers or by fixed sites in the membrane
3. Membrane surface reactions are not the rate-controlling step of a drug's action.

Two possibilities can be envisioned. In the first, the agonist is transported across the membrane by the carrier and, in the process, depolarizes the membrane. In the second, the drug cannot penetrate the membrane and, thus, cannot depolarize it; however, it can combine with the carrier and compete with agonist molecules for carrier sites. If the drug–carrier reaction is written as,

$$\mathrm{A} + \mathrm{C} \underset{k_2}{\overset{k_1}{\rightleftharpoons}} \mathrm{AC}$$

and the net influx (J) of drug is given by

$$J = DC(A_o - A_L)/L,$$

where D is the diffusion coefficient for agonist with concentration gradient $A_0 - A_L$ across the width of the membrane (L), then

$$J = J_{\max}\left[\frac{A_o}{K + A_o} - \frac{A_L}{K + A_L}\right]. \tag{8.12}$$

The similarity of equation (8.12) to equation (8.7) of classical theory prompted the suggestion that the diffusion coefficient of a drug through a membrane might be the physical meaning of Ariëns "intrinsic activity." Such a model might also explain tachyphylaxis as follows. Washing a drug from an isolated tissue preparation would preferentially remove extracellular drug, leaving a pool of intracellular drug undisturbed. Subsequent dose of drug would produce less of an effect than the first dose, because accumulated intracellular would reduce the transmembrane concentration gradient of drug. Tissue responsiveness would return to normal levels only when intracellular drug concentration could be reduced to low levels.

Antagonistic Agonism

Szabadi[47] proposed a mechanism by which a single agonist could activate mutually antagonistic receptor populations, producing opposing stimuli, S(+) and S(−), according to the scheme

$$A + R(+) \rightleftharpoons AR(+) \rightarrow S(+)$$

$$A + R(-) \rightleftharpoons AR(-) \rightarrow S(-)$$

Such a model describes a situation analogous to physiological antagonism. It is interesting that the relationship between S and drug concentration in this model incorporates parts of both Ariëns' and Stephenson's theories. The stimulus is assumed proportional to the fraction of receptors occupied (as in Stephenson's theory), but the proportionality constant is the intrinsic activity of Ariëns:

$$S = \frac{\alpha A}{A + K_A}$$

Dose–response curves of almost any shape can be explained using this model. It offers more freedom, in this respect, than does classical theory. Further, shifts in dose–response curves by antagonists simply reflect the preference of the antagonist for the "dominant," R(+), or "masked," R(−), receptor populations.

Statistical Models

Several analyses, such as that of Homer,[29] treat the drug–receptor interaction as a stochastic problem. For the case of r drug molecules competing for a single receptor site, the probability of the receptor being empty, $P(0)$, or occupied by a drug molecule, $P(i)$, is given by

$$\sum_{i=0}^{r} P(i) = 1.0,$$

and receptor occupancy is related to drug concentration, A, by

$$P(i) = \frac{b(i)A}{1 + b(i)A},$$

where $b(i)$ is a constant. This equation is of a form not too different from occupation theory, especially if $b(i)$ is equated to K. An interesting aspect of this type of analysis is the ability to handle nonhomogeneous receptor populations. Although this added level of sophistication yields a somewhat complicated mathematical expression, the theory at least allows for such an analysis if desired.

Solid-State Model

An analogy is often made between the drug-receptor interaction and enzyme-substrate reactions. Classical receptor theory benefited from such an analogy and from mathematical models of enzyme kinetics developed by Michaelis and Menten and others. The traditional models of enzyme-substrate reactions, however, described the situation of reactants at low concentrations dissolved in, and free to move in, a liquid of low viscosity. Such an approach may not be appropriate for reactions between drugs and receptors for several reasons. First, several reasons. First, actions involving membrane-bound receptors are perhaps more accurately viewed as occurring at liquid–solid interfaces rather than in dilute solutions. Second, a survey of the biochemical literature for the period 1965 to 1976 revealed more than 900 papers (a high percentage of the total) reporting enzyme-reaction data that did not fit Michaelis-Menten kinetics.[28]

Cope[10–13] found that a single mathematical expression can be used to describe reactions at liquid-solid interfaces (e.g., electrodes), photobiological interactions (e.g., certain actions of eye melanin, photosynthetic particles, etc), certain chemoreceptors (e.g., blowfly sucrose receptor), and experimental data in solid-state physics. The forward reaction rate, v_f, is assumed to be proportional to intensity, I,

$$v_f = k_1 I,$$

for example, light, sound, or pressure. In drug receptor terms, I might be the concentration of drug–receptor complex (classical theory) or biological stimulus (Stephenson's theory). The reverse reaction rate, v_f, is assumed to be described by the Elovich equation (borrowed from solid-state physics),

$$v_r = \frac{k_2 E}{(C - E)},$$

where E is observed effect, and k and c are constants. At steady state, $v_f = v_r$, hence,

$$E = \frac{CI}{K + I},$$

where $K = k_2/k_1$. This equation closely resembles those of Ariëns (if $C = \alpha$ and $S = A$) and Stephenson (if $C = \varepsilon E$). Thus, while it has not yet specifically been done, the application of this approach to drug receptor theory could be promising, especially in light of recent speculations that the drug–receptor interaction involves the transfer or the induced-movement of electrons and/or protons across or through the membrane.

Dissociation Constants

For the reaction

$$\mathrm{A} + \mathrm{R} \underset{k_2}{\overset{k_1}{\rightleftharpoons}} \mathrm{AR}$$

The dissociation constant is defined as the ratio of reactant and product concentrations at equilibrium

$$K = \frac{[\mathrm{A}][\mathrm{R}]}{[\mathrm{AR}]},$$

which is also the ratio of the reverse to forward rate constants of this reaction (k_2/k_1). Note that the dissociation constant is simply the reciprocal of the equilibrium constant commonly used in chemical and enzyme kinetics applications.

The pharmacologic dissociation constant, like an equilibrium constant, uniquely characterizes the interaction between reactants. In chemical applications, the nature and concentration of reactants are usually known. This is not always the case in pharmacologic applications. The drug–receptor interaction can be quantitated through the use of dissociation constants despite the fact that the receptor has not been measured, isolated, or even identified.

It is now generally accepted that there are pharmacologic methods presently existing that enable one to measure the dissociation constant of the reaction between drug and receptor. The measurement is limited somewhat by the inability, in many cases, to measure precisely the concentration of drug at the receptor site (biophase), so, for this reason, the determination of dissociation constants yields an approximate value referred to as an "apparent *K*." Even so, such determination provides a quantitative means of classifying receptors. For example, if an agonist produces two effects, E_1 and E_2, each believed to be mediated by the same receptor, then the same competitive blockers would be expected to antagonize both effect. Such a finding would at least identify the receptors as qualitatively the same. If the values of *K* for the antagonist, as determined from each effect, could be shown to be equal, then the receptors could logically be assumed to be also quantitatively similar. If two different *K*'s are obtained for the antagonist, the agonists probably act on different receptors. Similar arguments hold for agonist dissociation constants.

As an example of the practical application of dissociation constants, Furchgott[17] used K_B values when reporting his studies on β-adrenoceptors. He measured K_B for the β-adrenoceptor antagonist action of pronethalol in the rabbit aorta and duodenum. The values of K_B were $10^{-7.5}$ *M* for aortic β-receptors and $10^{-6.4}$ for the duodenal β-receptors. In other words, the β-receptors at both anatomical locations are antagonized by the same agent, pronethalol, but the affinities as determined by the K_B values suggest a quantitative difference. This difference in K_B values was among the first quantitative evidence for the existence of subtypes of β-receptors and, thus, highlights the importance of this measure in receptor differentiation. Other investigators have followed this type of approach (e.g., reference 6).

There are two methods of measuring dissociation constants of agonists: (1) by irreversible blockade of fraction of the receptor pool[17,19] and (2) by a method in which the dissociation constant of a partial agonist can be obtained.[4,57] For competitive antagonists, there is the dose-ratio method of Arunlakshana and Schild.[3] Certain drug–effector systems lend themselves to analysis by more than one of the above methods, and since each method is thoroughly independent of the other, the use of a second method reinforces the validity of the *K* value obtained.

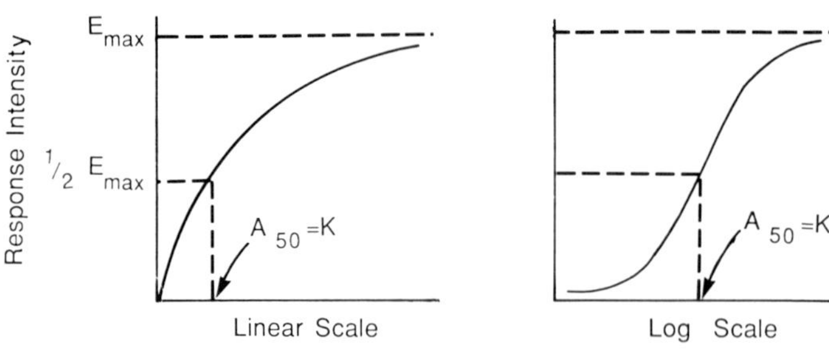

FIGURE 8.4. According to classical theory, the drug–receptor dissociation constant is numerically equal to the concentration that produces a half maximal response.

DISSOCIATION CONSTANTS IN CLASSICAL THEORY

Classical theory permits what is perhaps the most straightforward technique of determining the dissociation constant of an agonist. If one accepts the assumptions of classical theory leading to equation (8.7),

$$E = \frac{E_{max}A}{A + K},$$

then K can be determined directly from dose–response data. Substitution of $E = E_{max}/2$ in equation (8.7) and solving for A yields $A = K$. Thus, K is numerically equal to A_{50}, the concentration of agonist that produces a half-maximal effect.

The procedure for determining K based on classical theory is as follows:

1. Plot the values of effect against concentration (in rectangular coordinates), using either a linear or logarithmic scale for concentrations.
2. Construct a smooth curve through the plotted points that best represents the trend, ideally including all the plotted points.
3. Use that curve to determine the concentration of drug that produces an effect equal to one-half the maximum. This concentration is numerically equal to K (Figure 8.2) in classical theory.

The determination of K by this method has some practical drawbacks in addition to the theoretical assumptions that produced equation (8.7) and already mentioned. One such drawback is that it may not be easy to produce a smooth curve through the actual data points, or it may not be easy to fit the appropriate curve to the points. Another difficulty is E_{max} is often not obtained in typical experiments. In such situations the data can be analyzed using one of several mathematical transformations of equation (8.7). One commonly used transformation is the double-reciprocal plot, that is, a plot of $1/E$ against $1/A$ on linear

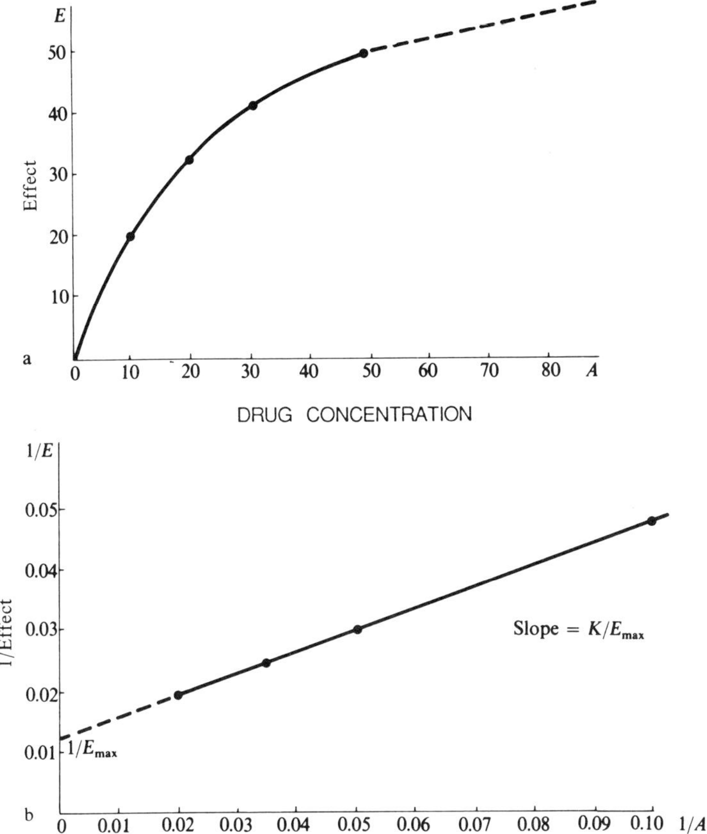

FIGURE 8.5. (a) Values of A and E graphed as a hyperbola. (b) Reciprocals of A and E graphed as a straight line. (Hypothetical concentration-effect data; arbitrary units.) From Tallarida RJ and Jacob LS: *The Dose-Response Relation in Pharmacology*. New York, Springer-Verlag, 1979, p. 55.

scales. The reason for graphing data in such a way is that this plot theoretically produces a straight line, as seen by inverting both sides of equation (8.7) to

$$\frac{1}{E} = \frac{K}{E_{max}} \cdot \frac{1}{A} + \frac{1}{E_{max}} \tag{8.13}$$

Equation (8.13) is in *linear form*, i.e., $y = mx + b$. A graph of reciprocated effect ($1/E$) against reciprocated concentrations ($1/A$) has a slope $= K/E_{max}$ and a y-intercept $= 1/E_{max}$. Such plots are commonly used in the analysis of enzyme–substrate kinetics and are generally referred to as Lineweaver-Burk plots. For the determination of K, a straight line is fitted to the reciprocated data and K is the product, (E_{max}).(slope) as displayed in Figure 8.5.

An obvious advantage of the double-reciprocal plot is that it is easier to fit a straight line to the reciprocated data than it is to fit the appropriate hyperbolic curve to the original data.

Another advantage is that the value of E_{max} may be approximated, even if it is not determined experimentally. This is done by extending the fitted straight line of a double-reciprocal plot to its intersection with the vertical axis.

It is important to note that the double-reciprocal plot is merely a convenient mathematical transformation of equation (8.7) and is valid in the analysis of drug–receptor data only under the assumption of classical theory.

Hypothetical values of drug concentration A and drug effect E are given in the table below and the same data are graphed in Figure 8.5a. From these values the reciprocals of E and A are calculated and graphed as in Figure 8.5b. The intercept of the double-reciprocal plot, obtained by extrapolation, is 0.012, from which $E_{max} = 83$. (i.e., 1/0.012).

A	E	$1/A$	$1/E$
10	21	0.10	0.048
20	33	0.050	0.030
30	41	0.033	0.024
50	50	0.020	0.020

The slope of the double-reciprocal plot is 0.36. Hence, K is $0.36 \times 83 = 30$ (two significant figures). Note that the largest measured effect is 50, a value much less than the calculated theoretical maximum of 83.

Hill Plot

Equation (8.7) can be rearranged such that,

$$\frac{E}{(E_{max} - E)} = \frac{A}{K}.$$

Taking logarithms,

$$\log\left(\frac{E}{E_{max} - E}\right) = \log A - \log K. \tag{8.14}$$

A plot of $\log[E/(E_{max} - E)]$ against $\log A$ is known as a Hill plot. Such a plot is linear with a slope of $+1.0$ and has a y-intercept of $-\log K$ (see Figure 8.6).

In certain situations, graphic representation of experimental data in the form of a Hill plot does not yield a slope of exactly 1.0. The implication of such results is that the drug–receptor interaction does not follow classical theory. Other explanations are possible; for example, the interaction of one drug molecule with one receptor molecule may not apply, that is, the kinetics would be of order other than two. If the drug–receptor interaction was such that n number of drug molecules per receptor were involved, then the interaction could be represented as

$$n\text{A} + \text{R} \rightleftharpoons \text{A}_n\text{R}.$$

FIGURE 8.6. The conventional Hill plot.

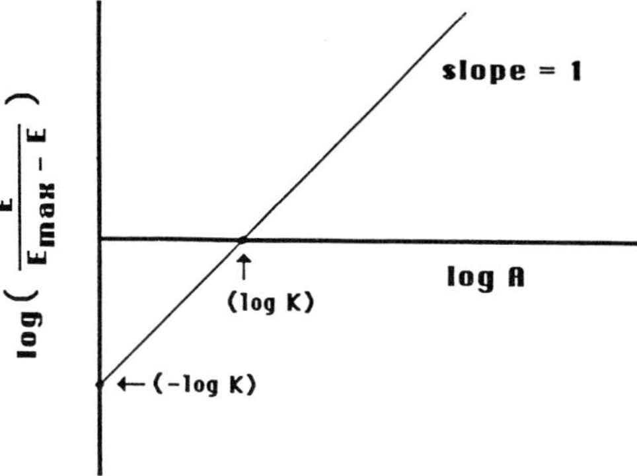

Equation (8.14) would be modified to

$$\log \frac{E}{E_{max} - E} = n \log A - \log K, \tag{8.15}$$

and the Hill plot would be of slope $= n$. Although nonlinear Hill plots or those that are linear with slopes $\neq 1.0$ suggest nonclassical reaction kinetics, the detailed molecular mechanism cannot be ascertained based on this information alone. The above reaction describes the situation of multiple drug molecules combining in a single receptor molecule or, just as likely, in a sequential type of binding scheme. In such situations the K value would be a composite of several binding parameters. Furthermore, it does not account for the possibility of more generalized mechanisms such as,

$$a\text{A} + r\text{R} \rightleftharpoons \text{A}_a\text{R}_r \tag{8.16}$$

Determination of Dissociation Constants: Competitive Antagonists

"It would obviously be of advantage if some common method of expressing drug antagonism could be agreed upon."

—H. O. Schild, 1947

The presence of a competitive antagonist in fixed concentration B produces a parallel displacement to the right of an agonist's log-dose response curve. The greater the concentration B, the greater the displacement (see Figure 8.7).

For a given concentration of competitive antagonist, B, the agonist "dose-ratio" for equal effects is defined as A'/A (see Figure 8.8) and is expressed by the relation

$$\frac{A'}{A} = 1 + \frac{B}{K_B} \tag{8.17}$$

where K_B is the dissociation constant of the competitive antagonist. The derivation of equation (8.17) is given below with no assumption made other than that

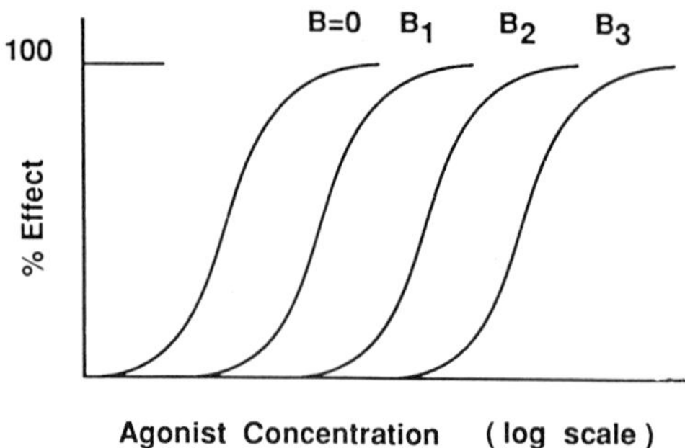

FIGURE 8.7. The concentration B of the competitive antagonist determines the amount of rightward shift of log dose-response curve of an agonist compound.

the magnitude of the agonist-induced effects depends on the amount of agonist–receptor complex, without specifying any particular functional relationship.

Example. In Figure 8.9 hypothetical log dose-response curves are shown for an agonist in the presence (curve 2) and absence (curve 1) of an antagonist at concentration B. The dose-ratio A'/A is obtained at half maximal effect ($E_{max}/2$). Since the calibration is logarithmic, the doses are $A = 10^{-8}\ M$ and $A' = 10^{-7}\ M$, yielding the ratio $A'/A = 10$. If, for example, $B = 5 \times 10^{-6}\ M$, we get from equation (8.17) $10 = 1 + 5 \times 10^{-6}/K_B$, from which $K_B = 5.5 \times 10^{-7}\ M$.

The value of K_B can be determined from equation (8.17) using a single concentration of antagonist B and a single dose-ratio A'/A. In practice, it is preferable to use several values of B and several dose-ratios. The dose-ratio A'/A for each of n antagonist concentrations B is obtained, i.e., $(A'/A)_i$ and B_i for $i = 1$ to $i = n$ and plotted in terms of logarithms: $\log (A'/A - 1)$ against $\log B$. By so doing, equation (8.17) is expressed in linear form: $(A'/A - 1) = \log B - \log K_B$. A

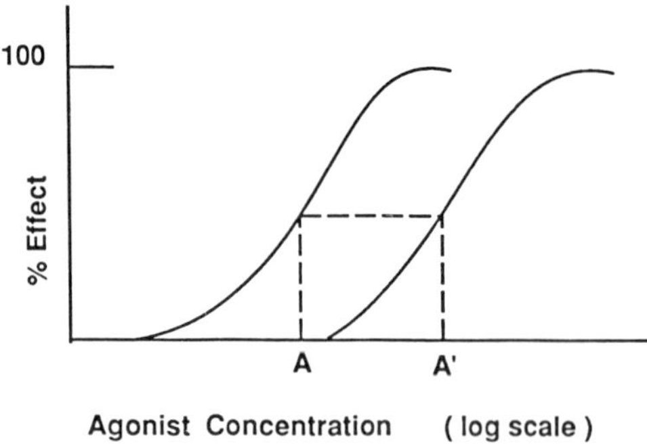

FIGURE 8.8. Graphical determination of the "dose–ratio," i.e., equieffective agonist concentration in the presence (A') and absence (A) of a surmountable antagonist.

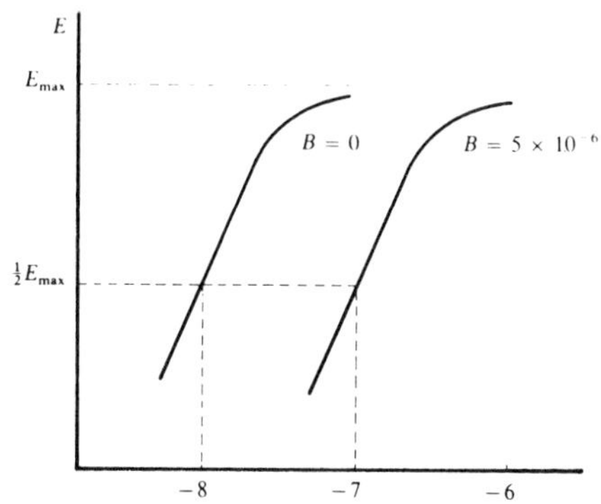

FIGURE 8.9. The dose-ratio in this example is $10^{-7}/10^{-8} = 10.0$. Note that the antagonist concentration does not enter into the calculation of the dose-ratio. The antagonist concentration is a factor, however, that is needed to calculate K_B [see equation (8.17)].

graph of log $(A'/A - 1)$ against log B theoretically yields a straight line of slope = 1.0 and intercept − log K_B. This method of plotting, used by Arunlakshana and Schild,[3] is preferred over the single dose-ratio determination since it minimizes the error inherent in a single determination. The plotted points should fit a straight line of slope unity; thus the method also provides an internal check on the applicability of the model (see Figure 8.10).

A commonly used way of expressing the dissociation constant of a competitive antagonist is the "pA_2."[3,43] The pA_2 is defined as the negative logarithm of (B) that yields a dose ratio of 2. Thus, log $(A'/A - 1) = 0$ and $-\log B$ (or pA_2) equals − log K_B. It is seen that the empirical constant, pA_2, is related theoretically to the more fundamental constant K_B of the competitive antagonist. This way of expressing the dissociation constant is analogous to pH and perhaps is more convenient than K_B. For example, if $K_B = 10^{-9}M$ (i.e., affinity $= 10^{+9}$), then pA_2 = 9. Changes in pA_2 occur in the same direction as changes in affinity, i.e., an increase in affinity is reflected as an increase in pA_2.

A graph of the kind illustrated in Figure 8.10 is called a Schild plot. When these plots are made using $-\log B$ on the abscissa, as is often done, the line should have slope = −1.0. Some curve-fitting procedure, such as the method of least squares, is usually used for constructing Schild plots. The slope of the resulting line may be different from −1.0 in some cases. If the discrepancy is not too great (usually a subjective appraisal), the fault is assumed to lie with the experimental data and not with the model. The intercept on the abscissa is the pA_2 value. Equating pA_2 to $-\log K_B$, however, is somewhat questionable, since competitive theory requires that both intercepts yield the same value. In some cases, the departure from unit slope, and even nonlinearity, can be explained and correction may be made as discussed by Furchgott.[18,21] An alternate method is to fit the data to the best line of unit slope using a least-square criteria.[50] The literature contains a number of articles that discuss several mathematical and pharmacologic methods for determining pA_2. See, for example, the treatments of Waud,[59] MacKay,[38] Stone and Angus,[46] and Tallarida et al.[50]

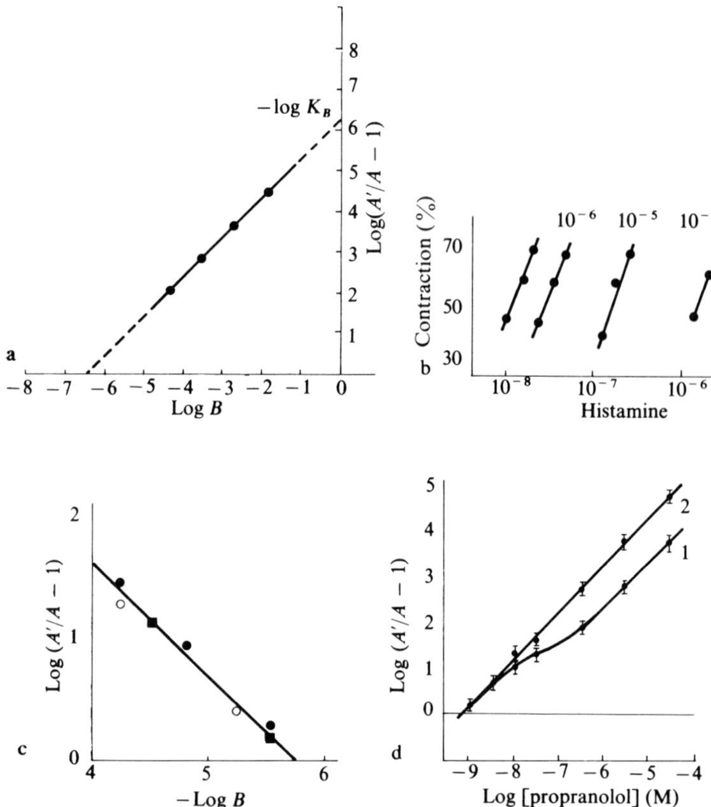

FIGURE 8.10. (a) Determination of K_B for a competitive antagonist using several concentrations of the antagonist (theoretical). Since the molar concentrations are negative powers of 10, such as 10^{-6}, 10^{-5}, etc, the values of log B are −6, −5, etc. Thus, the plotted values in the graph are in the negative domain. The intercept 6.2 equals $-\log K_B$; hence, $K_B = 10^{-6.2}$. (b) Dose-response data showing effect of histamine on guinea-pig ileum and the shifts produced by different concentrations of the antagonist atropine (A)[3]. (c) Schild plots from experiments of the kind shown in (b)[3]. (d) Illustration of the nonlinearity of Schild plots (curve 1) and the effect of blocking the extraneuronal uptake (curve 2) responsible for the nonlinearity.[18] Curves in (b) and (c) redrawn with permission of *British Journal of Pharmacology*; curve (d) redrawn with permission of *Federation Proceedings* (Bethesda, MD). From Tallarida RJ and Jacob LS: *The Dose–Response Relation in Pharmacology*, New York, Springer-Verlag, 1979, p. 63.

Competitive Antagonism: Rate Equations

In competitive antagonism the agonist, A, and the antagonist, B, react reversibly with a common receptor R:

$$\mathrm{A} + \mathrm{R} \underset{k_{2A}}{\overset{k_{1A}}{\rightleftharpoons}} \mathrm{AR}$$

$$\mathrm{B} + \mathrm{R} \underset{k_{2B}}{\overset{k_{\mathrm{B}}}{\rightleftharpoons}} \mathrm{BR}$$

The total receptor population will be denoted by r_t. At any time t let the number of AR complexes be given by x and BR complexes by y. These combinations reduce the unoccupied receptor population to $(r_t - x - y)$. The available agonist is therefore, $A - x$; also the available antagonist is $B - y$. As $A \gg x$ and $B \gg y$, we have $A - x \doteqdot A$ and $B - y \doteqdot B$. Application of the mass action law to these simultaneous reactions yields the equations for rates of formation

$$\frac{dx}{dt} = k_{1A}\,\mathrm{A}(r_t - x - y) - k_{2\mathrm{A}}\,x \tag{8.18}$$

and

$$\frac{dy}{dt} = k_{1B}\,B(r_t - x - y) - k_{2B}\,y. \tag{8.19}$$

At equilibrium $dx/dt = dy/dt = 0$, and equations (8.18) and (8.19) give

$$A(r_t - x - y) = K_{\mathrm{A}}\,x \tag{8.20}$$

and

$$B(r_t - x - y) = K_{\mathrm{B}}\,y \tag{8.21}$$

where $K_{\mathrm{A}} - k_{2A}/k_{1A}$ and $K_{\mathrm{B}} - k_{2B}/k_{1B}$.

From equation (8.21) we obtain Y, the concentration of BR at equilibrium:

$$y = \frac{B(r_t - x)}{B + K_{\mathrm{B}}}. \tag{8.22}$$

Substituting of Y from equation (8.22) into equation (8.20), and rearranging, we obtain x, the equilibrium concentration of AR:

$$x = \frac{Ar_t}{A + K_{\mathrm{A}}[1 + (B/K_{\mathrm{B}})]}. \tag{8.23}$$

In absence of the antagonist, $B = 0$, and equation (8.23) gives the usual equation

$$x = \frac{Ar_t}{A + K_{\mathrm{A}}}. \tag{8.24}$$

A salient feature of equation (8.23) is that for any value of A, x is less than it would be according to equation (8.24) in which there is no antagonist. Hence, for equal values of

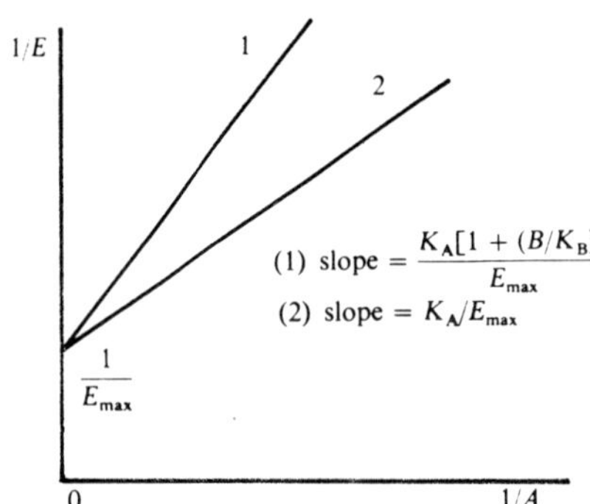

FIGURE 8.11. Double-reciprocal plot for a competitive antagonist. According to the classical theory, the intercept is the same. In the presence of antagonist, the slope is greater by the factor $(1 + B/K_B)$. Curve 1, antagonist and agonist; curve 2, agonist alone. From Tallarida RJ and Jacob LS: *The Dose–Response Relation in Pharmacology.* New York, Springer-Verlag, 1979, P. 67.

x, which means equal responses, the concentration of A in equation (8.23) would have to be increased to A'. Thus,

$$\frac{Ar_t}{A + K_A} = \frac{A' r_t}{A' + K_A[1 + (B/K_B)]}$$

from which it follows that

$$\frac{A'}{A} - 1 = \frac{B}{K_B} \tag{8.25}$$

which is the dose-ratio equation previously expressed in equation (8.17).

Equation (8.17) is derived with no assumption of direct proportionality between effect E and agonist–receptor complex x. If this assumption *is* made (i.e., $E = \alpha x$ and $E_{max} = \alpha r_t$), then $E = E_{max}A/(A + K_A)$ is the unblocked case and $E = AE_{max}/[A + K_A(1 + B/K_B)]$ in the presence of a competitive antagonist. The double-reciprocal (Lineweaver-Burk) relation for this case is

$$\frac{1}{E} = \frac{1}{E_{max}} + \frac{K_A(1 + B/K_B)}{E_{max}} \cdot \frac{1}{A}. \tag{8.26}$$

Note that if $B = 0$ (unblocked case), equation (8.26) reduces to

$$\frac{1}{E} = \frac{1}{E_{max}} + \frac{K_A}{E_{max}} \cdot \frac{1}{A}, \tag{8.27}$$

which is the same as equation (8.13). Equations (8.26) and (8.27) both have y-intercepts of $1/E_{max}$. The slope from equation (8.26) is $K_A\ (1 + B/K_B)/E_{max}$ and is larger than the slope from equation (8.27) by the factor $(1 + B/K_B)$. [See Figure 8.11 for a graphical representation of equations (8.26) and (8.27).] It should be emphasized that the double-reciprocal plots of effect against dose yield values for K_A and K_B only if one accepts the assumption of classical theory.

In vivo pA_2

The dissociation constant of a pure competitive antagonist (denoted K_B) is determined from the competitive equation (8.17) $A'/A - 1 = B/K_B$. It is seen that the unit of K_B is the same as that of B, namely concentration. When experiments are conducted in vivo, it may not be possible to determine B at equilibrium [a requirement of equation (8.17)] because the antagonist concentration, like the agonist concentration, is a time-varying function. Thus, the concentration of B at the receptor site is usually unknown.

At equilibrium, however, the tissue concentration of a drug is theoretically proportional to the administered dose (see Chapter 3, Pharmacokinetics). Accordingly, administered dose has been used instead of B, A, and A' in the calculation of K_B. Under appropriate experimental conditions the "in vivo pA_2" has shown to be a replicable constant.[48,49] Therefore, the analysis of competitive antagonism using Schild plots that are constructed using administered dose and effects at peak (or steady state) drug concentration is now common, particularly in experiments with narcotic agonist–antagonist pairs.

Constrained Schild Plot

Theoretically, the slope of a Schild plot is -1.0 (see p. 173). In many experiments, however, the actual slope of the Schild plot, as determined by standard linear regression, is different from unity. This is especially true for experiments conducted on intact animals.[34]

If the body of evidence regarding an agonist-antagonist pair suggests that the antagonism is truly competitive, then it is reasonable to *constrain* the Schild plot to the theoretically required slope of 1.0.* The regression analysis of log $(A'/A - 1)$ against $-\log(B)$, the constrained Schild plot,[50] will in this case yield identical values of the intercept on both the vertical and horizontal axes. Each intercept is the pA_2 value. Regression of y on x, when the slope is constrained to -1.0 gives the intercept b and standard error of the mean (SEM) from the following:

$$b = \bar{x} + \bar{y}$$

$$\text{SEM} = s/\sqrt{n}\,,$$

where x and y are the mean values of x_i and y_i; respectively, n is the number of points, and s is computed from

$$s^2 = \frac{1}{n-1} \sum_{i=1}^{n} \left\{(y_i - \bar{y}) + (x_i - \bar{x})\right\}^2 .$$

For a more detailed discussion, see references 50, 54a and 55.

---

*The slope of the linear regression plot should not differ significantly from unity prior to using the constraint.

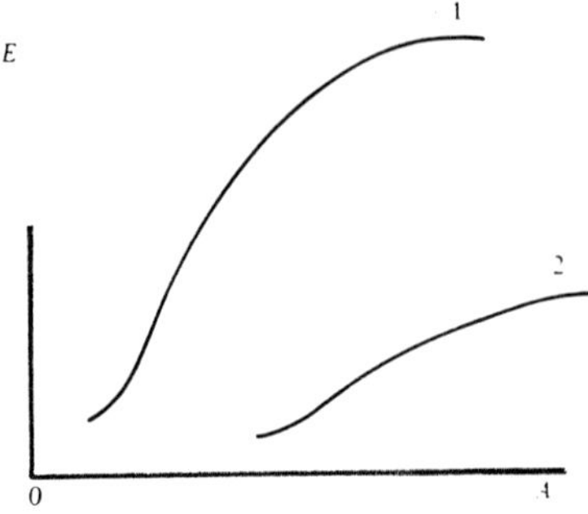

FIGURE 8.12. Partial irreversible blockade. Curve 2 represents the dose–response curve for the agonist after pretreatment with the noncompetitive antagonist. Curve 2 does not achieve the same maximum as curve 1, which is the agonist dose–response curve in the unblocked situation. From Tallarida RJ and Jacob LS: *The Dose–Response Relation in Pharmacology.* New York, Springer-Verlag, 1979, p. 68.

DISSOCIATION CONSTANTS OF AGONISTS

Method of Partial Irreversible Blockade

According to classical theory, one may determine the dissociation constant K of an agonist directly from the dose–response curve (A_{50} value). The value so obtained, however, is only as accurate as are the assumptions underlying classical theory. Perhaps the most questionable of these assumptions is the direct proportion between drug–receptor complex and effect. K can be obtained without this assumption, but the methodology is more involved and the determination cannot be made for all agonists. Nevertheless, where applicable, it remains the method of choice.

The method that is generally accepted is that proposed by Furchgott[17,19] in which the assumptions of classical theory are circumvented. The only assumption is that the effect depends on the amount of agonist–receptor complex such that equal effects, whether in the presence or absence of antagonist, imply equal amounts of agonist–receptor complex. The method uses an irreversible antagonist that combines with the same receptor as the agonist and, in so doing, reduces the total-receptor population.

The dose-response curves that are obtained in a typical experiment involving an irreversible antagonist are shown in Figure 8.12. The dose-response curve of an agonist is characteristically shifted to the right and downward by an irreversible antagonist. For analysis of the data, some number of equal effects are taken corresponding to agonist concentrations (A_1, A_1'), (A_2, A_2'), . . . , (A_N,A'_N). These pairs of concentrations are plotted as reciprocals ($1/A$ vs $1/A'$), according to the straight line equation,

$$\frac{1}{A} = \frac{1}{q}\,\frac{1}{A'} + \frac{1/q - 1}{K_A}. \tag{8.28}$$

where q is the fraction of receptors that remains unblocked by the antagonist. Since the slope in equation (8.28) is $1/q$ and the intercept on the vertical axis is $(1/q - 1)/K$, it follows that K may be determined from such a plot as

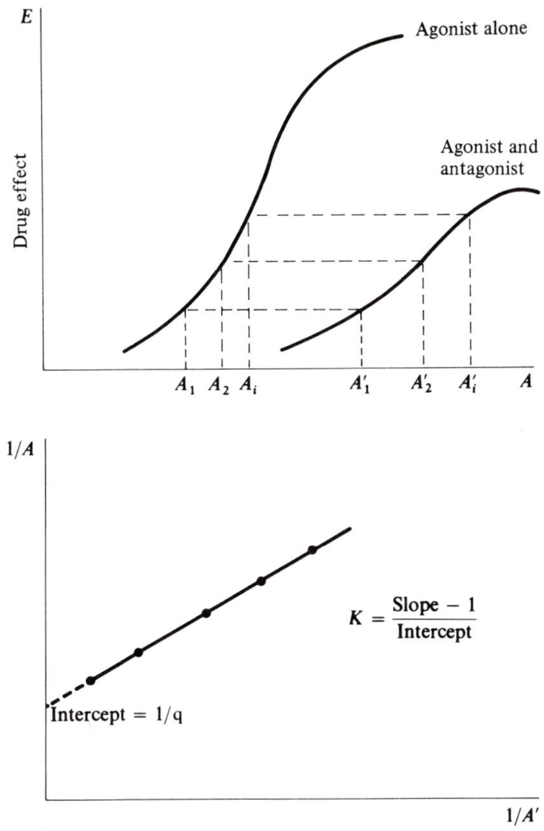

FIGURE 8.13. The method of partial irreversible blockade for determining the dissociation constant of an agonist. From Tallarida RJ and Jacob LS: *The Dose–Response Relation in Pharmacology.* New York, Springer-Verlag, 1979, p. 69.

$$K_A = \frac{\text{slope} - 1.0}{\text{intercept}}. \tag{8.29}$$

This method is shown illustratively in Figure 8.13 and with actual data in Figure 8.14.

The K for the vasoconstrictor effect of some catecholamines on the α-adrenoceptor in isolated strips of rabbit thoracic aorta has been determined by several independent investigators. The values (shown in Table 8.1) give some idea of the sensitivity of the method to variations in experimental protocol. The individual references should be consulted for details.

The method of partial irreversible blockade has become the standard method for determining agonist dissociation constants from functional studies since, unlike the classical theory, it does not assume linearity between drug effect and

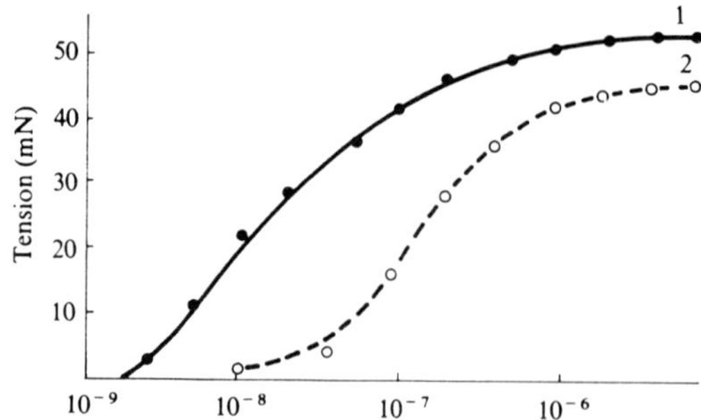

FIGURE 8.14. Norepinephrine concentration–response curve obtained on a spirally cut strip of rabbit thoracic aorta in the absence of (curve 1) and in the presence of (curve 2) phenoxybenzamine. Data for curve 2 were obtained after washing to zero baseline followed by incubation with 5×10^{-9} M phenoxybenzamine. Responses are recorded as isometric tension. (Redrawn from Tallarida et al[53] with permission © 1975 IEEE.)

the concentration of drug–receptor complex. A second method for determining the dissociation constant of certain agonists (partial agonists) is discussed subsequently.

Example. The derivation of equation (8.28) follows from the relation between the amount of drug–receptor complex x and the agonist concentration A and receptor concentration r_t, [equation (8.4)],

$$x = \frac{Ar_t}{A + K}.$$

In the presence of an irreversible antagonist, a fraction of the receptors is blocked, leaving qr_t ($q < 1$) available for interaction with agonist molecules. An increased agonist concentration, (A') assuming equal effects at equal receptor occupancy, must be in order to achieve the preblockade effect. Assuming equal effects at equal receptor occupancy,

$$\frac{A'qr_t}{A' + K} = \frac{Ar_t}{A + K}.$$

TABLE 8.1. Dissociation constants (±SEM) in molar units for several catecholamines in rabbit aortic strips.

Investigator	l-Norepinephrine	l-Epinephrine
Besse and Furchgott[5]	$(3.39 \pm 0.15) \times 10^{-7}$	$(2.07 \pm 0.31) \times 10^{-7}$
Sheys and Green[44]	$(1.31 \pm 0.54) \times 10^{-7}$	$(2.94 \pm 0.84) \times 10^{-7}$
Jacob and Tallarida[30]	$(0.84 \pm 0.16) \times 10^{-7}$	
	l-Phenylephrine	Dopamine
Besse and Furchgott[5]	$(1.13 \pm 0.14) \times 10^{-6}$	$(6.36 \pm 0.42) \times 10^{-5}$
Sheys and Green[44]	$(1.27 \pm 0.13) \times 10^{-6}$	$(1.53 \pm 0.66) \times 10^{-5}$

TABLE 8.2. Equiactive molar concentrations of norepinephrine in the absence (case 1) and presence (case 2) of a fixed concentration of blocker.

A(Case 1)	A′(Case 2)
0.20×10^{-7}	1.1×10^{-7}
0.14×10^{-7}	0.71×10^{-7}
0.12×10^{-7}	0.50×10^{-7}
0.091×10^{-7}	0.38×10^{-7}
0.076×10^{-7}	0.32×10^{-7}
0.067×10^{-7}	0.26×10^{-7}
0.055×10^{-7}	0.22×10^{-7}
0.048×10^{-7}	0.17×10^{-7}

Rearrangement of the above equation yields equation (8.28). In practice, the reciprocated data are fitted to a straight line using a curve-fitting procedure such as the method of least squares. (Confidence limits should be cautiously interpreted since reciprocated data do not fulfill the theoretical basis of regression analysis.)

Example. In a study by Tallarida et al[53] (Figure 8.14) rabbit aorta was contracted by norepinephrine alone (case 1) and by norepinephrine after exposure of the strip to the noncompetitive antagonist phenoxybenzamine (case 2). Equieffective responses were obtained for concentrations of norepinephrine and are given in Table 8.2. A plot of $1/A$ against $1/A'$ gave a straight line with slope 3.1 and intercept 2.5×10^7. Thus from equation (8.29):

$$K = (3.1 - 1)/(2.5 \times 10^7)$$
$$= 0.84 \times 10^{-7} M.$$

Stimulus–Effect Curves

Once the dissociation constant of an agonist has been determined, the value can be used to construct a stimulus–effect curve as discussed below. The advantage of such a graph is that it reveals the mathematical relation between drug-induced stimulus and observed effect, i.e., events occurring distal to the receptor. It is difficult to elucidate this information in any other way. Such a graph is useful in dissecting the relative importance of pre- and postreceptor events in situations where the overall processes are known to change (e.g., opiate tolerance). For the interested reader, an application of this theory is given in the example below.

Example. In an experiment on isolated rabbit thoracic aorta, measurements were made of the isometric tension developed in response to graded doses of norepinephrine.[53] In one set of experiments, preload was set at 10 g. In another set of experiments, preload was set at only 0.25 g. The dose-response curves for both preloads are shown in Figure 8.15. The values of A_{50}, determined directly from the curves, were 0.18×10^{-7} M for condition I (small stretch) and 0.052×10^{-7} M for condition II (large stretch). The values of K were

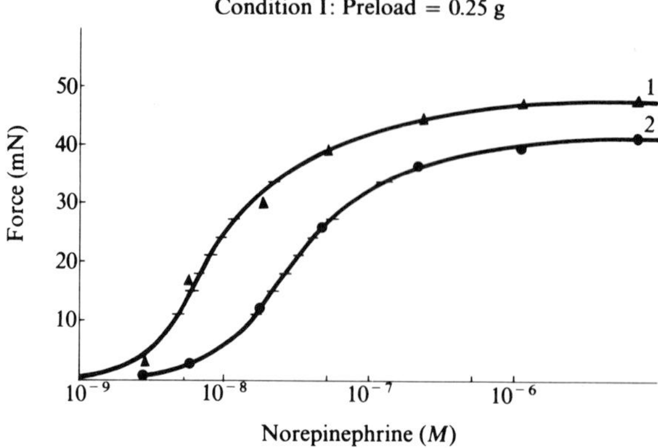

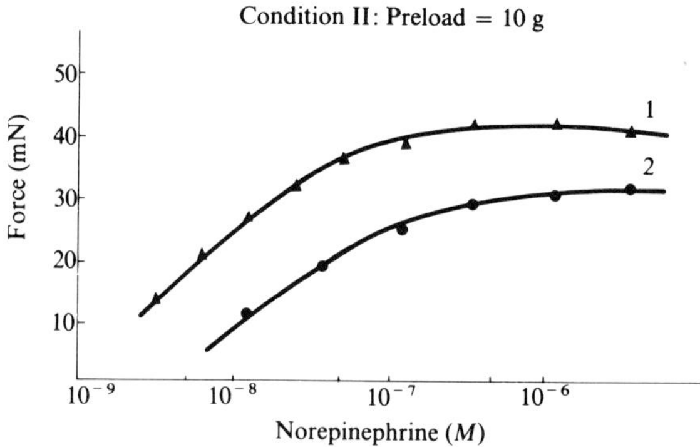

FIGURE 8.15. Effect of preload on the dissociation constant. Condition I: Dose–response curves to norepinephrine (curve 1) and norepinephrine after partial block with phenoxybenzamine (curve 2). Preload 0.25 g. Condition II: Dose–response curves as above under a preload of 10 g. (Reprinted by permission from *Arch. Int. Pharmacodyn Ther*[54]).

determined, by the method of partial irreversible blockade. The K values were found to be 0.84×10^{-7} M for condition I and 0.24×10^{-7} M for condition II.

From equation (8.9) the efficacy could be calculated: $\varepsilon_A = 5.7$ (condition I) and $\varepsilon_A = 5.6$ (condition II). The agreement in the values of the efficacy is compatible with Stephenson's concept of the efficacy as a link between a drug and the stimulus it produces. Further, this experiment illustrates the separation of the process into drug-dependent and drug-independent parts. Changing the conditions by adjusting preload (stretching the muscle) affected the stimulus-response relation (the drug-independent part), but it did not change the efficacy (the drug-dependent part).

Once the values of efficacy and K are known, the function f between stimulus and effect may be determined. Values of S and A are obtained using equation (8.8), and values of E and A are known from the experimental data. Then, for each A, the corresponding E and S values are paired. This process is illustrated in Table 8.3 for the present example of small (condition I) and large (condition II) stretch.

TABLE 8.3. Concentration-effect and stimulus values for norepinephrine under two different preload conditions in rabbit aorta.

Condition I			Condition II		
$S = \dfrac{5.7A}{A + 0.84 \times 10^{-7}}$			$S = \dfrac{5.6A}{A + 0.24 \times 10^{-7}}$		
A	E	S	A	E	S
5×10^{-9}	11	0.32	5×10^{-9}	17	0.97
10^{-8}	24	0.63	10^{-8}	22	1.6
5×10^{-8}	38	2.1	5×10^{-8}	35	3.8
10^{-7}	41	3.1	10^{-7}	39	4.5
5×10^{-7}	45	4.9	5×10^{-7}	40	5.3
10^{-6}	47	5.3	10^{-6}	40	5.5

The stimulus–effect functions are shown in Figure 8.16. In each case the function is clearly nonlinear, in contrast to predictions of classical theory and highlighting the value of Stephenson's approach. Gero[25] performed a similar analysis of the stimulus-effect relation for several cholinergic drugs on the fundus of the rabbit stomach.

Method of Partial Agonists

For the special case of partial agonists, two methods of determining dissociation constants are available. The first, partial irreversible blockade, has been dis-

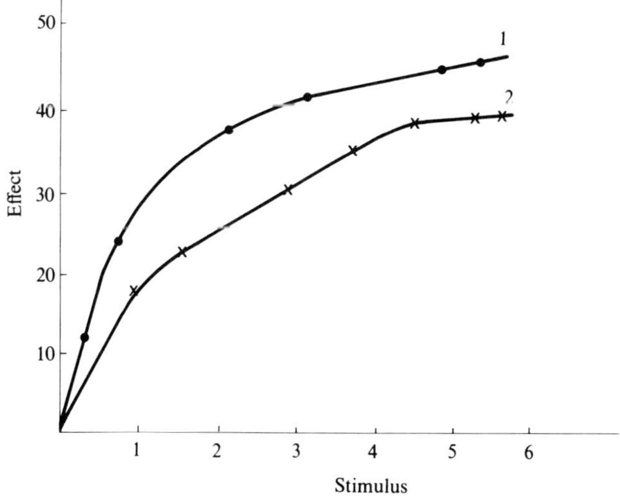

FIGURE 8.16. Stimulus–effect relations for isolated rabbit thoracic aorta. From Tallarida RJ and Jacob LS: *The Dose–Response Relation in Pharmacology.* New York, Springer-Verlag, 1979, p. 60.

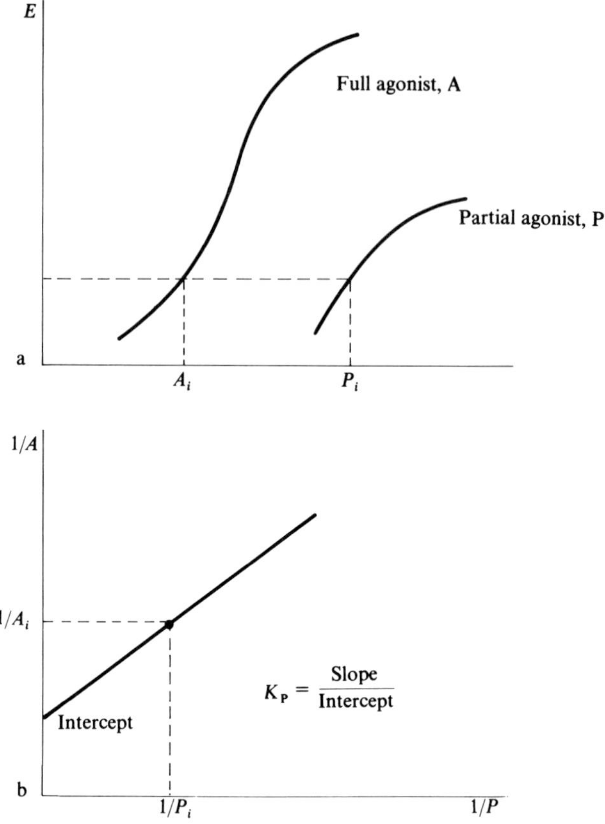

FIGURE 8.17. Method used for the determination of K_P for the concentration of a partial agonist, P. (a) Equieffective concentrations of a weak agonist (P_i) and a strong agonist (A_i). (b) A straight line is fitted to the reciprocals of equiactive concentrations from curve (a). From Tallarida RJ and Jacob LS: *The Dose–Response Relation in Pharmacology.* New York, Springer-Verlag, 1979, p. 73.

cussed previously and is applicable to all agonists for which an irreversible antagonist is available. The second (Barlow et al[4]; Waud[58]) is only applicable to partial agonists. Partial agonists are those that appear to require an appreciable receptor occupancy to cause effects and, even with full receptor occupancy, may not achieve the tissue's maximum response. This is in contrast to full (or "strong") agonists, which have a large spare receptor capacity.

In the method of partial agonists, dose-response curves for a partial agonist and a full agonist are obtained and graphed. Equieffective concentrations are selected using isoboles as shown in Figure 8.17. Each pair of concentrations A_i, P_i) is used in a plot of reciprocal full-agonist concentrations ($1/A_i$) against reciprocal partial-agonist concentration ($1/P_i$). A plot of $1/A$ against $1/P$ is theoretically linear with slope, y-intercept, and K_P (for the partial agonist) related by the expression

$$K_P = \frac{\text{slope}}{y\text{-intercept}} \tag{8.30}$$

When this method was applied to certain muscarinic agents, using carbachol as the full agonist, the values of K agreed well with those obtained by the method of irreversible blockage. The theory underlying this method utilizes Stephenson's[45] modification of classical theory (see p. 158).

We start with the equation relating the concentration of drug–receptor complex X to the drug concentration D:

$$X = (r_t A)/(A + K).$$

For this particular application, it is convenient to use fractional occupancy $Y = X/r_t = A/(A + K)$. A strong agonist, drug A, produces effects at low-receptor occupancy and at concentrations $\ll K_A$. Hence, the fraction Y_A of occupied receptors is given by the approximate equation

$$Y_A \doteqdot \frac{A}{K_A}.$$

In contrast, a partial agonist drug P, requires high-receptor occupancy to produce an effect and concentrations sufficiently high that one must use the full relation

$$Y_P = \frac{P}{P + K_P}.$$

For both types of drug, strong agonists and partial agonists, the effect of each is a function of the fractional occupancy

$$E_A = g(e_A Y_A) \text{ and } E_P = g(e_P Y_P)$$

where each e represents the "efficacy" in Stephenson's formulation. Equating equal responses, $E_A = E_P$, we get

$$e_A \frac{A}{K_A} = e_P \frac{P}{P + K_P}.$$

Reciprocating,

$$\frac{K_A}{e_A} \cdot \frac{1}{A} = \frac{1}{e_P} + \frac{K_P}{e_P} \cdot \frac{1}{P}. \tag{8.31}$$

or

$$\frac{1}{A} = \frac{e_A}{e_A K_A} + \frac{e_A}{K_A} \cdot \frac{K_P}{e_P} \cdot \frac{1}{P}. \tag{8.32}$$

Again, this equation is in linear form so that a plot of $1/A$ against $1/P$ is a straight line with slope $= e_A/e_P \cdot K_P/K_A$ and intercept $= e_A/e_P K_A$. Hence, slope/intercept $= K_P$, which is equation (8.30).

TABLE 8.4. Equiactive concentrations of a strong agonist (A) and a partial agonist (P)*.

A(butyl-TMA)	P(nonyl-TMA)
3.0×10^{-7}	4.5×10^{-6}
4.0×10^{-7}	6.6×10^{-6}
5.0×10^{-7}	8.0×10^{-6}
8.0×10^{-7}	14.0×10^{-6}
10.0×10^{-7}	50.0×10^{-6}

*Data from Stephenson.[45]

Example. Table 8.4 reproduces the equiactive concentrations of a representative experiment in which a strong agonist, butyl-trimethylammonium (TMA), and a partial agonist, nonyl-trimethylammonium (TMA), produced contractions of the guinea-pig ileum. A plot of $1/A$ against $1/P$ produced a line with slope 13 and intercept 0.046×10^7. From equation (8.30) we get $K_P = 2.8 \times 10^{-5}$.

Note that this method of determining K for a partial agonist requires that the full agonist produces an effect at low fractional receptor occupancy so that the condition $K_A \gg A$ is satisfied. If the full agonist does not have this property, the method is not applicable, in which case an alternative method is required. Gero and Tallarida[26] considered this case, and this alternative method also involves matching the responses of P with those of a full agonist A. With reference again to Figure 8.18, A_P denotes the concentration of A, which produces a tissue response equal to the maximum tissue response produced by drug P. Any other pair of concentrations P and A is selected which yields equal effect E. With no assumptions regarding the relative values of K_A, A_P, and A, it can be shown that K_P and K_A are related as

$$K_P = \frac{K_A(A_P - A_i) \cdot P_i}{(A_P + K_A) \cdot A_i}. \tag{8.33}$$

(See derivation below.) Hence, if K_A is known for the full agonist, K_P may be calculated from equation (8.33).

From the notion of a partial agonist as an agent that requires full receptor occupancy to produce maximum effect, it follows (from the formula $S = \varepsilon Y$) that the maximum stimulus produced by P is ε_P, its efficacy. This same value of stimulus can be achieved by a strong agonist with something less than full receptor occupancy at concentration A_P so that for drug A, $S_A = \varepsilon_A A_P/(A_P + K_A)$. Equating ε_P to S_A gives $\varepsilon_P = \varepsilon_A A_P/(A_P + K_A)$ or

$$\frac{\varepsilon_A}{\varepsilon_P} = 1 + \frac{K_A}{K_P}. \tag{8.34}$$

For any other level of effect E_i produced by A and P, their stimuli must be the same, or

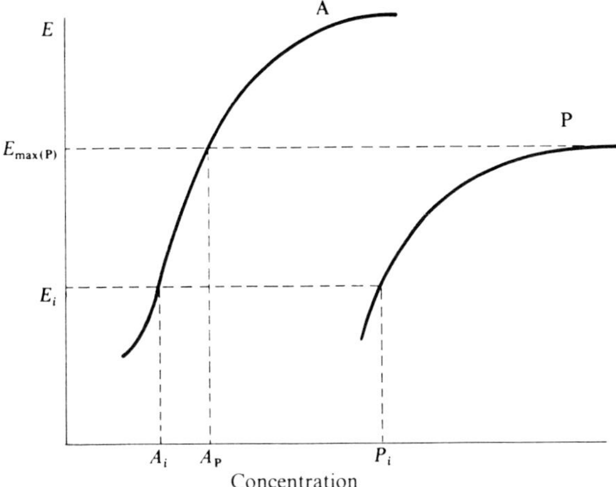

FIGURE 8.18. Graphical analysis of hypothetical dose–response curves of a full agonist (A) and a partial agonist (P) required for the determination of the dissociation constant of a partial agonist. Details of the technique are described in the text. From Tallarida RJ and Jacob LS: *The Dose–Response Relation in Pharmacology.* New York, Springer-Verlag, 1979, p. 75.

$$\frac{\varepsilon_A A_i}{A_i + K_A} = \frac{\varepsilon_P P_i}{P_i + K_P}$$

from which

$$\frac{\varepsilon_A}{\varepsilon_P} = \frac{P_i}{P_i + K_P} \cdot \frac{A_i + K_A}{A_i}. \tag{8.35}$$

Equating the right-hand sides of equations (8.34) and (8.35) gives

$$1 + \frac{K_A}{A_P} = \frac{P_i}{P_i + K_P} \cdot \frac{A_i + K_A}{A_i},$$

and solving for K_P

$$K_P = \frac{K_A(A_P - A_i) \cdot P_i}{A_i(A_P + K_A)},$$

which is equation (8.33).

Example. In an experiment with full and partial adrenergic agonists the following (molar) values were obtained: $A_i = 10^{-9}$; $A_P = 5 \times 10^{-9}$; $P_i = 10^{-7}$. The full agonist was known to have the value $K_A = 5 \times 10^{-8}$ (determined by the method on p. 178). The value of K_P is from equation (8.33).

$$K_P = \frac{5 \times 10^{-8}(5 \times 10^{-9} - 10^{-9})10^{-7}}{10^{-9}(5 \times 10^{-9} + 5 \times 10^{-8})}$$

$$= 3.6 \times 10^{-7}\ M.$$

Allosteric Model

As seen above, occupation theory provides methods for determining the dissociation constant for a strong agonist, a partial agonist, and a competitive antagonist.

The question that arises is, can dissociation constants be determined in the framework of some of the more sophisticated theories of drug action, such as the allosteric model? Without practical application, these theories would be mainly of academic interest.

C. D. Thron[56] and D. Calquhoun,[7] acting independently, considered this question and arrived at essentially the same conclusion, viz, that the allosteric model yields the same value for dissociation constants as does the occupation model in at least two major cases: (1) the case of competitive antagonism and (2) the case of partial agonism. The equivalency can be demonstrated by noting that allosteric theory defines efficacy as the relative affinities of a compound for the R and T forms of the receptor. The efficacy of an agonist is defined to be

$$\varepsilon_A = \frac{K_{AT}}{K_{AR}} - 1, \tag{8.36}$$

where all terms have the same meaning as previously described.

For an antagonist the "efficacy" is defined to be

$$\varepsilon_B = \frac{K_{BT}}{K_{BR}} - 1. \tag{8.37}$$

Note that "efficacy" of an antagonist has meaning in allosteric theory, but not in traditional occupation theory.

With this definition of efficacy, the allosteric model yields the same value for the dissociation constant of a partial agonist as does equation (8.30), and for a competitive antagonist as does equation (8.17). In the symbolism of allosteric theory, the K's so determined are K_{AT} and K_{BT}, respectively.

Quite a different situation arises for the dissociation constant of full agonists. In this case the equation relating equiactive agonist concentrations before and after partial irreversible blockade of a fraction of receptors is

$$\frac{1}{A} = \frac{1}{q}\,\frac{1}{A'} + \frac{(1-q)}{q}\left(\frac{1}{K_{AT}} + \frac{1}{A_{AR} \cdot \mathrm{L}}\right), \tag{8.38}$$

where all the symbols have been defined previously. Comparison of equation (8.38) to equation (8.28),

$$\frac{1}{A} = \frac{1}{q}\,\frac{1}{A'} + \frac{(1-q)}{q}\,\frac{1}{K_{AT}},$$

reveals the difference. If allosteric theory is used to analyze the data from a graph of $1/A$ against $1/A'$, the quantity (slope − 1)/intercept is interpreted as $1/[(K_{AT})^{-1} + (K_{AR}L)^{-1}]$ rather than K_{AT}. Unfortunately, the experimental evidence to date does not clearly favor one interpretation over the other.

Returning to the definition of efficacy used in allosteric theory, equations (8.36) and (8.37), some departure from Stephenson's original notion of this quantity should be noted. First, efficacy, according to allosteric theory, may be less than zero. Second, nonparallel shifts in the log-concentration response curves are permitted for competitive antagonism under certain conditions. Hence, allosteric theory provides some provocative ideas regarding the analysis and interpretation of dose–response curves. For further details, the interested reader is referred to the papers of Thron,[56] Colquhoun,[7] and others cited earlier as being associated with allosteric theory.

The validity of allosteric theory might be tested in a kind of experiment in which dissociation constants are determined using the methods described above. Specifically, the K of a partial agonist is determined in three different ways, and the values obtained are then compared.

The first determination compares the dose-response curve of the partial agonist to that of a full agonist acting on the same receptor. The K of the partial agonist can be determined using the method of equation (8.30).

The second determination of the K of the partial agonist makes use of the fact that it can be used as an antagonist to a full agonist that acts on the same receptor. The K for the partial agonist can be determined as described for the dose-ratio method [equation (8.17)].

The third determination employs the method of partial irreversible blockade (see p. 178).

Allosteric theory predicts that the dissociation constant determined by partial irreversible blockade will be smaller than the K determined by the first two methods.

Perturbation Methods

The method of partial irreversible receptor blockade is generally considered to be the method of choice for determining the dissociation constant of a full agonist. Fewer a priori assumptions need be made regarding drug action with this method than with most others. Unfortunately, an irreversible antagonist is not readily available for all agonists. Indeed, it may be the exception rather than the rule. Hence, the problem of determining pharmacologic dissociation constants of agonists depends on the availability of appropriate second drugs, or it involves the assumptions of classical theory ($K_A = A_{50}$). As we have seen, the assumption of a direct proportion between effect and concentration is a questionable one and to be avoided if possible. It is not surprising, therefore, that researchers have sought other methods of determining dissociation constants, even if such methods have limited application. A case in point is the perturbation or "relaxation" method.

In this method the steady-state interaction between drug and receptor is perturbed, and the kinetics of the restoration to equilibrium are monitored. Analysis of the restoration process yields the dissociation constant and, in addition, the forward and reverse rate constants of the drug–receptor equilibrium reaction.

The perturbation model is developed as follows. For a given agonist concentration, A, the concentration of drug–receptor complex at equilibrium is some value x_e. If the steady-state concentration is disturbed some small amount μ, the concentration of drug–receptor complex changes from x_e to $(x_e + \mu)$. The excursion from steady state occurs over a finite time and, thus, μ is a function of time. If the maximum deviation from steady state is denoted μ_{max}, it can be shown[52] that the equilibrium restoration is described by

$$\mu = \mu_{max} \left\{ \exp[-(k_1 A + k_2)t] \right\}. \tag{8.39}$$

During the period of perturbation, the pharmacologic effect will follow the alteration in concentration of drug–receptor complex and change from E to $E + \Delta E$. For sufficiently small μ, it can be shown that the change in pharmacologic response obeys the equation

$$\Delta E = \Delta E_{max} \left\{ \exp[-(k_1 A + k_2)t] \right\}, \tag{8.40}$$

where ΔE_{max} is the maximum observed change in pharmacologic effect caused by the perturbation from steady-state effect.

It is convenient to define a time constant for the exponential term of equation (8.40) as

$$\tau = (k_1 A + k_2)^{-1}. \tag{8.41}$$

Equation (8.40) then becomes, more simply,

$$\Delta E = \Delta E_{max} \cdot \exp(-t/\tau). \tag{8.42}$$

From equation (8.42) it follows that when $t = \tau$, $\Delta E = \Delta E_{max} \cdot \exp(-1) = 0.37\ \Delta E_{max}$. Thus, *the time constant is that time necessary for* ΔE *to change from* ΔE_{max} *to* $(0.37)\Delta E_{max}$, as shown in Figure 8.19.

With reference to Figure 8.19, a steady-state level of pharmacologic effect is disrupted by a perturbation introduced at the instant marked with an asterisk. The perturbation is a time-variant function that reaches a maximum at ΔE_{max} and then returns to zero (i.e., the effect returns to steady-state level) at a measurable rate. The time constant, τ, of the restoration to steady state is determined from the recovery record as shown in the figure.

Recall τ is related to the agonist concentration that produces the initial steady-state pharmacologic effect by equation (8.41). Hence, if perturbations are made at two different agonist concentrations, A_1 and A_2, the pairs A_1, τ_1, and A_2, τ_2 can be used in equation (8.41) to yield two equations from which k_1 and k_2 may be determined. The dissociation constant K is then obtained as $K = k_2/k_1$. Note that in the process of determining K, the forward and reverse rate constants (k_1 and k_2) of the drug–receptor interaction are also obtained. These quantities are not

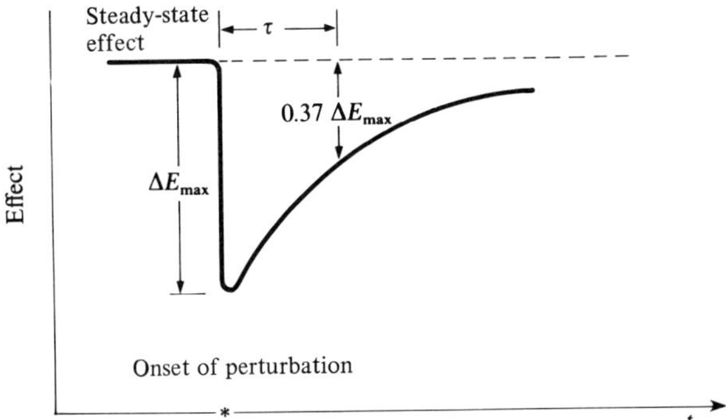

FIGURE 8.19. Perturbation method for determining rate constants of the drug-receptor reaction. The time constant is the time required for the system to recover to (0.37) ΔE_{max}. From Tallarida RJ and Jacob LS: *The Dose–Response Relation in Pharmacology.* New York, Springer-Verlag, 1979, p. 77.

obtained in the other methods described above. If perturbations are made at several values of concentration A and the corresponding time constants are measured then a graph of $1/\tau$ versus A is linear

$$\frac{1}{\tau} = k_1 A + k_2,$$

so that slope $= k_1$ and intercept $= k_2$

The use of equilibrium perturbation for the purpose of studying reaction kinetics is a standard practice in chemistry and has recently been extended to the study of the drug–receptor interaction. Two properties of equilibrium are specifically used in the application of the perturbation method to chemical equilibrium. First, for each set of external conditions such as temperature and pressure, there is a corresponding set of forward and reverse rate constants. Second, if an equilibrium is disturbed by altering the temperature or the pressure, the perturbation is transient, but finite. Since the reaction cannot regain equilibrium infinitely fast, the restoration to equilibrium may be monitored. An excellent review of relaxation methods in chemistry is given by Larry Faller.[16] A more complete account is contained in the book by Czerlinski.[14]

Tallarida and co-workers,[52] in a theoretical paper, considered the application of perturbation methods to pharmacologic systems in equilibrium and later applied this method to the determination of K for norepinephrine acting on isolated aortic strips of the rabbit.[53] The perturbing stimulus was ultraviolet light that was shown by Furchgott and co-workers to relax strips placed in a state of drug-induced contraction.[20] A basic assumption in this application is that ultraviolet light upsets the equilibrium between drug and receptor. Although not directly proved, this assumption has support, since the results of these experiments yielded a value of K for norepinephrine that agrees with that determined by the method of partial irreversible blockade. Another line of supportive evidence is that the time constant for restoration is different in the presence of antagonists[30] in agreement with theoretical predictions.[51]

Example. An isolated strip of rabbit aorta is contracted with a vasoconstricting drug in concentration $A_1 = 10^{-8}\ M$. Upon reaching an equilibrium tension, ultraviolet photoflash is applied, causing a brief loss of tension that recovers with time constant $\tau_1 = 35$ s. After recovery from the flash-induced relaxation, this same strip is given additional drug, bringing the total drug concentration to $A_2 = 10^{-6}\ M$ and producing a new level of equilibrium tension. Ultraviolet flash is applied at this time, causing less relaxation and a more rapid restoration given by the time constant $\tau_2 = 6$ s. From this experiment we can obtain the rat constants k_1 and k_2 for this drug by substituting equation (8.41): $35 = (k_1 10^{-8} + k_2)^{-1}$ and $6 = (k_1 10^{-6} + k^2)^{-1}$. Simultaneous solution yields $k_1 = 1.4 \times 10^5$ and $k_2 = 0.027$ from which $K = k_2/k_1 = 1.9 \times 10^{-7}$.

Drug Combinations: Isoboles

In contrast to the kinds of antagonism discussed in this chapter many combinations of drugs produce qualitatively similar effects. This was discussed in chapter two, and we saw there that some combinations produce superadditive effects. We now consider combinations of drugs in more detail. Toward that end, consider a level of effect, such as the half maximal effect, and say dose a of drug A acting alone or dose b of drug B acting alone produces this intensity of effect. We now consider combinations x of A and y of B that yield this level of effect. The locus of points (x,y) is an *isobole* for this situation. The straight line (I) of Figure 8.20 is an isobole that represents pure additivity. For all such points it is seen that $y + (b/a)\,x = b$. For example, if drug A were merely a dilution of drug B (so that dose a is larger than dose b) then the combinations represented by the straight line isobole (I) are the predictable amounts (x,y) of the mixture that are needed to be equivalent to a of A acting alone or b of B acting alone. This line is then a reference for graphically distinguishing subadditive and super additive combinations. Thus, point P in the figure denotes a superadditive combination of two different drugs, for $y + (b/a)\,x < b$; that is, the amount x of A allows less of B than is expected from pure addition. Stated differently, the presence of A has made B a more potent drug (or B has made drug A more potent), a phenomenon called *potentiation*.* In contrast, a combination such as point Q represents a reduction in potency or $y + (b/a)\,x > b$, a subadditive combination.

For the sake of completeness we consider also a situation in which drug A is devoid of efficacy. In this case the line of additivity is then horizontal through b such as curve II of Figure 8.20, and thus combinations (points) below the horizontal line are indicative of superadditivity or potentiation, whereas points above the horizontal are subadditive mixtures of the two drugs. If drug A were a pure competitive antagonist of drug B, this kind of plot would yield line III of the figure.

---

*No particular mechanism for potentiation is implied here.

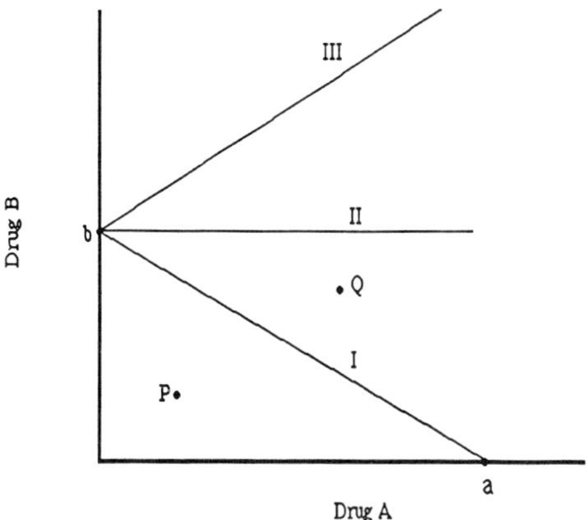

FIGURE 8.20. Isoboles are loci of points representing combinations of doses of each drug that yield the same intensity of effect or the same percentage of subjects that experience an end point. Courtesy of Tom Parry, Temple University School of Medicine.

Because equieffective doses, such as a and b and combinations x,y are determined experimentally, these are values of random variables and they must be subjected to proper statistical analysis in a rigorous demonstration of super or sub additivity. It is especially noteworthy that in the comparison of the quantity, $y + (b/a)\,x$, with b, the ratio (b/a) arises. Confidence limits for such potency ratios are often wide when determined by the usually employed experiments. (See Tallarida and Murray[55]). Accordingly, a relatively large number of experiments and good precision may be needed to distinguish among the different kinds of synergism.

A Changing Receptor Concentration: Modification of Rate Equations

The model for the interaction of a drug molecule with a receptor is the basis for most of the usual methods employed in the analysis of dose–response data. This model assumes a fixed number of receptors that at any time are either bound by one or more kinds of ligands or they are not, but they remain available for such binding if concentrations or other conditions change. We have seen in Chapter 5, however, that some receptors may become internalized and thus be unavailable for binding unless they are recycled to the cell surface. It is evident that a rapid and appreciable net rate of such receptor endocytosis will affect the equations previously developed. Interest in this phenomenon continues because of its possible relation to drug tolerance, tachyphyllaxis, partial agonism, etc. Additional studies are needed to assess the impact of receptor internalization on our interpretations of dose-response data.

Some idea of how a changing receptor concentration could modify theories of drug action was considered in a theoretical study by Raffa and Tallarida.[42a] For an initial receptor number R_t, the occupancy rate is $dx/dt = k_1 D(R_t - x)$ for drug in amount D that greatly exceeds R_t. If receptors are internalized at a net rate that is proportional to occupancy (proportionality constant a), then the rate equation is given by $dx/dt = k_1 D(R_t - x - ax)$ and the steady-state amount of complex is

$$x_{ss} = \frac{D\,R_t}{(1 + a)D + K}$$

Thus the steady-state amount of complex is less than it would be in the absence of endocytosis, yet the reduction in effect is not readily predictable since the effect of an agonist is an unknown function of occupancy. Experiments with competitive antagonists, in which the pA_2 is determined, may, however be subject to re-interpretation. It has been shown [54a] that if the competitive antagonist also promotes receptor endocytosis at a rate proportional to occupancy (proportionality constant b), then the pA_2 is no longer equal to $-\log(K)$; instead $pA_2 = -\log(K) + \log(1 + b)$.

References

1. Ariëns EJ: Affinity and intrinsic activity in the theory of competitive inhibition: problems and theory. *Arch Int Pharmacodynam* 1954;99:32.
2. Ariëns EJ: *Molecular Pharmacology.* New York, Academic Press, 1964.
3. Arunlakshana O, Schild HO: Some quantitative uses of drug antagonists. *Br J Pharmacol* 1959;14:48.
4. Barlow RB, Scott NC, Stephenson RP: The affinity and efficacy of onium salts on frog rectus abdominus. *Br J Pharmacol* 1967;31:188.
5. Besse JC, Furchgott RF: Dissociation constants and relative efficacies of agonists acting on alpha adrenergic receptors in rabbit aorta. *J Pharmacol Exp Ther* 1976;197:66.
6. Broadley KJ, Nicholson CD: Estimation of dissociation constants and relative efficacies of isoprenaline, orciprenaline and terbutaline in guinea pig isolated atria by use of functional antagonism. *Br J Pharmacol* 1978;64:420P.
7. Colquhoun D: in *Drug Receptors* (HP Rang, ed.) London, Macmillan, 1973.
8. Changeux JP, Thiery J, Tung Y, Kittel C: On cooperativity of biological membranes. *Proc. US Natl Acad Sci* 1967;57:335.
9. Clark AJ: *The Mode of Action of Drugs on Cells.* Baltimore, Williams & Wilkins, 1933.
10. Cope FW: A theory of enzyme kinetics based on electron conduction through the enzymatic particles with applications to cytochrome oxidases and to free radical decay in melanin. *Arch Biochem Biophys* 1963;103:352.
11. Cope FW: I melanin free radical kinetics and mechanism in relation to the Roginski Elovich equation and the adsorption of oxygen by semiconductors. *J Chem Physics* 1964;440:2653.
12. Cope FW: A review of the applications of solid state physics concepts to biological systems. *J Biol Physics* 1975;3:1.
13. Cope FW: Derivation of the Weber-Fechner Law and the Lowenstein equation as the steady-state response of an Elovich solid state biological system. *Bull Math Biol* 1976;38:111.

14. Czerlinski GH: *Chemical Relaxation*. New York, Marcel Dekker, 1966.
15. Ehrlich P: in *The Collected Papers of Paul Ehrlich*. vol III, *Chemotherapy* (F. Himmelweit, ed.). London, Pergamon, 1960.
16. Faller L: Relaxation methods in chemistry. *Sci Am*, p. 30, 1969.
17. Furchgott RF: The pharmacological differentiation of adrenergic receptors. *Ann NY Acad Sci* 1967;139:553.
18. Furchgott RF: Pharmacological characterization of receptors: Its relation to radioligand binding studies. *Fed Proc* 1978;37:115.
19. Furchgott RF, Bursztyn P: Comparisons of dissociation constants and relative efficacies of selected agonists acting on parasympathetic receptors. *Ann NY Acad Sci* 1967;144:882.
20. Furchgott RF, Ehrreich SJ, Greenblatt E: The photoactivated relaxation of smooth muscle of rabbit aorta. *J Gen Physiol* 1961;44:499.
21. Furchgott RF, Jurkiewicz A, Jurkiewicz NF: in *Frontiers of Catecholamine Research* (E. Usdin and S. Snyder, eds.) New York, Pergamon, p. 295, 1973.
22. Gaddum JH: The quantitative effects of antagonistic drugs. *J Physiol (Lond)* 1937;89:7.
23. Gaddum JH: Biologic aspects: The antagonism of drugs. *Trans Faraday Soc* 1943;39:323.
24. Gero A: in *Drill's Pharmacology in Medicine*, 4th ed. (J.R. Di Palma, ed.) New York, McGraw-Hill, 1971, p. 71.
25. Gero A: Use of the biological stimulus in determining parameters of drug action and its relationship to the drug effect: A contribution to the theory of drug action. *J Theor Biol* 1978;74:469.
26. Gero A, Tallarida RJ: Biological stimulus and drug effect. *J Theor Biol* 1977;69:265.
27. Guldberg CM, Waage P: Forhandlinger i Videnskabs i Christiania. *Etudes Affi Chem* 1864;35:92,111.
28. Hill CM, Waight RD, Bardsley WG: Does any enzyme follow the Michaelis-Menten equation? *Mol Cell Biol* 1977;15:173.
29. Homer LD: Receptor occupation theory of drug responses. *J Theor Biol* 1967; 17:399.
30. Jacob LS, Tallarida RJ: Further studies on the action of ultraviolet light on vascular smooth muscle: Effect of partial irreversible receptor blockade. *Arch Int Pharmacodyn* 1977;225:166.
31. Jenkinson DH: The antagonism between tubocurarine and substances which depolarize the endplate. *J Physiol* 1960;152:309.
32. Karlin AJ: On the application of a plausible model of allosteric proteins to the receptor for acetylcholine. *J Theor Biol* 1967;16:306.
33. Katz B, Thesleff S: A study of the desensitization produced by acetylcholine at the motor endplate. *J Physiol* 1957;138:63.
34. Kenakin TP, Black JW: The pharmacological classification of practolol and chlorpractolol. *Mol Pharmacol* 1978;14:607.
35. Langley JN: On the physiology of the salivary secretion. *J Physiol* 1878;1:339.
36. Langley JN: On the reaction of cells and nerve endings to certain poisons. *J Physiol* 1905;33:374.
37. Langmuir J: The constitution and fundamental properties of solids and liquids: I, solids. *J Am Chem Soc* 1916;38:2221.
38. MacKay D: How should pA_2 and affinity constants for pharmacological competitive antagonists be estimated? *J Pharm Pharmacol* 1978;30:312.

39. Monod J, Changeux JP, Jacob J: Allosteric proteins and control systems. *J Mol Biol* 1963;6:306.
40. Monod J, Wyman J, Changeux JP: On the nature of allosteric transitions: A plausible model. *J Mol Biol* 1965;12:88.
41. Nickerson M: Receptor occupancy and tissue response. *Nature* 1956;178:697.
42. Paton WDM: A theory of drug action based on the rate of drug-receptor combination. *Proc R Soc [Biol]* 1961;54:21.
42a. Raffa RB, Tallarida RJ: The concept of a changing receptor concentration: Implications for the theory of drug action. *J Theor Biol* 1985;115:625.
43. Schild HO: pA_2, a new scale for the measurement of drug antagonists. *Br J Pharmacol* 1947;2:189.
44. Sheys EM, Green RD: A quantitative study of alpha adrenergic receptors in the spleen and aorta of the rabbit. *J Pharmacol Exp Ther* 1972;180:317.
45. Stephenson RP: A modification of receptor theory. *Br J Pharmacol* 1956;11:379.
46. Stone M, Angus JA: Development of computer-based estimation of pA_2 values and associated analysis. *J Pharmacol Exp Ther* 1978;207:705.
47. Szabadi E: A theoretical study of two functionally opposite receptor populations. *Br J Pharmacol* 1975;55:311P.
48. Takemori AE, Kupferberg J, Miller JW: Quantitative studies of the antagonism of morphine by nalorphine and naloxone. *J Pharmacol Exp Ther* 1969;169:39.
49. Takemori AE, Hyashi G, Smits SE: Studies on the quantitative antagonism of analgesics by naloxone and diprenorphine. *Eur J Pharmacol* 1972;20:85.
50. Tallarida RJ, Cowan A, Adler MW: pA_2 and receptor differentiation: A statistical analysis of competitive antagonism. *Life Sci* (minireview) 1979;25:637.
51. Tallarida RJ, Laskin O, Jacob LS: Perturbation of drug receptor equilibrium in the presence of competitive blocking agents. *J Theor Biol* 1976;61:211.
52. Tallarida RJ, Sevy RW, Harakal C: Relaxation methods for the determination of drug receptor affinities. *Bull Math Biophysics* 1970;32:65.
53. Tallarida RJ, Sevy RW, Harakal C, Loughnane M: Characteristics of photorelaxation in vascular smooth muscle: Evidence supporting the hypothesis of drug–receptor equilibrium disturbance. *IEEE Trans Biomed Engineering* 1975;22:493.
54. Tallarida RJ, Sevy RW, Harakal C, Bendrick J, Faust R: The effect of preload on the dissociation constant of norepinephrine in isolated strips of rabbit thoracic aorta. *Arch Int Pharmacoyn* 1974;210:67.
54a. Tallarida RJ, Raffa RB, Aceto JF: Receptor down regulation, competitive antagonism and pA_2. *FASEB*, April, 1986.
55. Tallarida RJ, Murray RB: *Manual of Pharmacologic Calculation with Computer Programs*, 2nd ed., New York, Springer-Verlag, 1987.
56. Thron CD: On the analysis of pharmacologic experiments in terms of an allosteric receptor model. *Mol Pharmacol* 1973;9:1.
57. Waud DR: Pharmacological receptors. *Pharmacol Rev* 1968;20:49.
58. Waud DR: On the measurement of affinity of partial agonists for receptors. *J Pharmacol Exp Ther* 1969;170:117.
59. Waud DR: in *Methods in Pharmacology 3. Smooth Muscle* (E.E. Daniel and D.M. Paton, eds.) New York, Plenum, 1975, Chapt. 27.

Additional Readings

Colquhoun D: How fast do drugs work? *Trends Pharmacol Sci* August, 1981.

Kenakin TP: The Classification of drugs and drug receptors in isolated tissues. *Pharmacol Rev* 36:165, 1984.

Klotz IM: Numbers of receptor sites from Scatchard graphs: Facts and fantasies. *Science* 217:24, 1982.

Limbird LE: *Cell surface receptors: A short course on theory and methods*. Martinus Nijhoff, Boston, 1986.

Poste G, Crooke ST: (eds.) *Mechanisms of receptor regulation*. Plenum, New York, 1985.

Raffa RB, Tallarida RJ: The concept of a changing receptor concentration: implications for the theory of drug action. *J Theor Biol* 1985;115:625.

Tallarida RJ, Jacob LS: *The dose response relation in pharmacology*. Springer-Verlag, New York, 1979.

9
Radioligand Binding

Introduction

The use of radioligands to study receptors originated with the development of radiolabeled peptide hormones. In 1970 it was reported that ^{125}I-angiotensin [25] and ^{125}I-adrenocorticotrophic hormone [23] could be used to directly study the interactions of hormones with specific binding sites in the membrane. The first successful radioligand binding assay for neurotransmitter receptors, reported in 1971, measured the nicotinic cholinergic receptors present in the electric organs of fish and eels[7,27]. In 1973 the stereospecific binding of radiolabeled opiates in mammalian brain was demonstrated.[33,38,41] Over the next ten years, quantitative radioligand binding assays were developed for a number of receptors. Currently, appropriate ligands radiolabeled with tritium or iodine are available for the study of many receptors, including adrenergic receptors, cholinergic receptors, dopaminergic receptors, serotonergic receptors, and opiate receptors. This widespread availability has led to a rapid growth in the use of radioligand binding assays to characterize receptors and receptor subtypes.

In general, a receptor performs two important functions. First, it selectively recognizes and binds only those hormones, transmitters or drugs that have a specific molecular structure. Thus, it discriminates between appropriate agonists and all of the other molecules to which it is routinely exposed. Second, the receptor also functions as a transducer, that is, when an agonist binds to it, a series of steps that results in a biological response must ensue. It is commonly thought that the binding of an agonist to a receptor induces a conformational change that initiates this reaction sequence. Before the advent of radioligand binding assays, the properties of the receptor were inferred only from the measurement of biological responses. This approach proved to be very productive in the classification of receptors and even led to the discrimination of subtypes of receptors. There are a number of potential problems, however, that can arise when measuring a biological response either in vivo or in vitro. For example, in vivo the tissue distribution of an administered drug may vary depending on its ability to cross diffusion barriers, such as the blood-brain barrier, or the extent to which the drug binds to plasma proteins. In vitro, the lipophilic or hydrophilic nature of a compound can determine whether or not it has equal access to all the receptors. Drugs can also be metabolized before they have an opportunity to interact with the receptor. Metabolic transformations can produce compounds that are either more or less active than the parent drug, and thus markedly alter the observed pharmacological specificity. Drugs that are not subject to structural alteration are often removed from the extracellular environment by neuronal and extraneuronal uptake mechanisms. In vivo, the response to a drug is frequently attenuated by the activation of compensatory feedback mechanisms. The interpretation of a measured biological response can also be difficult if the drug has multiple sites of action. This phenomenon can occur in vitro with tissues that contain multiple receptor subtypes. When the receptor subtypes are linked to the same effector system, the observed pharmacological response is affected by the degree of selectivity of the drug. In general, the most reliable characterization of receptors results from simple isolated tissue preparations that exhibit reproducible graded dose-response curves. Even with such preparations, it is often impossible to measure accurately the kinetic characteristics of drug–receptor interactions.

The application of radioligand-binding techniques to the study of receptors has overcome many of the limitations inherent to studies that rely only on the measurement of biological responses. Radioligands provide precise probes that permit specific examination of the initial interaction between drug and receptor. For example, the kinetics of the association and dissociation of radioligand–receptor complex can be accurately determined from a simple tissue homogenate preparation. A pharmacological profile that is based on the equilibrium dissociation constants of a series of unlabeled ligands can be constructed by measuring the inhibition of the binding of a radioligand by these unlabeled compounds. Radioligand binding also permits a characterization of receptors without the need of a measurable effect, a fact of importance, for example, in the study of central nervous system receptors, where the effects of neurotransmitters are complex, and isolated tissue preparations are unfeasible. Only radioligand-binding assays can estimate the number or density of receptors in a particular tissue. Consequently, changes in receptor density resulting from pathological conditions or pharmacological intervention can be monitored. Radioligand binding assays can also be used to discriminate multiple receptor subtypes in a single tissue and provide an estimate of their relative proportions. These advantages must, however, be weighed against certain difficulties. Radioligand-binding studies are commonly performed on tissue homogenates rather than on cellularly intact tissues, and it is generally impossible to measure the physiological response mediated by the receptor in this homogenate preparation. In addition, radioligand-binding assays cannot adequately discriminate full agonists that elicit maximal physiological responses from partial agonists that cannot elicit this maximal response.

Many receptors, including α- and β-adrenergic receptors, mediate their effects via stimulation or inhibition of the enzyme adenylate cyclase. Studies utilizing radioligand-binding assays have been important in identifying the individual steps of this reaction. It is now generally accepted that the agonist binds to a receptor, then the resulting agonist-receptor complex binds to a membrane-bound regulatory protein to form a ternary complex before the enzyme is either stimulated or inhibited. The combination of radioligand-binding techniques with autoradiography can lead to the quantitative localization and visualization of receptors. For example, the use of these techniques has resulted in a map of the distribution of β-adrenergic receptor subtypes throughout the rat brain.[35] One of the more promising applications for radioligand-binding assays is in following receptors during solubilization, purification, and reconstitution. Ultimately, these procedures may lead to the complete elucidation of the molecular structures of receptors.

A receptor is defined as the site in or on the cell with which an agonist interacts to produce a response. For a specific binding site for a radioligand to be considered a receptor, it must be shown that this site mediates a biological response. This demonstration requires that a good correlation exists between the dissociation constants of a series of antagonists and agonists measured by radioligand-binding studies and the dissociation constants of the same series of agents derived from an appropriate pharmacological study. A comparison of the dissociation constants derived from radioligand-binding assays, and the measurement of smooth-muscle contraction, resulted in good correlation for both muscarinic and α-adrenergic receptors.[13] More recently, an excellent correlation between dissociation values was reported for the α_1-adrenergic receptor when the pharmacological and binding assays were performed with the same tissue.[28]

There are two basic types of assays that use radioligands. The first type is the direct binding assay in which the direct interaction of the radioligand with the receptor is measured. This assay permits the determination of both kinetic and equilibrium properties and provides an estimate of the density of receptors. It is also used to set the conditions and choose the appropriate radioligand for the second type of assay. The second type, an indirect binding assay, uses the inhibition of the binding of a radioligand by an unlabeled ligand to indirectly measure its interaction with the receptor. This assay is particularly useful in the pharmacological characterization of the receptor because of the vast selection of unlabeled ligands available.

Direct Binding

The simplest model describing the interaction of a radioligand, L, with a receptor, R, to form a complex, RL, is the bimolecular reaction

$$\mathrm{L} + \mathrm{R} \underset{k_{-1}}{\overset{k_1}{\rightleftharpoons}} \mathrm{RL} \tag{9.1}$$

where k_1 and k_{-1} are the rate constants for association and dissociation, respectively.

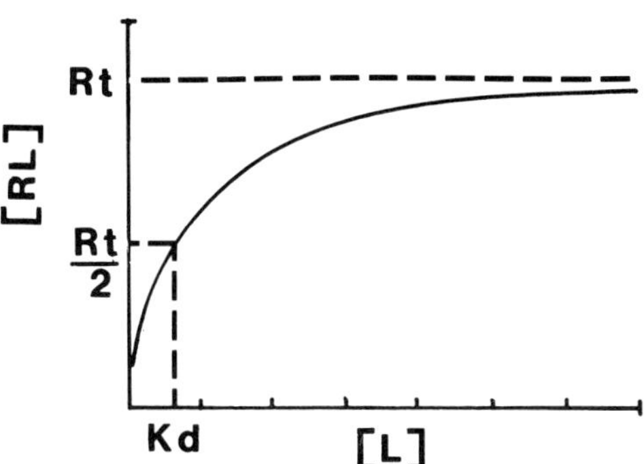

FIGURE 9.1. Theoretical saturation curve. The amount of radioligand bound to the receptor (RL) increases as a function of radioligand concentration until virtually all of the receptors are occupied, i.e., $RL = R_t$.

According to the laws of mass action, at equilibrium

$$K_d = \frac{[R][L]}{[RL]} \tag{9.2}$$

where K_d is the equilibrium dissociation constant, and [R], [L], and [RL] are the concentration of free receptor, free ligand, and ligand–receptor complex, respectively. The kinetic rate constants, k_1 and k_{-1}, and the equilibrium dissociation constant, K_d, are related such that

$$K_d = \frac{K_{-1}}{K_1} \tag{9.3}$$

The total concentration of receptors (R_t), also referred to as B_{max}, is equal to (R) + (RL). Substitution for (R) in equation (9.2) yields

$$K_d = \frac{[(R_t) - (RL)](L)}{(RL)} \tag{9.4}$$

which can be rearranged to form

$$(RL) = \frac{(R_t)(L)}{(L) + (K_d)} \tag{9.5}$$

In a typical saturation experiment, the radioligand is added in a range of concentrations to a fixed concentration of receptor, and the amount of radioligand bound to the receptor, (RL), is measured as a function of radioligand concentration. The concentration of radioligand is increased until virtually all the receptors are occupied or saturated. Figure 9.1 illustrates that the K_d value is equal to the radioligand concentration at which half the receptors are occupied, i.e., $(RL) = (R_t)/2$. Nonlinear regression analysis can be used to fit equation (9.5) to actual saturation data in order to provide estimates of both K_d and R_t. In practice, the radioligand not only binds to the receptor, but also binds to other nonspecific components of the system, including glass, paper, and other cellular membrane structures. The exact nature of nonspecific binding is unknown; however, it is generally nonsaturable and usually occurs instantaneously. It is essential to discriminate between specific and nonspecific binding since typically 5% to 50% of total binding is nonspecific. Moreover, an incorrect definition of

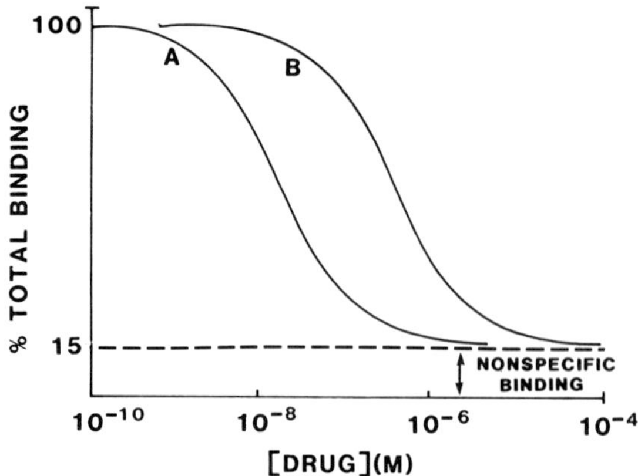

FIGURE 9.2. Determination of nonspecific binding. At high concentrations of unlabeled ligand, the displacement curves reach a plateau value that defines nonspecific binding. In this example, nonspecific binding represents 15% of total binding. Note that although drug A is more potent than drug B, both displacement curves plateau at the same level of binding.

this nonspecific component is a common source of error in the analysis of radioligand-binding data. Nonspecific binding is defined with high concentrations of an unlabeled competing ligand. When the binding of a radioligand is displaced by large concentrations of unlabeled ligand, the amount of radioligand bound should decrease until it reaches a plateau at high concentrations of unlabeled ligand (Figure 9.2). The amount of radioligand that remains bound in the presence of the high concentration of unlabeled ligand is defined as nonspecific binding. In a saturation experiment, the nonspecific component of binding at each radioligand concentration is subtracted from the total amount of radioligand bound to yield the amount of radioligand specifically bound to the receptor. Ideally, the definition of nonspecific binding should be the same for a variety of unlabeled ligands, including both agonists and antagonists.

SCATCHARD ANALYSIS

A very useful method for analyzing saturation binding data is to construct a Scatchard plot.[37] Rearrangement of the equilibrium binding equation (9.4) yields the Scatchard equation:[37]

$$\frac{(\mathrm{LR})}{(\mathrm{L})} = \frac{-(\mathrm{LR})}{K_\mathrm{d}} + \frac{(\mathrm{R_t})}{K_\mathrm{d}} \qquad (9.6)$$

A plot of the ratio of bound to free ligand against the concentration of bound ligand, (LR), is a straight line that has a slope equal to the negative reciprocal of the dissociation constant, $(-1/K_\mathrm{d})$, and an intercept on the abscissa equal to the total concentration of receptors, $(\mathrm{R_t})$(Figure 9.3).

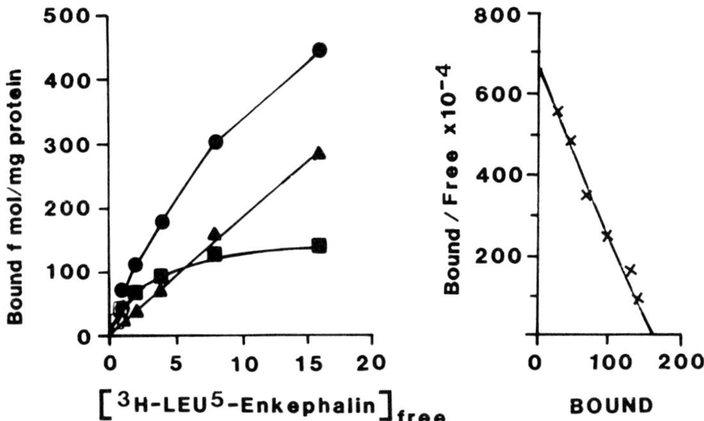

FIGURE 9.3. Typical saturation experiment. Total (●), nonspecific (▲), and specific (■) bindings are plotted as a function of radioligand concentration in the left panel. The specific-binding data are transformed into a Scatchard plot in the right panel. The K_d from the Scatchard plot is 2.4 nM and the B_{max} is 163 fmol/mg protein.

An advantage of the use of Scatchard analysis, as opposed to a nonlinear regression analysis, is that the Scatchard plot is theoretically linear, thereby permitting a reasonably accurate estimate of the total receptor concentration without the use of saturating concentrations of radioligand. This estimate of receptor concentration is determined by simply extrapolating the straight line to the abscissa. This is particularly important in systems with high levels of nonspecific binding since at saturating concentrations the proportion of nonspecific binding increases with increasing concentration of radioligand (Figure 9.2). Another advantage of the Scatchard plot is that visual inspection provides some insight into whether or not a simple bimolecular reaction adequately describes the interaction between ligand and receptor. Curvature in the Scatchard plot implies that this interaction is more complex. A nonlinear Scatchard plot can result from a heterogeneous population of receptors, a multiple step/multiple component binding reaction, or negative or positive cooperativity between the binding sites. Curvilinear Scatchard plots can also be produced artificially by a variety of factors that are discussed in detail by Boeynaems and Dumont.[2] Some of the more common factors include an incorrect definition of nonspecific binding, incomplete separation of bound and free ligand and dissociation during the separation of bound and free ligand. In addition, the reaction may not be at equilibrium for all concentrations of the ligand, since the time to reach equilibrium is a function of the concentration of ligand. To confirm that a simple bimolecular reaction is an accurate model for the system, the dissociation constant should be determined kinetically by measuring the rates of association and dissociation and then comparing their ratio with the equilibrium dissociation constant.

Rate of Association

The rate of association for the interaction of a radioligand with a receptor is determined by measuring the amount of bound ligand, (RL), as a function of time. At time $t = 0$, a specific concentration of radioligand, (L), is added to the receptors and the amount bound (RL) is measured at various times until equilibrium is reached. The amount of radioligand bound depends on the two simultaneously occurring processes of association and dissociation. In the simple bimolecular reaction described in equation (9.1), the rate of association of ligand receptor complex is k_1 (L)(R), and the rate of dissociation of this complex is k_{-1}(RL). Thus, the measured rate of formation of RL is

$$\frac{d(\mathrm{RL})}{dt} = k_1(\mathrm{L})(\mathrm{R}) - k_{-1}(\mathrm{RL}) \tag{9.7}$$

At equilibrium,

$$\frac{d(\mathrm{RL})}{dt} = 0$$

and

$$k_1(\mathrm{L})(\mathrm{R}) = k_{-1}(\mathrm{RL}) \tag{9.8}$$

The values (L) and (R) can be expressed in terms of equilibrium measurements as follows:

$$(\mathrm{L}) = (\mathrm{L}_t) - (\mathrm{RL}_e)$$

$$(\mathrm{R}) = (\mathrm{R}_t) - (\mathrm{RL}_e)$$

where L_t is the total ligand concentration, R_t is the total receptor concentration, and RL_e is the amount of ligand receptor complex at equilibrium. Substitution into equation (9.8) yields

$$k_1[(\mathrm{L}_t) - (\mathrm{RL}_e)][(\mathrm{R}_t) - (\mathrm{RL}_e)] = k_{-1}(\mathrm{RL}_e) \tag{9.9}$$

which can be rearranged to form

$$k_{-1} = k_1 \frac{[(\mathrm{L}_t) - (\mathrm{RL}_e)][(\mathrm{R}_t) - (\mathrm{RL}_e)]}{(\mathrm{RL}_e)} \tag{9.10}$$

Then, substitution for k_{-1} in equation (9.7) yields

$$\frac{d(\mathrm{RL})}{dt} = k_1[(\mathrm{L}_t) - (\mathrm{RL}_e)][(\mathrm{R}_t) - (\mathrm{RL}_e)] - k_1(\mathrm{RL}) \frac{[(\mathrm{L}_t) - (\mathrm{RL}_e)][(\mathrm{R}_t) - (\mathrm{RL}_e)]}{(\mathrm{RL}_e)} \tag{9.11}$$

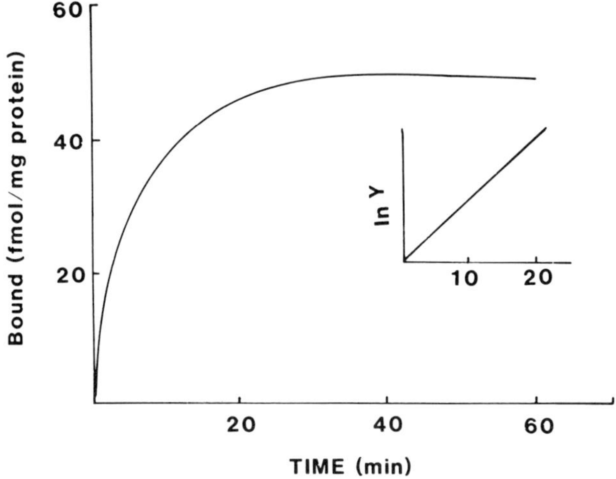

FIGURE 9.4. Rate of association. Time course of ^{125}I-iodopindolol association with β-adrenergic receptors. The reaction reaches equilibrium after 20 minutes. *Inset:* Association is plotted according to the integrated form of the second-order rate equation (9.12). The association constant, k_1, is equal to slope/$[(L_tR_t)/RL_e - RL_e]$.

which is an equation for the formation of ligand–receptor complex in terms of only the association rate constant k_1. The second-order rate equation (9.11) can be integrated to give

$$ln\left[\frac{(RL_e)[(L_t) - (RL)(RL_e)/(R_t)]}{(L_t)[(RL_e) - (RL)]}\right] = k_1t\left[\frac{(L_t)(R_t)}{(RL_3)} - (RL_e)\right] \quad (9.12)$$

The kinetic association constant can be determined from the slope of a plot of the expression on the left side of equation (9.12) against time (Figure 9.4). If the reaction obeys simple bimolecular kinetics, this plot will result in a straight line. Although this expression may seem complicated, only RL actually varies with time. L_t is the total amount of radioligand added at each time point and RL_e is the amount of radioligand bound at equilibrium. R_t is the number of receptors determined by Scatchard analysis of a saturation experiment performed with the same tissue. One disadvantage of this analysis is that the association rate constant is not totally independent of the equilibrium dissociation constant K_d because of the inclusion of R_t in equation (9.12). An advantage in using the full second-order equation is that no assumptions are made about the relative concentrations of radioligand and receptor.

In many radioligand-binding studies the total concentration of radioligand, (L_t), is much greater than the total concentration of receptors, (R_t). Under these conditions there is little or no change in the concentration of free ligand, (L), as the reaction proceeds to equilibrium. Even at equilibrium, only a small fraction

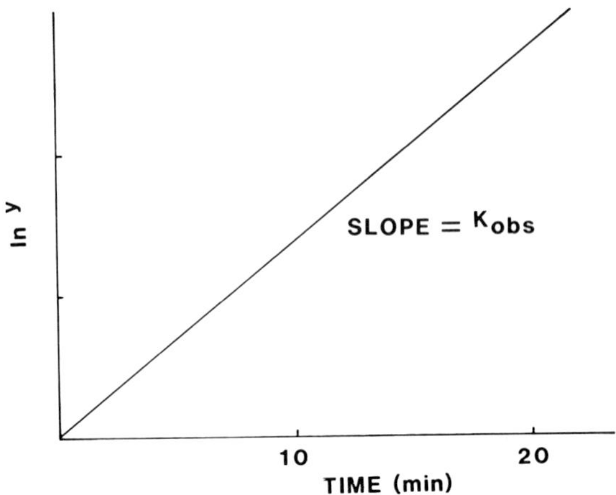

FIGURE 9.5. Pseudo-first-order plot. Association is plotted according to the pseudo-first-order rate equation (9.13).

of the total ligand concentration, (L_t), is bound to the receptor. For all practical purposes, (L) is a constant and the reaction can be considered a "pseudo-first-order" reaction. Thus, equation (9.12) can be simplified to:

$$\ln\left[\frac{(RL_e)}{(RL_e - (RL)}\right] = k_1 t\left[\frac{(L_t)(R_t)}{(RL_e)}\right] \tag{9.13}$$

(See reference 44.) A plot of the term on the left side of equation (9.13) versus time is called a pseudo-first-order plot (Figure 9.5). The association rate constant, k_1, is related to the slope of the pseudo-first-order plot, k_{obs}, as follows:

$$k_1 = \frac{k_{obs}}{(L_t)(R_t)/(RL_e)} \tag{9.14}$$

where L_t, R_t, and RL_e are all constants. In addition to the assumption that $L_t >> RL_e$, the determination of k_1 again depends on the equilibrium measurement of R_t.

One method of analyzing pseudo-first-order time courses eliminates the need for an independent determination of R_t. This method requires the measurement of the slopes of pseudo-first-order plots (k_{obs}) over a range of ligand concentrations.[40] It can be shown (for derivation see reference 44) that the slope of the pseudo-first-order plot, k_{obs}, is related to the ligand concentration, (L), as follows:

$$k_{obs} = k_1(L) + k_{-1} \tag{9.15}$$

A plot of k_{obs} versus ligand concentration results in a straight line with a slope equal to k_1 and an intercept on the ordinate equal to k_{-1} (Figure 9.6).

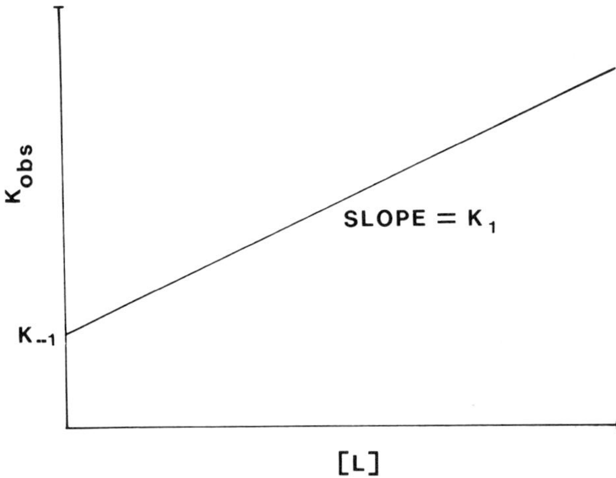

FIGURE 9.6. Determination of rate constants. k_{obs} is plotted as a function of radioligand concentration. From equation (9.15), the slope of the line is equal to k_1 and the intercept on the ordinate is equal to k_{-1}.

The association and dissociation rate constants determined by this method can be compared with the rate constants determined at a single ligand concentration to confirm their accuracy. Curvilinear second-order plots and pseudo-first-order plots imply that a simple bimolecular reaction is inadequate to describe the interaction between the ligand and the receptor. More complex kinetics may result from the same factors that are listed above for curvilinear Scatchard plots.

Rate of Dissociation

The rate of dissociation is determined by stopping the association of the ligand and receptor and measuring the amount of radioligand that remains bound as a function of time. In practice, the reaction between receptor and ligand is allowed to reach equilibrium, and the forward reaction is stopped by "infinite dilution" by the addition of a high concentration of unlabeled competing ligand. The rate of change of ligand-receptor complex concentration becomes

$$\frac{d(\mathrm{RL})}{dt} = -\,k_{-1}\,(\mathrm{RL}) \tag{9.16}$$

so that k_{-1} is a simple, first-order rate constant. Integration of equation (9.16) yields

$$ln\,[(\mathrm{RL})/(\mathrm{RL}_0)] = -\,k_{-1}t \tag{9.17}$$

where (RL) is the concentration of ligand-receptor complex at time t, and (RL_0) is the concentration of ligand receptor complex just prior to dilution by the addi-

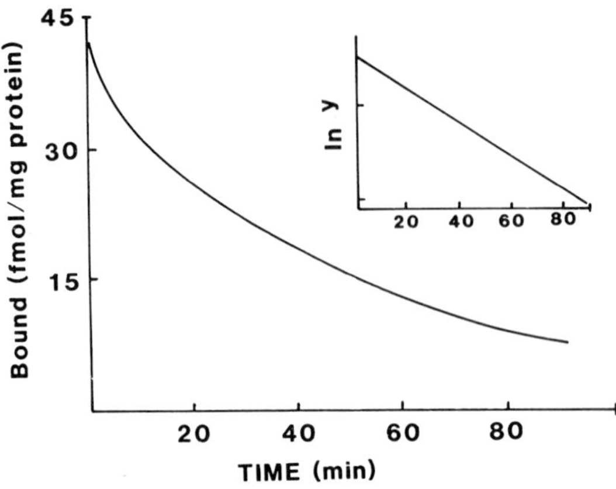

FIGURE 9.7. Rate of dissociation. Time course of ^{125}I-iodopindolol dissociation from β-adrenergic receptors. Dissociation is initiated after the reaction has reached equilibrium (Figure 9.4). *Inset:* Dissociation is plotted according to the integrated first-order rate equation (9.17). The dissociation constant, k_{-1}, is equal to the negative of the slope.

tion of a competing ligand. The dissociation rate constant, k_{-1}, is the negative of the slope in a plot of *l*n [(RL)/(RL$_0$)] versus time (Figure 9.7). A simple bimolecular reaction should be completely reversible; therefore, if the experiment is carried out for a sufficiently long time, the ligand should completely dissociate from the receptor.

The dissociation rate constant has important methodological implications. The most common radioligand-binding technique utilizes vacuum filtration to separate bound from free ligand. This process involves a 15-second exposure to buffer during dilution, filtration, and rinsing of the filter. If the dissociation is too fast, as indicated by a low rate constant, there will be a measurable loss of ligand-receptor complex during the filtration. This can sometimes be prevented by measuring and stopping the reaction at a lower temperature.

Once the association and dissociation rate constants have been determined, the kinetic dissociation constant can be calculated ($K_d = k_{-1}/k_1$). This independently determined dissociation constant can be compared with the equilibrium dissociation constant derived from saturation experiments to verify its accuracy and to validate the assumptions made during the analysis. The kinetic dissociation constant is impossible to determine in functional assays, which must rely solely on equilibrium measurements of K_d.

Two-Site Analysis

Tissue homogenates used in radioligand-binding assays do not always contain a homogeneous population of binding sites for the ligand. This often results from the existence of receptor subtypes, as seen in mammalian heart tissue that con-

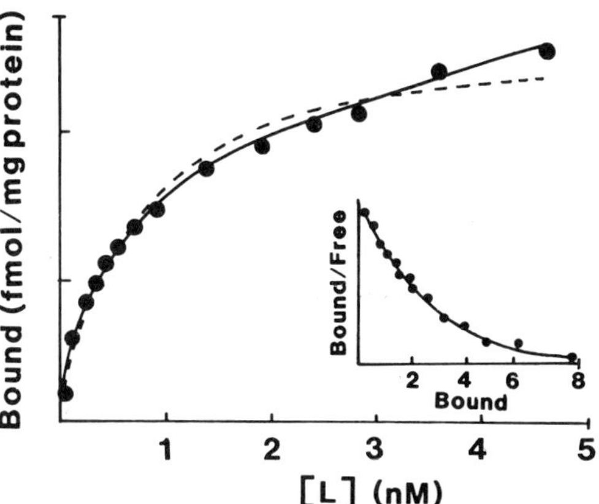

FIGURE 9.8. Two-site saturation analysis. Specific binding of a selective radioligand is plotted as a function of increasing concentrations of radioligand. The dashed line is the best one-site fit and the solid line is the best two-site fit to the data. *Inset:* Scatchard transformation of the saturation data results in a curvilinear plot.

tains both β_1- and β_2-adrenergic receptor subtypes.[3,30] It is also possible for the radioligand to have a high affinity for different receptors. For example, the neuroleptic spiroperidol has high affinity for both dopamine and serotonin receptors in mammalian brain tissue.[24] Multiple populations of receptors or receptor subtypes can be detected in a saturation experiment if the radioligand is selective, i.e., it has a significantly lower dissociation constant for its interaction with one of the receptors. The interaction of a radioligand with two types of receptors is modeled as two independent bimolecular reactions. At equilibrium, the total amount of radioligand bound, B, is

$$B = \frac{(\mathrm{L})(\mathrm{R}_{t1})}{(\mathrm{L}) + (K_{d1})} + \frac{(\mathrm{L})(\mathrm{R}_{t2}}{(\mathrm{L}) + (K_{d2})} \tag{9.18}$$

where (L) is the concentration of radioligand, R_{t1} and R_{t2} are the densities of each population of receptor, and K_{d1} and K_{d2} are the dissociation constants for the interaction of the ligand with each receptor. Nonlinear least-squares regression analysis can be used to fit equation (9.18) to the saturation data (Figure 9.8) in order to provide estimates of the dissociation constants and the receptor densities of each population of receptors. The validity of the two-site model is tested by comparing the goodness of fit of the one-site and two-site models. The improvement of fit is estimated statistically from an F-test on the sum of squares of the residuals. The F value for this test is

$$F = \frac{(SS_1 - SS_2)/(df_1 - df_2)}{SS_2/df_2} \tag{9.19}$$

where SS_1 and SS_2 are the sums of squares of the residuals for the one-site and two-site fits, respectively, and df_1 and df_2 are the degrees of freedom for each fit.[15] Results from this analysis should be interpreted with caution since the above listed factors that lead to curvilinear Scatchard plots also cause complex saturation curves. Scatchard transformation of the saturation data for the interaction of a selective radioligand with multiple receptor subtypes will result in a curvilinear plot (Figure 9.8). It is difficult to use this transformed data to provide estimates of the parameters K_d and R_t of the two subtypes. The dependent variable, ligand bound, appears on both the abscissa and the ordinate; therefore, the individual Scatchard equations cannot be simply added together. Moreover, any error in the measurement of the amount of radioligand bound is propagated from the abscissa to the ordinate. In the presence of multiple receptor subtypes, the Scatchard plot is most effectively used to provide quick visual confirmation of the existence of a heterogeneous population of binding sites. A comprehensive approach to establishing the existence of multiple subtypes of receptors is described in the section on indirect binding studies.

Indirect Binding

The interactions of unlabeled ligands with a receptor can be indirectly characterized by studying their ability to inhibit the binding of a radioligand. Since unlabeled ligands are far more numerous than radioligands, indirect binding assays are essential to completely characterize a population of receptors. Classically, receptors have been classified by the order of potency of various compounds that either stimulate or antagonize the functional response. Indirect binding assays permit the measurement of an analogous "pharmacological profile" based on the dissociation constants for several compounds determined from the inhibition of radioligand binding. This pharmacological profile may actually be more accurate than one determined in a functional assay, since factors such as spare receptors and partial agonism, which complicate the interpretation of results from functional assays, often have no effect on radioligand-binding assays. Another important use of indirect binding assays is to define the level of nonspecific binding, as described earlier. This definition of nonspecific binding is used in the analysis of both direct and indirect binding data and should be established prior to the measurement of the kinetic and equilibrium properties of the radioligand. In a typical competition experiment, the binding of a fixed concentration of radioligand is inhibited by increasing concentrations of unlabeled ligand. The amount of radioligand that remains bound to the receptor, (RL), is

$$\mathrm{RL} = (\mathrm{RL}_t) - \frac{(\mathrm{RL}_t)(I)}{(I) + IC_{50}} \tag{9.20}$$

where RL_t is the amount of radioligand bound to the receptor in the absence of the unlabeled competing ligand, I is the concentration of free unlabeled ligand, and IC_{50} is the concentration of unlabeled ligand that inhibits 50% of the specific binding of the radioligand. Equation (9.20) can be rearranged to a simpler form:

$$\mathrm{RL} = \frac{(\mathrm{RL}_t)}{1 + [(I)/IC_{50}]} \tag{9.21}$$

Nonlinear regression analysis can be used to fit this equation to the inhibition data and provide an estimate of the IC_{50} value (Figure 9.9). The level of non-

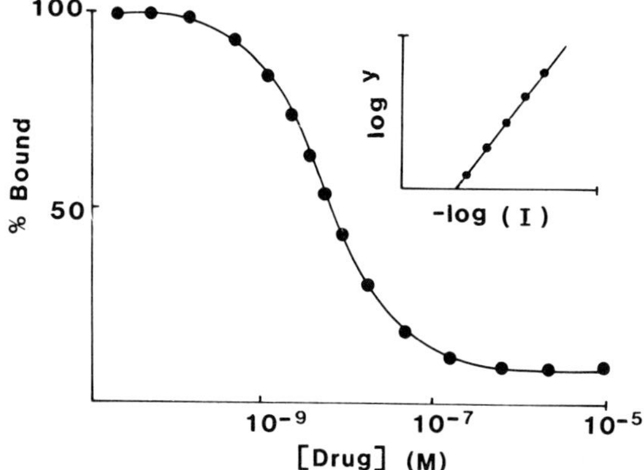

FIGURE 9.9. Typical competition curve. The amount of radioligand that remains bound to the receptor is plotted as a function of increasing inhibitor concentration. *Inset:* The indirect Hill plot constructed from the competition data has a slope equal to the Hill coefficient and an intercept on the abscissa equal to $-\log(\mathrm{IC}_{50})$.

specific binding can be determined experimentally, or it can be determined from the regression analysis by adding a term for nonspecific binding to both sides of equation (9.21). The equilibrium dissociation constant (K_I) of the unlabeled competing ligand, I, is related to the IC_{50} value by the Cheng and Prusoff[8] equation:

$$K_I = \frac{IC_{50}}{1 + (\mathrm{L})/K_L} \tag{9.22}$$

where L is the concentration of free radioligand and K_L is the equilibrium dissociation constant of the radioligand. Since the concentration of free unlabeled ligand is difficult to determine experimentally, it is approximated by the total concentration of unlabeled ligand in the assay. This is usually valid if the concentration of receptors is much less than the dissociation constant for the unlabeled ligand. Furthermore, the amount of radioligand bound should be much less than the total concentration of radioligand to prevent a significant change in the concentration of free radioligand by the addition of high concentrations of unlabeled competing ligand. Note, if $(\mathrm{L})/K_L << 1$, then $K_I = IC_{50}$.

Hill Plot

Another useful method for analyzing indirect binding data is the construction of an indirect Hill plot[18] from the following equation:

$$\log\left[\frac{(\mathrm{RL}_t)}{(\mathrm{RL}) - (\mathrm{RL}_I)}\right] = -\mathrm{n}\log(I) + \mathrm{n}\log(IC_{50}) \tag{9.23}$$

where RL_I is the amount of radioligand bound to the receptor in the presence of unlabeled ligand, RL is the amount of radioligand bound in the absence of unlabeled ligand, I is the concentration of unlabeled ligand, and IC_{50} is the concentration of unlabeled ligand that inhibits 50% of specific binding. A plot of log $[(RL_I)/(RL) - (RL_I)]$ versus log (I) has a slope value of $-n$, which is the apparent Hill coefficient, and an intercept on the abscissa of log (IC_{50}). The Hill coefficient is also referred to as the Hill slope, and it provides a convenient index of the steepness of slope of the inhibition curve (Figure 9.9). Only those concentrations of unlabeled ligand that inhibit between 10% and 90% of specific binding are included, since the Hill plot deviates from linearity at the extremes. If the reaction follows mass-action principles at equilibrium, the apparent Hill coefficient will be equal to one. A Hill coefficient significantly different from one indicates a more complex interaction between ligand and receptor. This may result from a heterogeneous population of binding sites, a two-step/three-component binding system, negative or positive cooperativity between sites or an incorrect definition of nonspecific binding. A heterogeneous population of binding sites may be indicative of multiple receptor subtypes, which is a topic that will be discussed in detail in a following section. It is important to note that the addition of a competing ligand increases the time required for the reaction to reach equilibrium. Thus, the incubation time of the indirect binding assay should be greater than the time to equilibrium determined for the radioligand in the direct binding assays.[44]

Ternary Complex Formation

A Hill coefficient less than one for the interaction of an agonist with a receptor often results from a two-step reaction that involves three components and leads to the formation of a ternary complex.[9,22] According to this reaction scheme, the agonist binds to the receptor and causes a conformational change. The agonist-receptor complex then interacts with a third component in the membrane to form a ternary complex. This ternary complex model appears to accurately describe agonist interactions in a number of receptor systems that are linked to the enzyme adenylate cyclase. For example, the interaction of agonists with the β-adrenergic receptor results in the formation of a high-affinity ternary complex composed of agonist, β-receptor, and guanine nucleotide-binding protein.[11] The formation of ternary complex appears to be a required step in the stimulation or inhibition of adenylate cyclase.[39] Addition of the nucleotide guanosine triphosphate (GTP) appears to destabilize the ternary complex so that only the initial interaction of the agonist with the receptor can be detected. In the presence of GTP, the affinity of the receptor for the agonist is decreased and the slope of the inhibition curve is increased.[26] Hegstrand et al[16] examined the effects of guanine nucleotides on agonist interactions in tissues known to contain only a single homogeneous population of β-adrenergic receptors. They demonstrated that the presence of guanine nucleotides increased the Hill coefficients from 0.7 to 0.8 to one. Similar effects of guanine nucleotides on agonist interactions have been reported for dopamine receptors[46] and α-adrenergic receptors.[42] Thus, in systems coupled to the enzyme adenylate cyclase, addition of GTP in radioligand-binding assays appears to pre-

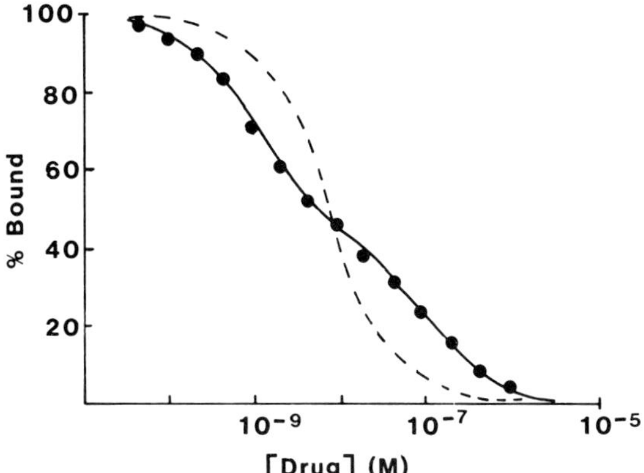

FIGURE 9.10. Two-site competition analysis. Inhibition of the binding of a nonselective radioligand by a selective competing drug. The dashed line is the best one-site fit to the data and the solid line is the best two-site fit. Improvement of fit, determined using equation (9.19), was significant at $p < .0001$.

vent the accumulation of ternary complex and permit the characterization of the initial reaction between agonist and receptor. The degree to which ternary complex formation changes the Hill coefficient in these systems appears to be a function of the ratio of guanine nucleotide-binding protein concentration to receptor concentration. If the ratio of binding protein to receptor is one or less, the Hill coefficient will be significantly less than one. Conversely, when there is a large excess of binding protein relative to receptor, there will be little or no change in the Hill coefficient.[44]

Two-Site Analysis

A Hill coefficient less than one can also result from the presence of multiple receptor subtypes. If an unlabeled competing ligand is selective for one of the subtypes, i.e., if it has a lower dissociation constant for one population of sites, the inhibition curve will be shallow and the Hill coefficient will be less than one. Inhibition of the binding of a nonselective radioligand by a selective competing ligand is described by the following equation:

$$\mathrm{RL} = \frac{(\mathrm{RL}_1)}{1 + [(I)/IC_1]} + \frac{(\mathrm{RL}_2)}{1 + [(I)/IC_2]} \tag{9.24}$$

where RL is the total amount of radioligand bound, RL_1 and RL_2 are the total number of sites of each subtype labeled by the radioligand in the absence of competing ligand, I is the concentration of competing ligand, and IC_1 and IC_2 are the concentrations of competing ligand that inhibit 50% of the binding to each receptor subtype, respectively. Nonlinear regression analysis is used to provide estimates for each of the parameters (Figure 9.10). This analysis assumes that the interaction of both the radioligand and the competing ligand with each receptor subtype follows mass-action principles. The improvement in the fit with the two-site model compared with the one-site model described by equation (9.21) is determined from the F value calculated with equation (9.19). Nonlinear regression analysis can be used to estimate all the parameters, including total binding ($RL_1 + RL_2$) and the level of nonspecific binding. This approach increases the number of parameters to be fit and consequently decreases the precision of the estimates of each parameter.* The accuracy of the determinations of total and nonspecific binding can be improved by increasing the number of measurements of these values. To ensure that only two receptor subtypes are being discriminated, a three-site model can be constructed by adding a third term to equation (9.24). If there are only two subtypes present, there should be no significant improvement in fit when the three-site model is compared with the two-site model.

Inhibition curves can also be analyzed by transforming the data according to the method of Eadie[12] and Hofstee.[19] This transformation involves the construction of a plot of the ratio of bound to free ligand versus bound ligand. The Hofstee plot is linear if there is a homogeneous population of receptors, or if the competing ligand is nonselective. In the presence of receptor subtypes, however, a selective competing ligand will produce a curvilinear Hofstee plot. Like the curvilinear Scatchard plot, a curvilinear Hofstee provides visual confirmation that the competing ligand is interacting with more than one population of receptors. Analysis of the curvilinear Hofstee plot is subject to the same statistical and mathematical limitations described for the analysis of curvilinear Scatchard plots.

Analysis of Receptor Subtypes

Radioligand-binding assays are routinely used to characterize the kinetic properties of receptor subtypes in a wide variety of tissues. This characterization is completely independent of the functional response elicited by the receptor. This is particularly important in the study of the central nervous system (CNS) because the effects mediated by neurotransmitter receptors are often complex behaviors that are not easily quantified. Under these circumstances, it is difficult to use classical pharmacological techniques to characterize these receptors. Accordingly, radioligand-binding techniques have been used extensively to localize and characterize CNS receptors. Further, these techniques have the specificity to discriminate subtypes of these receptors. Classification of receptors is also complicated by the existence of multiple subtypes of receptors in a single tissue.† Both β_1- and β_2-adrenergic receptors are present[30] but only β_1-receptors have

*Alternatively, total and nonspecific binding can be determined experimentally.

†For example, beta-adrenergic receptors are present in the heart (1) where they mediate the chronotropic and inotropic effects of catecholamines (4).

been shown to mediate the inotropic effects of catecholamines.[5] The inotropic effect elicited by any β-adrenergic drug is heavily influenced by its selectivity for the β_1- or β_2-receptor subtype and the relative proportions of these subtypes in the heart. A characterization of β-receptors based on inotropic effects would clearly be inadequate, whereas radioligand-binding studies can provide a pharmacological profile for each subtype in this tissue and a measure of the relative proportion of each.

Two approaches have been developed to study receptors in tissues that contain multiple receptor subtypes. The first approach uses the direct binding assay with a radioligand that is selective for one of the subtypes. If the radioligand is completely selective, the density of a single receptor subtype can be determined from a saturation experiment, and the pharmacological profile for this receptor subtype can be determined from the inhibition of the binding of this radioligand. There are only a few radioligands that are known to be completely selective. These include prazosin at the α_1-receptor, clonidine at the α_2-receptor, and spiroperidol at the D-2 (dopaminergic) receptor. If, as is more common, the radioligand is partially selective, nonlinear regression analysis of the saturation data provides estimates of the relative densities of the subtypes and their different affinities for the radioligand. Since the number of selective radioligands is limited, a second approach was developed to take advantage of the availability of numerous selective unlabeled ligands. The second approach involves the inhibition of the binding of a nonselective radioligand by unlabeled competing ligands. The relative proportions of the subtypes and their affinities for each ligand can be determined by nonlinear regression analysis of the inhibition curves. Regardless of the ligand used for the determination, the number and relative proportions of the subtypes in a specific tissue should always be the same. In practice, it is usually impossible to discriminate more than two, at most three, receptor subtypes on the basis of nonlinear regression analysis. It takes at least 15 to 18 concentrations of competing ligand to define two subtypes reliably and precisely.[31] The limits of resolution of nonlinear regression analysis also depend on the relative proportions of the subtypes present and the selectivity of the ligands. For example, these limits were experimentally determined in the β-adrenergic system by combining various proportions of previously characterized pure β_1- and β_2-adrenergic receptor preparations.[10] A mixture of 90:10 or 10:90 high- and low-affinity receptor subtypes was resolved with ligands that were at least 70-fold selective. Alternatively, a ligand that was only sixfold selective discriminated a 50:50 mixture of receptor subtypes.[10] It is also important to verify that all of the ligands are interacting with the receptors according to the principles of mass action. This is accomplished by performing indirect binding assays in tissues that contain only one receptor subtype. Analysis of inhibition data from these tissues should yield Hill coefficients equal to one and linear Hofstee plots. This has been demonstrated for subtypes of the β-adrenergic receptor from studies of ^{125}I-iodohydroxybenzylpindolol binding in rat cortex, rat liver, and guinea-pig ventricle. The rat cortex contains both β_1- and β_2-receptor subtypes, and the selective antagonists zinterol and IPS-339 both produced markedly curvilinear Hofstee plots. In contrast, in the guinea-pig ventricle, which contains only β_1-receptors, and the rat liver, which contains only β_2-receptors, each antagonist produced linear Hofstee plots and Hill coefficients of one.[29] If the concept of a receptor is to have any meaning, the properties of the receptor should be conserved in different tissues. Thus, the pharmacological profile of a receptor subtype should be the same, regardless of whether it is derived from tissues that contain a single subtype or tissues that contain multiple subtypes. This has been demonstrated in the β-adrenergic system where the dissociation constants for seven selective drugs measured in heterogeneous and homogeneous tissues were compared. The correlation coefficient for both β_1- and β_2-receptors for heterogeneous against homogeneous tissues was found to be 0.99.[29]

Radioligand-Binding Techniques

The development of reliable ligand-binding assays has led to rapid advances in our understanding of receptors and receptor-mediated mechanisms. Despite the diversity exhibited by receptors, they share certain fundamental properties that result in common difficulties in their measurement. Consequently, a limited number of techniques have been found to be generally applicable in studying many different types of receptors. For example, virtually all membrane receptors are present in extremely small quantities and in a highly impure state. Thus, specific and sensitive techniques are required for their detection and characterization. All of the methods described in this section capitalize on the ability of the receptors to bind specific ligands with high specificity. Moreover, precise measurement of such small quantities of receptor is permitted by using highly radioactive ligands. This section is intended to provide a brief overview of current radioligand binding methodology and additional detail may be obtained by consulting the literature cited.

Tissue Preparations

Cell-free tissue homogenates are the most common preparation used in the study of radioligand binding. These homogenates are obtained by placing a tissue sample into a buffer solution, homogenizing and subjecting the homogenate to differential centrifugation. The centrifugation usually results in a fraction consisting of membrane fragments that are partially enriched in plasma membrane. This enrichment is desirable, since most receptors are located on the plasma membrane. The final membrane fraction is then resuspended in the desired volume of buffer solution and ready for incubation with radioligand. Some tissues are more amenable to this preparation than others. For example, brain tissue often contains high densities of receptors and is easily homogenized whereas vascular tissue has lower densities of receptors and is difficult to homogenize because of the presence of the structural protein collagen. One advantage of this preparation is that in many tissues, the adenylate cyclase response is preserved.

For receptor systems that are linked to adenylate cyclase, this permits the measurement of a functional response and radioligand binding under virtually identical conditions in vitro. A good correlation between the action of drugs on the cyclase response and their binding characteristics would support the contention that the binding site is indeed a functional receptor.

In addition to membrane preparations, radioligand-binding assays are also carried out with isolated intact cells. An obvious advantage of working with intact cells is that the structural and metabolic environments of the cell are more similar to in vivo conditions. The disadvantage is that the isolation of these cells is more difficult than the preparation of membrane fragments. The problems associated with isolation of intact cell have been circumvented by growing cells in tissue culture. One notable example is the S-49 mouse lymphoma cell that contains a high density of β-adrenergic receptors that are coupled to adenylate cyclase.[21,36] Mutant cell lines of these S-49 cells have been developed that lack functional guanine nucleotide-binding protein[36] or are uncoupled from the receptor.[14] These mutant cell lines have been valuable in elucidating the role of ternary complex in the regulation of adenylate cyclase. Both isolated and grown cells have also been used to investigate the phenomenon of desensitization in vitro.

Radioligand-binding assays are used to follow the receptors during their solubilization, purification, and reconstitution. Receptors are solubilized by the addition of a detergent, such as digitonin, to a homogenate of membrane fragments. The detergent destabilizes the membrane and releases the receptor into solution. The solubilized receptor is initially purified by column chromatography. An affinity column is constructed which contains a high-affinity ligand as a component of its adsorbent material. When the solubilized receptor is run over the column, it is preferentially retained, whereas the majority of nonspecific proteins are eluted. The receptors are eluted off the column with a media that contains an excess of high-affinity ligand. This procedure has resulted in a 2,000-fold purification of the β-receptor.[43] The final step in the purification procedure is sodium dodecyl sulfate (SDS)-polyacrilimide gel electrophoresis, which separates the remaining proteins on the basis of molecular weight and charge distribution. This has resulted in a 55,000-fold purification of the β-receptor.[6] Ideally, after the receptor has been purified, it can be reconstituted into an intact cell or vesicle to determine whether or not it has retained its functional properties. Ultimately, purification of the receptor will lead to the elucidation of its molecular structure.

Radioisotopes

Radioligands used in the study of receptors are most frequently labeled with either iodine or tritium. The major advantage of iodinated ligands is their high specific activity. Incorporation of one atom of ^{125}I per molecule of ligand would produce a compound with a specific radioactivity of 2,175 Ci/mmol. The high specific activity means that low concentrations of radioligand can be detected and, consequently, that low concentrations of receptors can be used in the assay.

This can be a very important consideration when the availability of tissue is limited. The disadvantages of iodinated ligands are the relatively short half-life (60 days) and the alteration in the biological properties of the ligand by incorporation of an iodine molecule. In contrast, tritiated compounds have a long half-life and are not biologically altered by incorporation of the isotope. The major disadvantage of tritiated ligands is the relatively low specific activity, which, assuming an ideal one to one incorporation, is 29 Ci/mmol. There are a number of criteria with which to judge the value of a radioligand.[45] It should have a high affinity for the receptors, so that the low concentrations will demonstrate minimal levels of nonspecific binding. The radioligand should have measurable biological activity. It should have a high specific activity, i.e., greater than 10 Ci/mmol. Finally, it should have a rate of dissociation that is slow enough to allow the separation of bound and free ligand.

Filtration

Any procedure to measure radioligand binding must include a method to separate bound from free ligand and a method to measure the bound radioactivity. The most commonly used technique is rapid filtration.[45] In this method the incubation sample is rapidly filtered (10 to 15 seconds) under reduced pressure through a small paper or fiberglass filter. Frequently, the incubation sample is diluted with cold wash buffer just before filtration to ensure the creation of a uniform vacuum. Following filtration, the filters are rinsed with cold buffer to remove any free ligand remaining on the filter. The amount of radioactivity trapped on the filter is measured with the aid of a gamma counter or liquid scintillation detector. One common difficulty with this method is that many ligands adsorb to the filter in a displaceable manner, thereby resulting in significant levels of nonspecific binding.

Centrifugation

An alternative method used to separate bound from free ligand is centrifugation.[45] In this method a small incubation aliquot (250 μl) is subjected to rapid centrifugation (1 minute) in a table-top centrifuge. The supernatant is discarded, and the resulting pellet is quickly rinsed with cold buffer without resuspension. The amount of radioactivity in the pellet is measured in a gamma counter or a liquid scintillation detector. Although this method obviously eliminates the problem of nonspecific binding to filters, high levels of nonspecific binding can result from the trapping of free ligand in the pellet. Both filtration and centrifugation procedures are sufficiently rapid to prevent any significant association or dissociation of ligand during the separation process.

Gel Filtration

Gel filtration has also been used to measure binding in soluble preparations of receptor.[20] In this assay the free radioligand and the radioligand-receptor complex migrate at different rates through the gel and are collected in separate fractions. The amount of radioactivity recovered in the collection fractions is then determined. Although this method is not rapid, it is performed at low temperature to reduce the dissociation of bound ligand during elution. The low temperature also prevents the degradation of the binding site.

AUTORADIOGRAPHY

An exciting new technique for the measurement of radioligand binding is quantitative autoradiography. This method permits the simultaneous characterization and visualization of receptors in a wide variety of tissues. In this method the tissue of interest is quickly frozen and cut into thin sections that are individually affixed to gelatin-coated slides. The slide-mounted tissue samples are incubated with radioligand and competing ligands by immersing the slide into incubation medium. The reaction is stopped by removing the slides from the incubation medium and rinsing with ice-cold buffer solution. The slides are rapidly dried with forced air to prevent dissociation and diffusion of bound ligand. If the tissue sample has been properly mounted, it will remain intact throughout this procedure. The amount of radioactivity bound to the tissue can be measured in one of two ways. If the tissue section is wiped off the slide with filter paper, the radioactivity can be measured as described for the filtration method. The unique advantage of this method, however, is that the radioactivity can also be measured by radiation-sensitive film. In this procedure the film is exposed by placing it directly on the radiolabeled tissue section. Tritium requires an exposure time of between 2 and 16 weeks whereas ^{125}I requires only 4 to 24 hours. When the film is developed, the localization of the radioactivity in the tissue section can be visualized. The amount of radioactivity, i.e., the amount of radioligand bound at any particular location can be quantitated by optical densitometry, since the optical density is functionally related to the amount of radioactivity. Following the exposure of the film, the tissue section can be stained for histological examination in order to correlate radioligand binding to morphology. This autoradiographic method has been successfully used to visualize and localize opiate receptors,[17] serotonin receptors,[34] and β-adrenergic receptors[32] in the brain.

References

1. Alexander RW, Williams LT, Lefkowitz RJ: Identification of cardiac beta-adrenergic receptors by (−)(^{3}H)-alprenolol binding. *Proc Natl Acad Sci USA* 1975; 72:1564–1568.
2. Boeynaems JM, Dumont JE: Quantitative analysis of the binding of ligands to their receptors. *J Cyclic Nucl Res* 1975;1:123–142.
3. Carlsson E, Ablad B, Brandstrom A, et al: Differentiated blockade of the chronotropic effects of various adrenergic stimuli in the cat heart. *Life Sci* 1972;11:953–958.

4. Carlsson E, Dahlof CG, Hedberg A, et al: Differentiation of cardiac chronotropic and inotropic effects of β-adrenoceptor agonists. *Naunyn Schmiedebergs Arch Pharmacol* 1977;300:101–105.
5. Carlsson E, Hedberg A: Are cardiac effects of noradrenaline and adrenaline mediated by different beta-adrenoceptors. *Acta Physiol Scand [Suppl]* 1976;440:47.
6. Caron MG, Srinivasan Y, Pitha J, et al: Affinity chromatography of the β-adrenergic receptor. *J Biol Chem* 1979;254:2923–2927.
7. Changeux JP, Meunier JC, Hucket M: Studies on the cholinergic receptor protein of *Electrophorus Electricus*. I. An assay *in vitro* for the cholinergic receptor site and solubilization of the receptor protein from electric tissue. *Mol Pharmacol* 1971;7:538–553.
8. Cheng YC, Prusoff WH: Relationship between the inhibition constant K_I and the concentration of inhibitor which caused 50% inhibition (IC_{50}) of an enzymatic reaction. *Biochem Pharmacol* 1973;22:3099–3108.
9. DeHean C: The non-stoichiometric floating receptor model for hormone sensitive adenylyl cyclase. *J Theor Biol* 1976;58:383–400.
10. DeLean A, Hancock AA, Lefkowitz RJ: Validation and statistical analysis of a computer modeling method for quantitative analysis of radioligand binding data for mixtures of pharmacological receptor subtypes. *Mol Pharmacol* 1982;21:5–16.
11. DeLean A, Stadel JM, Lefkowitz RJ: A ternary complex model explains the agonist-specific binding properties of the adenylate cyclase-coupled β-adrenergic receptor. *J Biol Chem* 1980;255:7108–7117.
12. Eadie GS: On the evaluation of the constants V_m and K_m in enzyme reactions. *Science* 1952;116:688.
13. Furchgott RF: Pharmacological characterization of receptors: its relation to radioligand binding studies. *Fed Proc* 1978;37:115–120.
14. Haga T, Ross EM, Anderson HJ, et al: Adenylate cyclase permanently uncoupled from hormone receptors in a novel variant of S49 mouse lymphoma cells. *Proc Natl Acad Sci USA* 1977;74:2016–2020.
15. Hancock AA, DeLean AL, Lefkowitz RJ: Quantitative resolution of beta-adrenergic receptor subtypes by selective ligand binding: Application of a computerized model fitting technique. *Mol Pharmacol* 1979;16:1–9.
16. Hegstrand LR, Minneman KP, Molinoff PB: Multiple effects of guanosine triphosphate on beta adrenergic receptors and adenylate cyclase activity in rat heart, lung and brain. *J Pharmacol Exp Ther* 1979;210:215–221.
17. Herkenham M, Pert CB: Light microscopic localization of brain opiate receptors: A general autoradiographic method which preserves tissue quality. *J Neurosci* 1982;2:1129–1149.
18. Hill AV: The possible effects of the aggregation of the molecules of haemoglobin on its dissociation curves. *J Physiol (Lond)* 1910;40:iv-vii.
19. Hofstee HJ: On the evaluation of the constants V_m and K_m in enzyme reactions. *Science* 1952;116:329–331.
20. Hollenberg MD, Nexo E: Receptor binding assays, in *Receptors and Recognition*, Series B, vol 11, 1981, pp 3–31.
21. Insel PA, Maguire ME, Gilman AG, et al: Beta adrenergic receptors and adenylate cyclase: products of separate genes? *Mol Pharmacol* 1976;12:1062–1069.
22. Jacobs S, Cuatrecasas P: The mobile receptor hypothesis and "cooperativity" of hormone binding: Application to insulin. *Biochim Biophys Acta* 1976;433:482–495.
23. Lefkowitz RJ, Roth J, Pricer W, et al: ACTH receptors in the adrenal: Specific binding

of ACTH-(^{125}I) and its relation to adenyl cyclase. *Proc Natl Acad Sci USA* 1970;65:745–752.
24. Leysen JE, Niemegeers CJE, Tollenaere JP, et al: Serotonergic component of neuroleptic receptors. *Nature* 1978;272:168–171.
25. Lin SY, Goodfriend TL: Angiotensin receptors. *Am J Physiol* 1970;218:1319–1328.
26. Maguire ME, Van Arsdale PM, Gilman AG: An agonist-specific effect of guanine nucleotides on binding to the beta adrenergic receptor. *Mol Pharmacol* 1976;12:335–339.
27. Miledi R, Molinoff P, Potter LT: Isolation of the cholinergic receptor protein of *Torpedo* electric tissue. *Nature* 1971;229:554–557.
28. Minneman KP, Fox AW, Abel PW: Occupancy of alpha$_1$-adrenergic receptors and contraction of rat vas deferens. *Mol Pharmacol* 1983;23:359–368.
29. Minneman KP, Hedberg A, Molinoff PB: Comparison of beta-adrenergic receptor subtypes in mammalian tissues. *J Pharmacol Exp Ther* 1979;211:502–508.
30. Minneman KP, Hegstrand L, Molinoff PB: The pharmacological specificity of beta-1 and beta-2 adrenergic receptors in rat heart and lung *in vitro. Mol Pharmacol* 1979;16:21–33.
31. Minneman KP, Hegstrand LR, Molinoff PB: Simultaneous determination of beta-1 and beta-2 adrenergic receptors in tissues containing both subtypes. *Mol Pharmacol* 1979;16:34–46.
32. Palacios JM, Kuhar MJ: Beta-adrenergic-receptor localization by light microscopic autoradiography. *Science* 1980;208:1378–1380.
33. Pert CB, Snyder SH: Opiate receptor: demonstration in nervous tissue. *Science* 1973;179:1011–1014.
34. Rainbow TC, Bleisch WV, Biegon A, et al: Quantitative densitometry of neurotransmitter receptors. *J Neurosci Methods* 1982;5:127–138.
35. Rainbow TC, Parsons B, Wolfe BB: Quantitative autoradiography of β_1 and β_2 adrenergic receptors in rat brain. *Proc Natl Acad Sci USA* 1984;81:1585–1589.
36. Ross EM, Maguire ME, Sturgill TW, et al: Relationship between the β-adrenergic receptor and adenylate cyclase. *J Biol Chem* 1977;252:5761–5775.
37. Scatchard G: The attractions of proteins for small molecules and ions. *Ann NY Acad Sci* 1949;51:660–672.
38. Simon EJ, Hiller JM, Edelman I: Stereospecific binding of the potent analgesic (^{3}H)-Etorphine to rat brain homogenate. *Proc Natl Acad Sci USA* 1973;70:1947–1949.
39. Stadel JM, DeLean A, Lefkowitz RJ: A high affinity agonist. β-adrenergic receptor complex is an intermediate for catecholamine stimulation of adenylate cyclase in turkey and frog erythrocyte membranes. *J Biol Chem* 1980;225:1436–1441.
40. Strickland S, Palmer G, Massay V: Determination of dissociation constants and specific rate constants of enzyme-substrate (or protein-ligand) interactions from rapid reaction kinetic data. *J Biol Chem* 1975;250:4048–4052.
41. Terenius L: Stereospecific interaction between narcotic analgesics and a synaptic plasma membrane fraction of rat cerebral cortex. *Acta Pharmacol Toxicol* 1973; 32:317–320.
42. Tsai BS, Lefkowitz RJ: Agonist-specific effects of guanine nucleotides on alpha-adrenergic receptors in human platelets. *Mol Pharmacol* 1979;16:61–68.
43. Vauquelin G, Geynet P, Hanoune J, et al: Isolation of adenylate cyclase-free, β-adrenergic receptor from turkey erythrocyte membranes by affinity chromatography. *Proc Natl Acad Sci USA* 1977;74:3710–3714.

44. Weiland GA, Molinoff PB: Quantitative analysis of drug-receptor interactions: I. Determination of kinetic and equilibrium properties. *Life Sci* 1981;29:313–330.
45. Williams LT, Lefkowitz RJ: *Receptor Binding Studies in Adrenergic Pharmacology.* New York, Raven Press, 1978.
46. Zahniser NR, Molinoff PB: Effect of guanine nucleotides on striatal dopamine receptors. *Nature* 1978;275:453–455.

Appendix
Mathematical Tables

TABLE A.1. Areas Under the Standard Normal Curve.

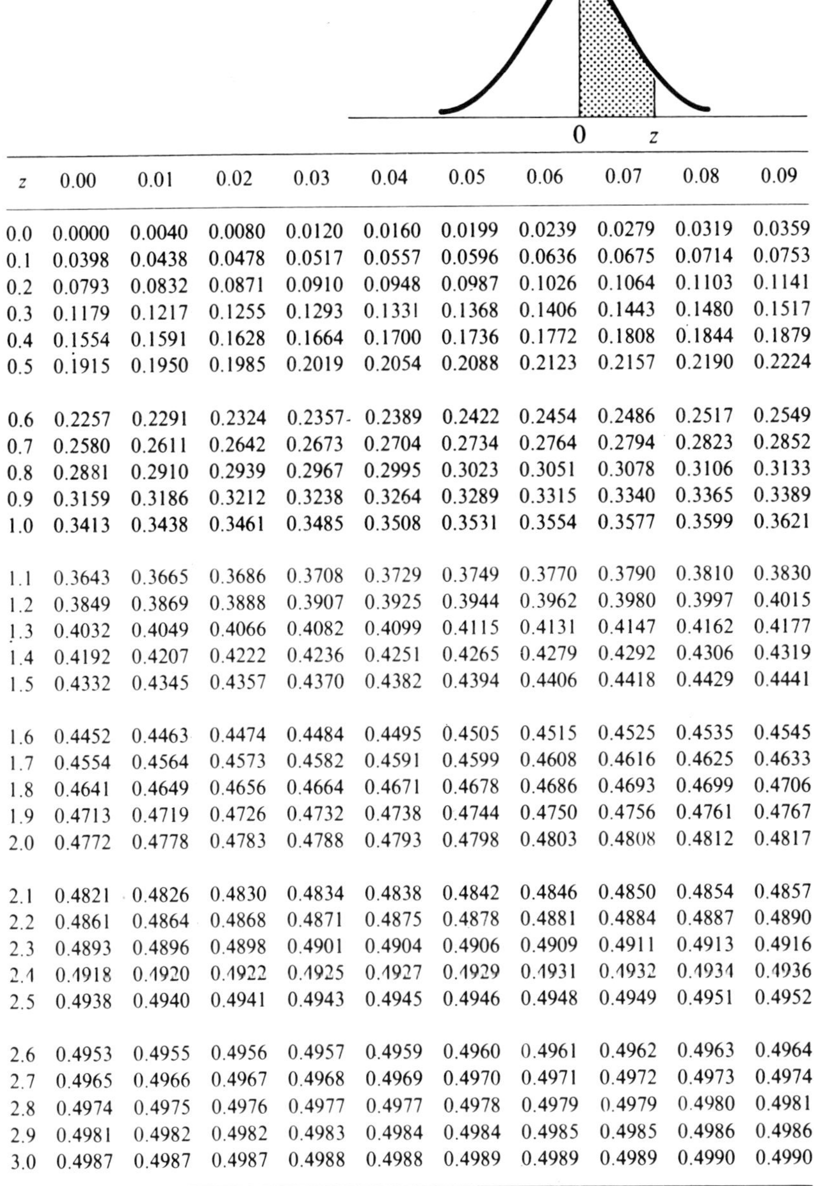

z	0.00	0.01	0.02	0.03	0.04	0.05	0.06	0.07	0.08	0.09
0.0	0.0000	0.0040	0.0080	0.0120	0.0160	0.0199	0.0239	0.0279	0.0319	0.0359
0.1	0.0398	0.0438	0.0478	0.0517	0.0557	0.0596	0.0636	0.0675	0.0714	0.0753
0.2	0.0793	0.0832	0.0871	0.0910	0.0948	0.0987	0.1026	0.1064	0.1103	0.1141
0.3	0.1179	0.1217	0.1255	0.1293	0.1331	0.1368	0.1406	0.1443	0.1480	0.1517
0.4	0.1554	0.1591	0.1628	0.1664	0.1700	0.1736	0.1772	0.1808	0.1844	0.1879
0.5	0.1915	0.1950	0.1985	0.2019	0.2054	0.2088	0.2123	0.2157	0.2190	0.2224
0.6	0.2257	0.2291	0.2324	0.2357	0.2389	0.2422	0.2454	0.2486	0.2517	0.2549
0.7	0.2580	0.2611	0.2642	0.2673	0.2704	0.2734	0.2764	0.2794	0.2823	0.2852
0.8	0.2881	0.2910	0.2939	0.2967	0.2995	0.3023	0.3051	0.3078	0.3106	0.3133
0.9	0.3159	0.3186	0.3212	0.3238	0.3264	0.3289	0.3315	0.3340	0.3365	0.3389
1.0	0.3413	0.3438	0.3461	0.3485	0.3508	0.3531	0.3554	0.3577	0.3599	0.3621
1.1	0.3643	0.3665	0.3686	0.3708	0.3729	0.3749	0.3770	0.3790	0.3810	0.3830
1.2	0.3849	0.3869	0.3888	0.3907	0.3925	0.3944	0.3962	0.3980	0.3997	0.4015
1.3	0.4032	0.4049	0.4066	0.4082	0.4099	0.4115	0.4131	0.4147	0.4162	0.4177
1.4	0.4192	0.4207	0.4222	0.4236	0.4251	0.4265	0.4279	0.4292	0.4306	0.4319
1.5	0.4332	0.4345	0.4357	0.4370	0.4382	0.4394	0.4406	0.4418	0.4429	0.4441
1.6	0.4452	0.4463	0.4474	0.4484	0.4495	0.4505	0.4515	0.4525	0.4535	0.4545
1.7	0.4554	0.4564	0.4573	0.4582	0.4591	0.4599	0.4608	0.4616	0.4625	0.4633
1.8	0.4641	0.4649	0.4656	0.4664	0.4671	0.4678	0.4686	0.4693	0.4699	0.4706
1.9	0.4713	0.4719	0.4726	0.4732	0.4738	0.4744	0.4750	0.4756	0.4761	0.4767
2.0	0.4772	0.4778	0.4783	0.4788	0.4793	0.4798	0.4803	0.4808	0.4812	0.4817
2.1	0.4821	0.4826	0.4830	0.4834	0.4838	0.4842	0.4846	0.4850	0.4854	0.4857
2.2	0.4861	0.4864	0.4868	0.4871	0.4875	0.4878	0.4881	0.4884	0.4887	0.4890
2.3	0.4893	0.4896	0.4898	0.4901	0.4904	0.4906	0.4909	0.4911	0.4913	0.4916
2.4	0.4918	0.4920	0.4922	0.4925	0.4927	0.4929	0.4931	0.4932	0.4934	0.4936
2.5	0.4938	0.4940	0.4941	0.4943	0.4945	0.4946	0.4948	0.4949	0.4951	0.4952
2.6	0.4953	0.4955	0.4956	0.4957	0.4959	0.4960	0.4961	0.4962	0.4963	0.4964
2.7	0.4965	0.4966	0.4967	0.4968	0.4969	0.4970	0.4971	0.4972	0.4973	0.4974
2.8	0.4974	0.4975	0.4976	0.4977	0.4977	0.4978	0.4979	0.4979	0.4980	0.4981
2.9	0.4981	0.4982	0.4982	0.4983	0.4984	0.4984	0.4985	0.4985	0.4986	0.4986
3.0	0.4987	0.4987	0.4987	0.4988	0.4988	0.4989	0.4989	0.4989	0.4990	0.4990

TABLE A.2. *t* Distribution.

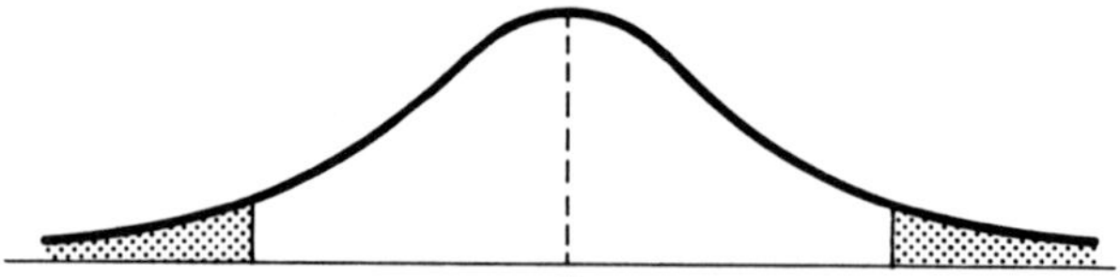

deg. freedom, ν	90% ($P = 0.1$)	95% ($P = 0.05$)	99% ($P = 0.01$)
1	6.314	12.706	63.657
2	2.920	4.303	9.925
3	2.353	3.182	5.841
4	2.132	2.776	4.604
5	2.015	2.571	4.032
6	1.943	2.447	3.707
7	1.895	2.365	3.499
8	1.860	2.306	3.355
9	1.833	2.262	3.250
10	1.812	2.228	3.169
11	1.796	2.201	3.106
12	1.782	2.179	3.055
13	1.771	2.160	3.012
14	1.761	2.145	2.977
15	1.753	2.131	2.947
16	1.746	2.120	2.921
17	1.740	2.110	2.898
18	1.734	2.101	2.878
19	1.729	2.093	2.861
20	1.725	2.086	2.845
21	1.721	2.080	2.831
22	1.717	2.074	2.819
23	1.714	2.069	2.807
24	1.711	2.064	2.797
25	1.708	2.060	2.787
26	1.706	2.056	2.779
27	1.703	2.052	2.771
28	1.701	2.048	2.763
29	1.699	2.045	2.756
inf.	1.645	1.960	2.576

TABLE A.3. Probit Transformation.[a]

%		%		%		%		%	
0		20	4.1584	40	4.7467	60	5.2533	80	5.8416
1	2.6737	21	4.1936	41	4.7725	61	5.2793	81	5.8779
2	2.9463	22	4.2278	42	4.7981	62	5.3055	82	5.9154
3	3.1192	23	4.2612	43	4.8236	63	5.3319	83	5.9542
4	3.2493	24	4.2937	44	4.8490	64	5.3585	84	5.9945
5	3.3551	25	4.3255	45	4.8743	65	5.3853	85	6.0364
6	3.4452	26	4.3567	46	4.8996	66	5.4125	86	6.0803
7	3.5242	27	4.3872	47	4.9247	67	5.4399	87	6.1264
8	3.5949	28	4.4172	48	4.9498	68	5.4677	88	6.1750
9	3.6592	29	4.4466	49	4.9749	69	5.4959	89	6.2265
10	3.7184	30	4.4756	50	5.0000	70	5.5244	90	6.2816
11	3.7735	31	4.5041	51	5.0251	71	5.5534	91	6.3408
12	3.8250	32	4.5323	52	5.0502	72	5.5828	92	6.4051
13	3.8736	33	4.5601	53	5.0753	73	5.6128	93	6.4758
14	3.9197	34	4.5875	54	5.1004	74	5.6433	94	6.5548
15	3.9636	35	4.6147	55	5.1257	75	5.6745	95	6.6449
16	4.0055	36	4.6415	56	5.1510	76	5.7063	96	6.7507
17	4.0458	37	4.6681	57	5.1764	77	5.7388	97	6.8808
18	4.0846	38	4.6945	58	5.2019	78	5.7722	98	7.0537
19	4.1221	39	4.7207	59	5.2275	79	5.8064	99	7.3263

[a] The percentages of the area under the normal distribution curve from negative infinity and the corresponding probits. The computer programs contain a subroutine that calculates probit values directly, thus avoiding interpolation of tabular values.

TABLE A.4. Common logarithms.

n	0	1	2	3	4	5	6	7	8	9
1.0	0.0000	0.0043	0.0086	0.0128	0.0170	0.0212	0.0253	0.0294	0.0334	0.0374
1.1	0.0414	0.0453	0.0492	0.0531	0.0569	0.0607	0.0645	0.0682	0.0719	0.0755
1.2	0.0792	0.0828	0.0864	0.0899	0.0934	0.0969	0.1004	0.1038	0.1072	0.1106
1.3	0.1139	0.1173	0.1206	0.1239	0.1271	0.1303	0.1335	0.1367	0.1399	0.1430
1.4	0.1461	0.1492	0.1523	0.1553	0.1584	0.1614	0.1644	0.1673	0.1703	0.1732
1.5	0.1761	0.1790	0.1818	0.1847	0.1875	0.1903	0.1931	0.1959	0.1987	0.2014
1.6	0.2041	0.2068	0.2095	0.2122	0.2148	0.2175	0.2201	0.2227	0.2253	0.2279
1.7	0.2304	0.2330	0.2355	0.2380	0.2405	0.2430	0.2455	0.2480	0.2504	0.2529
1.8	0.2553	0.2577	0.2601	0.2625	0.2648	0.2672	0.2695	0.2718	0.2742	0.2765
1.9	0.2788	0.2810	0.2833	0.2856	0.2878	0.2900	0.2923	0.2945	0.2967	0.2989

(Continued)

TABLE A.4. *(Continued)*.

n	0	1	2	3	4	5	6	7	8	9
2.0	0.3010	0.3032	0.3054	0.3075	0.3096	0.3118	0.3139	0.3160	0.3181	0.3201
2.1	0.3222	0.3243	0.3263	0.3284	0.3304	0.3324	0.3345	0.3365	0.3385	0.3404
2.2	0.3424	0.3444	0.3464	0.3483	0.3502	0.3522	0.3541	0.3560	0.3579	0.3598
2.3	0.3617	0.3636	0.3655	0.3674	0.3692	0.3711	0.3729	0.3747	0.3766	0.3784
2.4	0.3802	0.3820	0.3838	0.3856	0.3874	0.3892	0.3909	0.3927	0.3945	0.3962
2.5	0.3979	0.3997	0.4014	0.4031	0.4048	0.4065	0.4082	0.4099	0.4116	0.4133
2.6	0.4150	0.4166	0.4183	0.4200	0.4216	0.4232	0.4249	0.4265	0.4281	0.4298
2.7	0.4314	0.4330	0.4346	0.4362	0.4378	0.4393	0.4409	0.4425	0.4440	0.4456
2.8	0.4472	0.4487	0.4502	0.4518	0.4533	0.4548	0.4564	0.4579	0.4594	0.4609
2.9	0.4624	0.4639	0.4654	0.4669	0.4683	0.4698	0.4713	0.4728	0.4742	0.4757
3.0	0.4771	0.4786	0.4800	0.4814	0.4829	0.4843	0.4857	0.4871	0.4886	0.4900
3.1	0.4914	0.4928	0.4942	0.4955	0.4969	0.4983	0.4997	0.5011	0.5024	0.5038
3.2	0.5051	0.5065	0.5079	0.5092	0.5105	0.5119	0.5132	0.5145	0.5159	0.5172
3.3	0.5185	0.5198	0.5211	0.5224	0.5237	0.5250	0.5263	0.5276	0.5289	0.5302
3.4	0.5315	0.5328	0.5340	0.5353	0.5366	0.5378	0.5391	0.5403	0.5416	0.5428
3.5	0.5441	0.5453	0.5465	0.5478	0.5490	0.5502	0.5514	0.5527	0.5539	0.5551
3.6	0.5563	0.5575	0.5587	0.5599	0.5611	0.5623	0.5635	0.5647	0.5658	0.5670
3.7	0.5682	0.5694	0.5705	0.5717	0.5729	0.5740	0.5752	0.5763	0.5775	0.5786
3.8	0.5798	0.5809	0.5821	0.5832	0.5843	0.5855	0.5866	0.5877	0.5888	0.5899
3.9	0.5911	0.5922	0.5933	0.5944	0.5955	0.5966	0.5977	0.5988	0.5999	0.6010
4.0	0.6021	0.6031	0.6042	0.6053	0.6064	0.6075	0.6085	0.6096	0.6107	0.6117
4.1	0.6128	0.6138	0.6149	0.6160	0.6170	0.6180	0.6191	0.6201	0.6212	0.6222
4.2	0.6232	0.6243	0.6253	0.6263	0.6274	0.6284	0.6294	0.6304	0.6314	0.6325
4.3	0.6335	0.6345	0.6355	0.6365	0.6375	0.6385	0.6395	0.6405	0.6415	0.6425
4.4	0.6435	0.6444	0.6454	0.6464	0.6474	0.6484	0.6493	0.6503	0.6513	0.6522
4.5	0.6532	0.6542	0.6551	0.6561	0.6571	0.6580	0.6590	0.6599	0.6609	0.6618
4.6	0.6628	0.6637	0.6646	0.6656	0.6665	0.6675	0.6684	0.6693	0.6702	0.6712
4.7	0.6721	0.6730	0.6739	0.6749	0.6758	0.6767	0.6776	0.6785	0.6794	0.6803
4.8	0.6812	0.6821	0.6830	0.6839	0.6848	0.6857	0.6866	0.6875	0.6884	0.6893
4.9	0.6902	0.6911	0.6920	0.6928	0.6937	0.6946	0.6955	0.6964	0.6972	0.6981
5.0	0.6990	0.6998	0.7007	0.7016	0.7024	0.7033	0.7042	0.7050	0.7059	0.7067
5.1	0.7076	0.7084	0.7093	0.7101	0.7110	0.7118	0.7126	0.7135	0.7143	0.7152
5.2	0.7160	0.7168	0.7177	0.7185	0.7193	0.7202	0.7210	0.7218	0.7226	0.7235
5.3	0.7243	0.7251	0.7259	0.7267	0.7275	0.7284	0.7292	0.7300	0.7308	0.7316
5.4	0.7324	0.7332	0.7340	0.7348	0.7356	0.7364	0.7372	0.7380	0.7388	0.7396
5.5	0.7404	0.7412	0.7419	0.7427	0.7435	0.7443	0.7451	0.7459	0.7466	0.7474
5.6	0.7482	0.7490	0.7497	0.7505	0.7513	0.7520	0.7528	0.7536	0.7543	0.7551
5.7	0.7559	0.7566	0.7574	0.7582	0.7589	0.7597	0.7604	0.7612	0.7619	0.7627
5.8	0.7634	0.7642	0.7649	0.7657	0.7664	0.7672	0.7679	0.7686	0.7694	0.7701
5.9	0.7709	0.7716	0.7723	0.7731	0.7738	0.7745	0.7752	0.7760	0.7767	0.7774

TABLE A.4. *(Continued).*

n	0	1	2	3	4	5	6	7	8	9
6.0	0.7782	0.7789	0.7796	0.7803	0.7810	0.7818	0.7825	0.7832	0.7839	0.7846
6.1	0.7853	0.7860	0.7868	0.7875	0.7882	0.7889	0.7896	0.7903	0.7910	0.7917
6.2	0.7924	0.7931	0.7938	0.7945	0.7952	0.7959	0.7966	0.7973	0.7980	0.7987
6.3	0.7993	0.8000	0.8007	0.8014	0.8021	0.8028	0.8035	0.8041	0.8048	0.8055
6.4	0.8062	0.8069	0.8075	0.8082	0.8089	0.8096	0.8102	0.8109	0.8116	0.8122
6.5	0.8129	0.8136	0.8142	0.8149	0.8156	0.8162	0.8169	0.8176	0.8182	0.8189
6.6	0.8195	0.8202	0.8209	0.8215	0.8222	0.8228	0.8235	0.8241	0.8248	0.8254
6.7	0.8261	0.8267	0.8274	0.8280	0.8287	0.8293	0.8299	0.8306	0.8312	0.8319
6.8	0.8325	0.8331	0.8338	0.8344	0.8351	0.8357	0.8363	0.8370	0.8376	0.8382
6.9	0.8388	0.8395	0.8401	0.8407	0.8414	0.8420	0.8426	0.8432	0.8439	0.8445
7.0	0.8451	0.8457	0.8463	0.8470	0.8476	0.8482	0.8488	0.8494	0.8500	0.8506
7.1	0.8513	0.8519	0.8525	0.8531	0.8537	0.8543	0.8549	0.8555	0.8561	0.8567
7.2	0.8573	0.8579	0.8585	0.8591	0.8597	0.8603	0.8609	0.8615	0.8621	0.8627
7.3	0.8633	0.8639	0.8645	0.8651	0.8657	0.8663	0.8669	0.8675	0.8681	0.8686
7.4	0.8692	0.8698	0.8704	0.8710	0.8716	0.8722	0.8727	0.8733	0.8739	0.8745
7.5	0.8751	0.8756	0.8762	0.8768	0.8774	0.8779	0.8785	0.8791	0.8797	0.8802
7.6	0.8808	0.8814	0.8820	0.8825	0.8831	0.8837	0.8842	0.8848	0.8854	0.8859
7.7	0.8865	0.8871	0.8876	0.8882	0.8887	0.8893	0.8899	0.8904	0.8910	0.8915
7.8	0.8921	0.8927	0.8932	0.8938	0.8943	0.8949	0.8954	0.8960	0.8965	0.8971
7.9	0.8976	0.8982	0.8987	0.8993	0.8998	0.9004	0.9009	0.9015	0.9020	0.9025
8.0	0.9031	0.9036	0.9042	0.9047	0.9053	0.9058	0.9063	0.9069	0.9074	0.9079
8.1	0.9085	0.9090	0.9096	0.9101	0.9106	0.9112	0.9117	0.9122	0.9128	0.9133
8.2	0.9138	0.9143	0.9149	0.9154	0.9159	0.9165	0.9170	0.9175	0.9180	0.9186
8.3	0.9191	0.9196	0.9201	0.9206	0.9212	0.9217	0.9222	0.9227	0.9232	0.9238
8.4	0.9243	0.9248	0.9253	0.9258	0.9263	0.9269	0.9274	0.9279	0.9284	0.9289
8.5	0.9294	0.9299	0.9304	0.9309	0.9315	0.9320	0.9325	0.9330	0.9335	0.9340
8.6	0.9345	0.9350	0.9355	0.9360	0.9365	0.9370	0.9375	0.9380	0.9385	0.9390
8.7	0.9395	0.9400	0.9405	0.9410	0.9415	0.9420	0.9425	0.9430	0.9435	0.9440
8.8	0.9445	0.9450	0.9455	0.9460	0.9465	0.9469	0.9474	0.9479	0.9484	0.9489
8.9	0.9494	0.9499	0.9504	0.9509	0.9513	0.9518	0.9523	0.9528	0.9533	0.9538
9.0	0.9542	0.9547	0.9552	0.9557	0.9562	0.9566	0.9571	0.9576	0.9581	0.9586
9.1	0.9590	0.9595	0.9600	0.9605	0.9609	0.9614	0.9619	0.9624	0.9628	0.9633
9.2	0.9638	0.9643	0.9647	0.9652	0.9657	0.9661	0.9666	0.9671	0.9675	0.9680
9.3	0.9685	0.9689	0.9694	0.9699	0.9703	0.9708	0.9713	0.9717	0.9722	0.9727
9.4	0.9731	0.9736	0.9741	0.9745	0.9750	0.9754	0.9759	0.9763	0.9768	0.9773
9.5	0.9777	0.9782	0.9786	0.9791	0.9795	0.9800	0.9805	0.9809	0.9814	0.9818
9.6	0.9823	0.9827	0.9832	0.9836	0.9841	0.9845	0.9850	0.9854	0.9859	0.9863
9.7	0.9868	0.9872	0.9877	0.9881	0.9886	0.9890	0.9894	0.9899	0.9903	0.9908
9.8	0.9912	0.9917	0.9921	0.9926	0.9930	0.9934	0.9939	0.9943	0.9948	0.9952
9.9	0.9956	0.9961	0.9965	0.9969	0.9974	0.9978	0.9983	0.9987	0.9991	0.9996

TABLE A.5. Natural Logarithms.

x	$\ln x$	x	$\ln x$	x	$\ln x$
		4.5	1.5041	9.0	2.1972
0.1	7.6974 − 10	4.6	1.5261	9.1	2.2083
0.2	8.3906 − 10	4.7	1.5476	9.2	2.2192
0.3	8.7960 − 10	4.8	1.5686	9.3	2.2300
0.4	9.0837 − 10	4.9	1.5892	9.4	2.2407
0.5	9.3069 − 10	5.0	1.6094	9.5	2.2513
0.6	9.4892 − 10	5.1	1.6292	9.6	2.2618
0.7	9.6433 − 10	5.2	1.6487	9.7	2.2721
0.8	9.7769 − 10	5.3	1.6677	9.8	2.2824
0.9	9.8946 − 10	5.4	1.6864	9.9	2.2925
1.0	0.0000	5.5	1.7047	10	2.3026
1.1	0.0953	5.6	1.7228	11	2.3979
1.2	0.1823	5.7	1.7405	12	2.4849
1.3	0.2624	5.8	1.7579	13	2.5649
1.4	0.3365	5.9	1.7750	14	2.6391
1.5	0.4055	6.0	1.7918	15	2.7081
1.6	0.4700	6.1	1.8083	16	2.7726
1.7	0.5306	6.2	1.8245	17	2.8332
1.8	0.5878	6.3	1.8405	18	2.8904
1.9	0.6419	6.4	1.8563	19	2.9444
2.0	0.6931	6.5	1.8718	20	2.9957
2.1	0.7419	6.6	1.8871	25	3.2189
2.2	0.7885	6.7	1.9021	30	3.4012
2.3	0.8329	6.8	1.9169	35	3.5553
2.4	0.8755	6.9	1.9315	40	3.6889
2.5	0.9163	7.0	1.9459	45	3.8067
2.6	0.9555	7.1	1.9601	50	3.9120
2.7	0.9933	7.2	1.9741	55	4.0073
2.8	1.0296	7.3	1.9879	60	4.0943
2.9	1.0647	7.4	2.0015	65	4.1744
3.0	1.0986	7.5	2.0149	70	4.2485
3.1	1.1314	7.6	2.0281	75	4.3175
3.2	1.1632	7.7	2.0412	80	4.3820
3.3	1.1939	7.8	2.0541	85	4.4427
3.4	1.2238	7.9	2.0669	90	4.4998
3.5	1.2528	8.0	2.0794	95	4.5539
3.6	1.2809	8.1	2.0919	100	4.6052
3.7	1.2083	8.2	2.1041		
3.8	1.3350	8.3	2.1163		
3.9	1.3610	8.4	2.1281		
4.0	1.3863	8.5	2.1401		
4.1	1.4110	8.6	2.1518		
4.2	1.4351	8.7	2.1633		
4.3	1.4586	8.8	2.1748		
4.4	1.4816	8.9	2.1861		

TABLE A.6. Powers of e: $\exp(x)$ and $\exp(-x)$.

x	e^x	e^{-x}	x	e^x	e^{-x}
0.00	1.00000	1.00000	1.60	4.95302	0.20189
0.01	1.01005	0.99004	1.70	5.47394	0.18268
0.02	1.02020	0.98019	1.80	6.04964	0.16529
0.03	1.03045	0.97044	1.90	6.68589	0.14956
0.04	1.04081	0.96078	2.00	7.38905	0.13533
0.05	1.05127	0.95122			
0.06	1.06183	0.94176	2.10	8.16616	0.12245
0.07	1.07250	0.93239	2.20	9.02500	0.11080
0.08	1.08328	0.92311	2.30	9.97417	0.10025
0.09	1.09417	0.91393	2.40	11.02316	0.09071
0.10	1.10517	0.90483	2.50	12.18248	0.08208
			2.60	13.46372	0.07427
0.11	1.11628	0.89583	2.70	14.87971	0.06720
0.12	1.12750	0.88692	2.80	16.44463	0.06081
0.13	1.13883	0.87810	2.90	18.17412	0.05502
0.14	1.15027	0.86936	3.00	20.08551	0.04978
0.15	1.16183	0.86071			
0.16	1.17351	0.85214	3.50	33.11545	0.03020
0.17	1.18530	0.84366			
0.18	1.19722	0.83527	4.00	54.95815	0.01832
0.19	1.20925	0.82696	4.50	90.01713	0.01111
0.20	1.22140	0.81873	5.00	148.41316	0.00674
0.30	1.34985	0.74081	5.50	224.69193	0.00409
0.40	1.49182	0.67032			
0.50	1.64872	0.60653	6.00	403.42879	0.00248
0.60	1.82211	0.54881	6.50	665.14163	0.00150
0.70	2.01375	0.49658			
0.80	2.22554	0.44932	7.00	1096.63316	0.00091
0.90	2.45960	0.40656	7.50	1808.04241	0.00055
1.00	2.71828	0.36787			
			8.00	2980.95799	0.00034
			8.50	4914.76884	0.00020
1.10	3.00416	0.33287			
1.20	3.32011	0.30119	9.00	8130.08393	0.00012
1.30	3.66929	0.27253	9.50	13359.72683	0.00007
1.40	4.05519	0.24659			
1.50	4.48168	0.22313	10.00	22026.46579	0.00005

TABLE A.7. Squares and Square Roots.

n	n^2	$\sqrt{n}$	$\sqrt{10n}$	n	n^2	$\sqrt{n}$	$\sqrt{10n}$
1	1	1.000	3.162	41	1681	6.403	20.248
2	4	1.414	4.472	42	1764	6.481	20.494
3	9	1.732	5.477	43	1849	6.557	20.736
4	16	2.000	6.325	44	1936	6.633	20.976
5	25	2.236	7.071	45	2025	6.708	21.213
6	36	2.449	7.746	46	2116	6.782	21.448
7	49	2.646	8.367	47	2209	6.856	21.679
8	64	2.828	8.944	48	2304	6.928	21.909
9	81	3.000	9.487	49	2401	7.000	22.136
10	100	3.162	10.000	50	2500	7.071	22.361
11	121	3.317	10.488	51	2601	7.141	22.583
12	144	3.464	10.954	52	2704	7.211	22.804
13	169	3.606	11.402	53	2809	7.280	23.022
14	196	3.742	11.832	54	2916	7.348	23.238
15	225	3.873	12.247	55	3025	7.416	23.452
16	256	4.000	12.649	56	3136	7.483	23.664
17	289	4.123	13.038	57	3249	7.550	23.875
18	324	4.243	13.416	58	3364	7.616	24.083
19	361	4.359	13.784	59	3481	7.681	24.290
20	400	4.472	14.142	60	3600	7.746	24.495
21	441	4.583	14.491	61	3721	7.810	24.698
22	484	4.690	14.832	62	3844	7.874	24.900
23	529	4.796	15.166	63	3969	7.937	25.100
24	576	4.899	15.492	64	4096	8.000	25.298
25	625	5.000	15.811	65	4225	8.062	25.495
26	676	5.099	16.125	66	4356	8.124	25.690
27	729	5.196	16.432	67	4489	8.185	25.884
28	784	5.292	16.733	68	4624	8.246	26.077
29	841	5.385	17.029	69	4761	8.307	26.268
30	900	5.477	17.321	70	4900	8.367	26.458
31	961	5.568	17.607	71	5041	8.426	26.646
32	1024	5.657	17.889	72	5184	8.485	26.833
33	1089	5.745	18.166	73	5329	8.544	27.019
34	1156	5.831	18.439	74	5476	8.602	27.203
35	1225	5.916	18.708	75	5625	8.660	27.386
36	1296	6.000	18.974	76	5776	8.718	27.568
37	1369	6.083	19.235	77	5929	8.775	27.749
38	1444	6.164	19.494	78	6084	8.832	27.928
39	1521	6.245	19.748	79	6241	8.888	28.107
40	1600	6.325	20.000	80	6400	8.944	28.284

(Continued)

TABLE A.7. *(Continued)*.

n	n^2	$\sqrt{n}$	$\sqrt{10n}$	n	n^2	$\sqrt{n}$	$\sqrt{10n}$
81	6561	9.000	28.460	91	8281	9.539	30.166
82	6724	9.055	28.636	92	8464	9.592	30.332
83	6889	9.110	28.810	93	8649	9.644	30.496
84	7056	9.165	28.983	94	8836	9.695	30.659
85	7225	9.220	29.155	95	9025	9.747	30.822
86	7396	9.274	29.326	96	9216	9.798	30.984
87	7569	9.327	29.496	97	9409	9.849	31.145
88	7744	9.381	29.665	98	9604	9.899	31.305
89	7921	9.434	29.833	99	9801	9.950	31.464
90	8100	9.487	30.000	100	10000	10.000	31.623

TABLE A.8. x^2 Distribution.

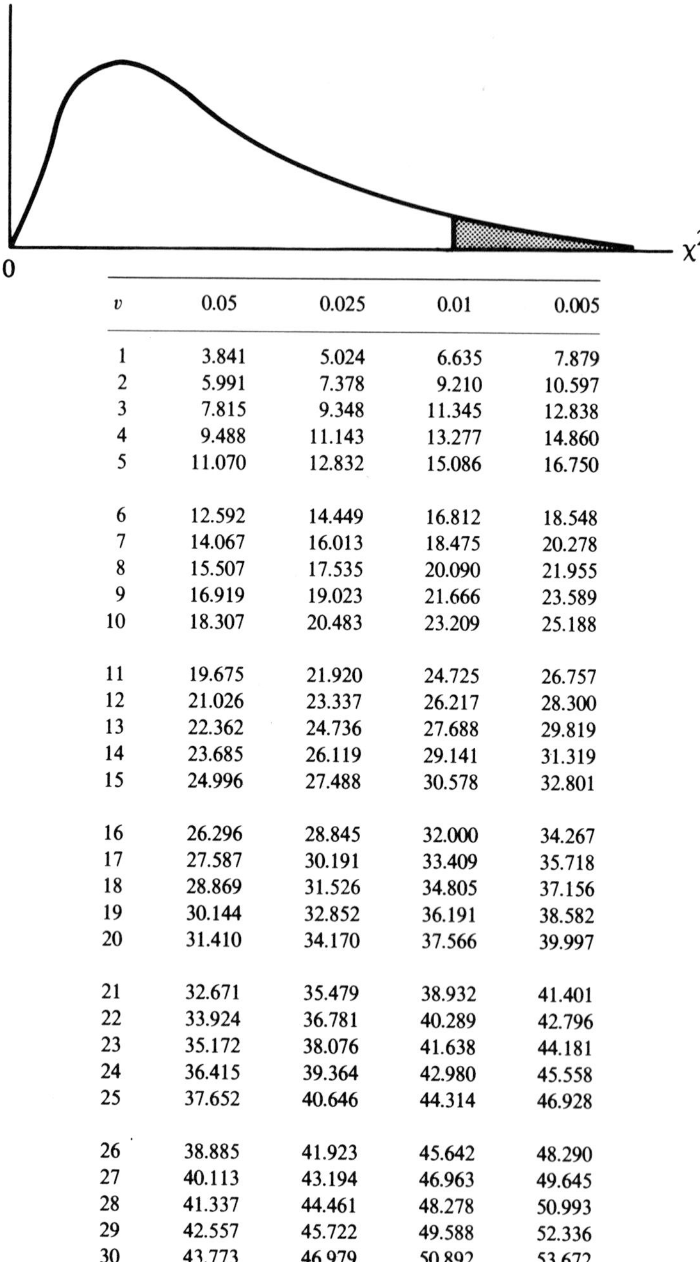

v	0.05	0.025	0.01	0.005
1	3.841	5.024	6.635	7.879
2	5.991	7.378	9.210	10.597
3	7.815	9.348	11.345	12.838
4	9.488	11.143	13.277	14.860
5	11.070	12.832	15.086	16.750
6	12.592	14.449	16.812	18.548
7	14.067	16.013	18.475	20.278
8	15.507	17.535	20.090	21.955
9	16.919	19.023	21.666	23.589
10	18.307	20.483	23.209	25.188
11	19.675	21.920	24.725	26.757
12	21.026	23.337	26.217	28.300
13	22.362	24.736	27.688	29.819
14	23.685	26.119	29.141	31.319
15	24.996	27.488	30.578	32.801
16	26.296	28.845	32.000	34.267
17	27.587	30.191	33.409	35.718
18	28.869	31.526	34.805	37.156
19	30.144	32.852	36.191	38.582
20	31.410	34.170	37.566	39.997
21	32.671	35.479	38.932	41.401
22	33.924	36.781	40.289	42.796
23	35.172	38.076	41.638	44.181
24	36.415	39.364	42.980	45.558
25	37.652	40.646	44.314	46.928
26	38.885	41.923	45.642	48.290
27	40.113	43.194	46.963	49.645
28	41.337	44.461	48.278	50.993
29	42.557	45.722	49.588	52.336
30	43.773	46.979	50.892	53.672

Reprinted from: John E. Freund and Frank J. Williams, *Elementary Business Statistics: The Modern Approach*, Second Edition, © 1972. By permission of Prentice-Hall, Inc., Englewood Cliffs, N.J.

TABLE A.9. Variance Ratio[a]

	$F(95\%)^b$									
	n_1									
n_2	1	2	3	4	5	6	8	12	24	∞
1	161.4	199.5	215.7	224.6	230.2	234.0	238.9	243.9	249.0	254.3
2	18.51	19.00	19.16	19.25	19.30	19.33	19.37	19.41	19.45	19.50
3	10.13	9.55	9.28	9.12	9.01	8.94	8.84	8.74	8.64	8.53
4	7.71	6.94	6.59	6.39	6.26	6.16	6.04	5.91	5.77	5.63
5	6.61	5.79	5.41	5.19	5.05	4.95	4.82	4.68	4.53	4.36
6	5.99	5.14	4.76	4.53	4.39	4.28	4.15	4.00	3.84	3.67
7	5.59	4.74	4.35	4.12	3.97	3.87	3.73	3.57	3.41	3.23
8	5.32	4.46	4.07	3.84	3.69	3.58	3.44	3.28	3.12	2.93
9	5.12	4.26	3.86	3.63	3.48	3.37	3.23	3.07	2.90	2.71
10	4.96	4.10	3.71	3.48	3.33	3.22	3.07	2.91	2.74	2.54
11	4.84	3.98	3.59	3.36	3.20	3.09	2.95	2.79	2.61	2.40
12	4.75	3.88	3.49	3.26	3.11	3.00	2.85	2.69	2.50	2.30
13	4.67	3.80	3.41	3.18	3.02	2.92	2.77	2.60	2.42	2.21
14	4.60	3.74	3.34	3.11	2.96	2.85	2.70	2.53	2.35	2.13
15	4.54	3.68	3.29	3.06	2.90	2.79	2.64	2.48	2.29	2.07
16	4.49	3.63	3.24	3.01	2.85	2.74	2.59	2.42	2.24	2.01
17	4.45	3.59	3.20	2.96	2.81	2.70	2.55	2.38	2.19	1.96
18	4.41	3.55	3.16	2.93	2.77	2.66	2.51	2.34	2.15	1.92
19	4.38	3.52	3.13	2.90	2.74	2.63	2.48	2.31	2.11	1.88
20	4.35	3.49	3.10	2.87	2.71	2.60	2.45	2.28	2.08	1.84
21	4.32	3.47	3.07	2.84	2.68	2.57	2.42	2.25	2.05	1.81
22	4.30	3.44	3.05	2.82	2.66	2.55	2.40	2.23	2.03	1.78
23	4.28	3.42	3.03	2.80	2.64	2.53	2.38	2.20	2.00	1.76
24	4.26	3.40	3.01	2.78	2.62	2.51	2.36	2.18	1.98	1.73
25	4.24	3.38	2.99	2.76	2.60	2.49	2.34	2.16	1.96	1.71
26	4.22	3.37	2.98	2.74	2.59	2.47	2.32	2.15	1.95	1.69
27	4.21	3.35	2.96	2.73	2.57	2.46	2.30	2.13	1.93	1.67
28	4.20	3.34	2.95	2.71	2.56	2.44	2.29	2.12	1.91	1.65
29	4.18	3.33	2.93	2.70	2.54	2.43	2.28	2.10	1.90	1.64
30	4.17	3.32	2.92	2.69	2.53	2.42	2.27	2.09	1.89	1.62
40	4.08	3.23	2.84	2.61	2.45	2.34	2.18	2.00	1.79	1.51
60	4.00	3.15	2.76	2.52	2.37	2.25	2.10	1.92	1.70	1.39
120	3.92	3.07	2.68	2.45	2.29	2.17	2.02	1.83	1.61	1.25
∞	3.84	2.99	2.60	2.37	2.21	2.10	1.94	1.75	1.52	1.00

[a] From R.A. Fisher and F. Yates, *Statistical Tables for Biological, Agricultural and Medical Research*. Oliver & Boyd, London, 1957, pp. 51 and 53, Table V. By permission of the authors and publishers.

[b] Five percent points of *F*. Lower 5% points are found by interchange of n_1 and n_2—that is, n_1 must always correspond with the greater mean square, where n_1 and n_2 are appropriate degrees of freedom.

[c] One percent points of *F*. Lower 1% points are found by interchange of n_1 and n_2—that is, n_1 must always correspond with the greater mean square, where n_1 and n_2 are appropriate degrees of freedom.

TABLE A.9. *(Continued)*.

	$F(99\%)^b$									
	n_1									
n_2	1	2	3	4	5	6	8	12	24	∞
1	4,052	4,999	5,403	5,625	5,764	5,859	5,982	6,106	6,234	6,366
2	98.50	99.00	99.17	99.25	99.30	99.33	99.37	99.42	99.46	99.50
3	34.12	30.82	29.46	28.71	28.24	27.91	27.49	27.05	26.60	26.12
4	21.20	18.00	16.69	15.98	15.52	15.21	14.80	14.37	13.93	13.46
5	16.26	13.27	12.06	11.39	10.97	10.67	10.29	9.89	9.47	9.02
6	13.74	10.92	9.78	9.15	8.75	8.47	8.10	7.72	7.31	6.88
7	12.25	9.55	8.45	7.85	7.46	7.19	6.84	6.47	6.07	5.65
8	11.26	8.65	7.59	7.01	6.63	6.37	6.03	5.67	5.28	4.86
9	10.56	8.02	6.99	6.42	6.06	5.80	5.47	5.11	4.73	4.31
10	10.04	7.56	6.55	5.99	5.64	5.39	5.06	4.71	4.33	3.91
11	9.65	7.20	6.22	5.67	5.32	5.07	4.74	4.40	4.02	3.60
12	9.33	6.93	5.95	5.41	5.06	4.82	4.50	4.16	3.78	3.36
13	9.07	6.70	5.74	5.20	4.86	4.62	4.30	3.96	3.59	3.16
14	8.86	6.51	5.56	5.03	4.69	4.46	4.14	3.80	3.43	3.00
15	8.68	6.36	5.42	4.89	4.56	4.32	4.00	3.67	3.29	2.87
16	8.53	6.23	5.29	4.77	4.44	4.20	3.89	3.55	3.18	2.75
17	8.40	6.11	5.18	4.67	4.34	4.10	3.79	3.45	3.08	2.65
18	8.28	6.01	5.09	4.58	4.25	4.01	3.71	3.37	3.00	2.57
19	8.18	5.93	5.01	4.50	4.17	3.94	3.63	3.30	2.92	2.49
20	8.10	5.85	4.94	4.43	4.10	3.87	3.56	3.23	2.86	2.42
21	8.02	5.78	4.87	4.37	4.04	3.81	3.51	3.17	2.80	2.36
22	7.94	5.72	4.82	4.31	3.99	3.76	3.45	3.12	2.75	2.31
23	7.88	5.66	4.76	4.26	3.94	3.71	3.41	3.07	2.70	2.26
24	7.82	5.61	4.72	4.22	3.90	3.67	3.36	3.03	2.66	2.21
25	7.77	5.57	4.68	4.18	3.86	3.63	3.32	2.99	2.62	2.17
26	7.72	5.53	4.64	4.14	3.82	3.59	3.29	2.96	2.58	2.13
27	7.68	5.49	4.60	4.11	3.78	3.56	3.26	2.93	2.55	2.10
28	7.64	5.45	4.57	4.07	3.75	3.53	3.23	2.90	2.52	2.06
29	7.60	5.42	4.54	4.04	3.73	3.50	3.20	2.87	2.49	2.03
30	7.56	5.39	4.51	4.02	3.70	3.47	3.17	2.84	2.47	2.01
40	7.31	5.18	4.31	3.83	3.51	3.29	2.99	2.66	2.29	1.80
60	7.08	4.98	4.13	3.65	3.34	3.12	2.82	2.50	2.12	1.60
120	6.85	4.79	3.95	3.48	3.17	2.96	2.66	2.34	1.95	1.38
∞	6.64	4.60	3.78	3.32	3.02	2.80	2.51	2.18	1.79	1.00

Index